CARDIO CORE 4×4

THE 20-MINUTE, NO-GYM WORKOUT THAT WILL TRANSFORM YOUR BODY!

JAY CARDIELLO
AND PETE WILLIAMS

RODALE.

© 2012 by Jay Cardiello and Pete Williams

All rights reserved. No part of this publication may be reproduced or transmitted in any form or by any means, electronic or mechanical, including photocopying, recording, or any other information storage and retrieval system, without the written permission of the publisher.

Rodale books may be purchased for business or promotional use or for special sales. For information, please write to: Special Markets Department, Rodale Inc., 733 Third Avenue, New York, NY 10017.

Printed in the United States of America

Rodale Inc. makes every effort to use acid-free ⊛, recycled paper ♺.

Book design by Christopher Rhoads

Photographs by Beth Bischoff

Library of Congress Cataloging-in-Publication Data.

Cardiello, Jay.
  Cardio core 4 x 4 : the 20-minute, no-gym workout that will transform your body! / Jay Cardiello, Pete Williams.
      p.   cm.
  Includes bibliographical references and index.
  ISBN 978–1–60961–402–7 hardcover
  1. Physical fitness.   2. Exercise.   I. Williams, Pete, 1969–   II. Title.   III. Title: Cardio core four by four.
  RA781.C316 2012
  613.7—dc23   2011040875

Distributed to the trade by Macmillan

2 4 6 8 10 9 7 5 3 1   paperback

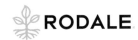

We inspire and enable people to improve their lives and the world around them.
www.rodalebooks.com

To my father. Thanks, Dad.

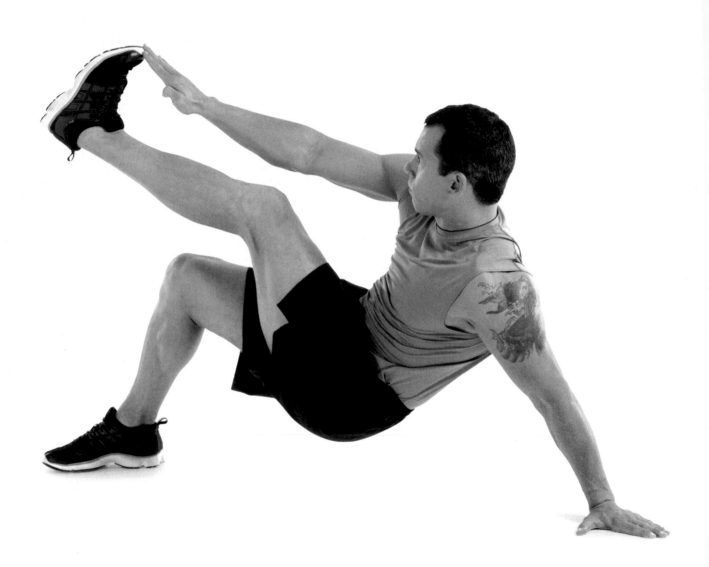

CONTENTS

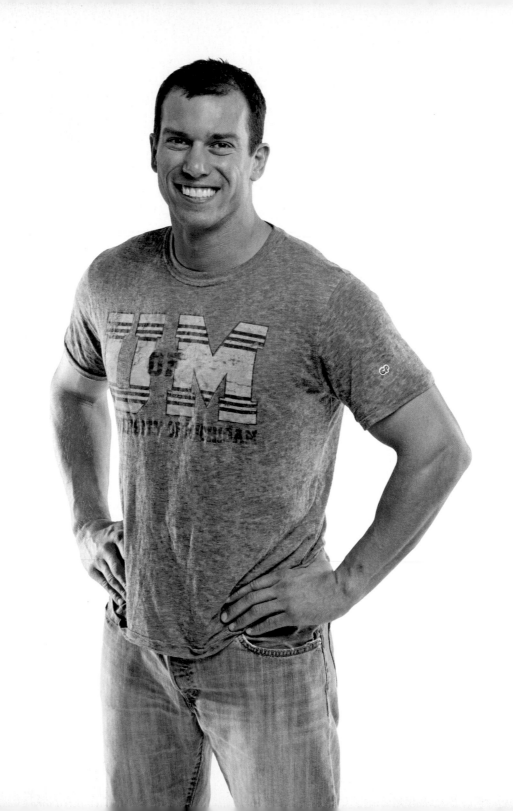

INTRODUCTION

AS A KID GROWING UP in Cedar Grove, New Jersey, I was an international martial arts champion, competing in tournaments as far away as Hawaii. Martial arts, like gymnastics or equestrian pursuits, takes place away from school, so I made it a point to stay in the loop by wrestling and playing football. During my senior year of high school, I went out for track and field, and even though I had little idea what I was doing, I excelled in the long jump and became a conference champion.

I ended up at the University of Arkansas, whose track and field program is the most successful in NCAA history in any sport. The Razorbacks have won 42 national titles in track and cross-country, producing a long line of Olympians. When new athletes arrive on campus, they're measured for championship rings. That's the standard of excellence.

My career as an Arkansas long jumper ended horrifically after just one season when I slipped on the runway prior to the national championships. My foot went out from under me, and I came down with so much force on my heel that as the foot kept sliding, the vertebrae went forward, a disk went backward, and I cracked my tailbone.

Realizing that my athletic career was over, I decided to transfer, seeking the best academic school that would have me. I enrolled at the College of William & Mary.

During my years at the historic campus in Williamsburg, Virginia, I helped coach the track and field team, pouring my passion into the athletes and living vicariously through them. The team set 16 school records, and other William & Mary athletes took notice. I trained a quarterback named Michael Cook, who, though undrafted by the NFL, latched on with the Cleveland Browns and later played in NFL Europe.

Shortly before graduation, I wrote more than 300 letters to pro sports teams and agents. I offered to work for free in exchange for the opportunity to prove myself as a strength coach. Thus began a series of valuable if low-paying jobs with teams in the Arena Football League, the NFL, Major League Baseball, and the XFL, the short-lived football league created by WWE founder Vince McMahon.

At no point did I make more than $300 a week. Most of the time, I earned less or nothing, quite literally paying my dues throughout my late twenties. In between gigs, I'd earn money however I could, at one point spraying Bloomingdale's customers with cologne and wondering how I'd ever make it in the field of athletic training. I thought of Kurt Warner, who stocked grocery store shelves when his football career stalled before emerging as one of the best NFL quarterbacks ever.

In the fall of 2001, not long after the XFL folded, the Cincinnati Reds hired me for $25 per diem to help with their instructional league players in Sarasota, Florida. One sunny morning, with 30 players lined up on the field before a workout, one of the coaches turned to me and said, "Okay, Cardiello. You have 20 minutes."

Twenty minutes? We had no equipment out on the field, little space, and I knew we couldn't just do sprints. I remembered some routines I had done with one of the pitchers that focused on hip stability and building lower lumbar strength.

I told the players to get down on all fours, and I put them through a series of movements to strengthen and stabilize their shoulders, midsections, and hips. Thus was born the Cardio Core 4×4, a 20-minute routine that could be done, as it was that day by the young Reds, in as little as a 4×4-foot space.

When that gig ended, the Reds offered me a job as head trainer and conditioning coach for their Class-A minor league ball club. Finally, I figured, a real title with real money. Instead, they offered just $1,500 a month, which would not go far in Southern California, where the team was located.

Frustrated, I returned home to Cedar Grove, or Cedar *Grave*, as I called it. You were born there and you died there, like in so many other American small towns. It's the type of place where guys in their late twenties get together at the local restaurant and reminisce about their high school football glory days.

That wasn't the life I wanted.

I walked into a boxing gym in Cedar Grove and saw Al Cole, the former cruiserweight champion, stretching.

I approached Cole and said, "Your hips are asymmetrical."

"Excuse me?"

"Your hips," I repeated, "are asymmetrical. You're imbalanced."

He raised an eyebrow. "I'm the cruiser-weight champion."

"*Former*," I said, smiling. "Look, I've watched you doing your moves here, and you're not training like a fighter. You're training for aesthetics."

Cole must have admired my brash approach or at least agreed with what I had to say. I came on board as one of his trainers and later worked with Jameel McCline, a top heavyweight.

During this time, my father suffered a fatal heart attack while attempting to start the lawn mower. What made his death even worse was that I was living nearby and had postponed going over to cut the grass.

I trained McCline for 13 weeks, but when it was over, I quit. The uncertainty and instability of the training profession were getting to me, and now I no longer had my father and mentor, the guy I most wanted to please.

So I moved to New York City, put on a suit, and went to work for ESPN in radio sales. I realized quickly I was not meant to sit behind a desk, and I sighed whenever I read a story about athletes I had trained whose careers were thriving. I was thrilled for them, but I wondered why I couldn't find similar success. Since there were other trainers building significant careers, I vowed to give myself one more year to make it in the business.

I went to work at Clay Fitness, which at the time was Manhattan's premier gym, attracting a who's who of celebrities and other successful professionals. I threw myself into the job, training as many as 16 clients a day over 18-hour shifts.

Clients appreciated my work ethic but also my unusual approach, inspired by knowledge I had gained between gigs in pro sports working with physical therapists. Since I knew what it took to rehab a surgically repaired knee or shoulder, I focused my program on "prehab," a proactive approach to preventing injuries by strengthening the many small stabilizer muscles of the hips, shoulders, and midsection.

The Cardio Core 4×4, hatched on the grass of the Cincinnati Reds ballpark in Sarasota, was now an integrated, efficient workout. Publications such as the *New York Times* took notice.

So did 50 Cent, the rapper and actor, who offered me a contract to train him full time.

For the next 4 years, I traveled the world with 50 Cent, helping him create one of the most impressive physiques in the world, producing the vehicle to drive his success. During 2-month breaks, I added other celebrity clients such as Val Kilmer.

I appeared on 50 Cent's reality series *The Money and the Power* and on *The Real Housewives of New York City*. My work was continually featured in magazines and in New York newspapers, and I began making regular appearances on television programs. I began spending summers in the Hamptons to be closer to my clients from the worlds of entertainment and finance and traveled to South Florida to train a prominent polo team.

These days, I'm around the money and the power all the time, and I'm referred to as a "celebrity trainer," as if I'm a celebrity who works as a trainer rather than a trainer who works with celebrities. I'm flattered, though a little startled, when I teach group fitness classes and someone asks for my autograph. I'm still the kid from Cedar Grove who just a few years ago was working for $25 a day for the Cincinnati Reds.

We tend to think of celebrities as people who excel in entertainment and perhaps business, but their success is due more to a mindset, a mind-set of people who want to improve. We all have goals and want to improve but just need the discipline and guidance to achieve those dreams.

I'm sometimes asked to name the most prominent celebrity I've trained. I point to a 5-year-old boy I taught to ride a bicycle. Long after my adult clients will have forgotten about me, that little boy will be teaching his children how to ride a bike and have at least a vague memory of me.

I bring this young man up to illustrate that I don't train celebrities; I train celebrations. There's something magical about seeing a child take off on a two-wheeler unassisted for the first time. That boy celebrated that day, as kids often do.

As adults, we forget how to celebrate the simple things, which often are life's greatest accomplishments. We tend to make everything too complicated, and that approach applies to our workout regimens.

What we need is a simple, effective, efficient program. That's where I can help. Anyone can join the ranks of the top 5 percent. Let's start celebrating together.

PLEDGE OF EXPECTATIONS

Whenever I begin working with new clients, I outline my expectations. No matter how famous they are, I ask them to make the same commitment to this program that they've made to other aspects of their lives.

I know you've been incredibly successful in other aspects of your life, so perhaps this statement I'm asking you to sign is simply a reaffirmation of sorts. Either way, this pledge is a powerful reminder awaiting your signature.

Dear Reader:

Five percent of the people in this world make things happen.

Fifteen percent of the people in this world watch them happen.

And 80 percent have no idea what's happening.

By embarking on this program, you've shown that you are willing to make things happen. By signing below, you have committed to making things happen.

YOUR SIGNATURE_____

JAY CARDIELLO

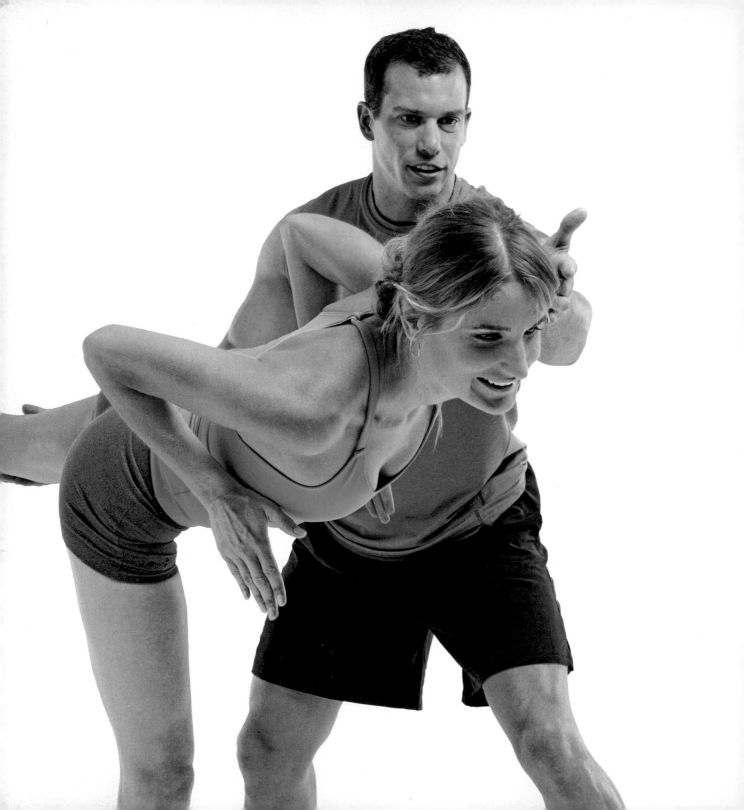

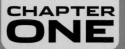

IT'S ALL ABOUT YOUR CORE

I'M A CELEBRITY TRAINER, the guy you see quoted in entertainment magazines with screaming headlines about how actors and entertainers shed pounds and produce incredible swimsuit physiques in a short amount of time. The magazines promise to "reveal the secret workouts" and show how you too can achieve similar results. After all, who doesn't want to look like a celebrity?

Here's the secret, though. Celebrities maintain their training regimens not just to produce a swimsuit-ready physique or prepare for a role. They do it because they discover how a lean, powerful physique provides the energy and stamina to deal with challenges, achieve the most ambitious of goals, and prevent injury and long-term deterioration.

Here's the other secret, and it's one you're going to love: Celebrities don't put in nearly as much time at this as you might think. They live in movie trailers, airplanes, and hotel rooms and sometimes have just 20-minute windows to train.

How do they make that work? And, more important, how can *you*?

That's where I come in. Working with entertainers and professional athletes for the past 15 years, I've developed a program tailored to the demands of their lives: They don't have a whole lot of spare time, and they need to be in peak shape year-round.

The result is Cardio Core 4×4, a totally effective, full-body workout that can be done with no equipment in little space and in just 20 minutes. You can do it in a tiny hotel room or an apartment, a movie trailer, an office, a group fitness class—even an airplane. I've integrated elements of yoga, Pilates, boxing, martial arts, and dance wrapped into one intense, efficient workout. The idea is to make things fun, simple, and effective.

Some of my clients are household names from the worlds of entertainment, sports, and business. Others are like you and me, stars of our own hectic, fast-paced lives.

The common denominator for everyone is that we're looking to create lean, powerful physiques that provide the energy and stamina to achieve personal and professional goals, preferably while balancing family, social lives, and hobbies.

IT'S STILL ALL ABOUT THE CORE

You don't have to spend a lot of time in New York and Los Angeles to see the influence of

FIT FOOD

Next time you get a cut, disinfect it with one of nature's best bacteria fighters: honey. Pour a dab of honey on a cut before covering it with a bandage. Because of its powerful antibacterial properties, honey is capable of destroying almost all strains of the most common wound-infecting bacteria.

celebrity culture in the gym. Guys want to be huge, and women generally want to get toned so they can look like the hot model or actress du jour.

A few years back, it appeared we were getting away from that with the popularization of "core" training. The idea was to shift from bodybuilding-based workouts to focus on strengthening and stabilizing all the muscles around the hips, midsection, and shoulders.

The idea was to build a solid framework for everyday functional movements and make the body resistant to the many ailments produced by a sedentary culture in which we spend most of our time slumped over computers and cramped into a car or an airline seat.

Unfortunately, core training was hijacked by magazine editors and others in the fitness world to refer to just another way to produce washboard abs. Gyms began to look a little like daycare centers, with all the big, colorful balls and plastic equipment geared toward building balance and stability through instability. But, for the most part, people returned to bodybuilding-based workouts to tone or produce big muscles along with the abs.

I figured there had to be a happy medium. Celebrities always will inspire people, for the better perhaps when it comes to fitness. Since I'm hired to motivate celebrities, I'm excited about the notion of developing a program that can get you celeblike results but will also give you a rock-solid, sustainable foundation that will keep you healthy and injury free.

BUILDING A STRONG FOUNDATION

The challenge, of course, never has been more formidable. Americans are getting bigger and fatter all the time. Thankfully, many try to lose the weight and get in shape, but that's where things get scary.

Whenever I travel, I visit gyms and ask for an introductory training session, preferably with the best trainer available. I never reveal my background; my goal is to learn what's being taught in different parts of the country.

Inevitably I'm sized up as someone in pretty good shape and immediately thrown into a crazy workout involving massive weights and potentially back-wrenching movements. Nobody ever stops to think that perhaps I've had 13 surgeries involving my knees, neck, and back. Through hard work, I've restored my body's natural movement patterns, but how would anyone know?

A few years ago, I was working at a gym in New York City when a relatively fit man in his thirties wandered in looking for an introductory training session. I had him walk and perform some arm rotations and other basic moves. It became clear he was becoming light-headed and dizzy. We took his pulse, and it registered at 170.

After lying down for 15 minutes and drinking some orange juice, the guy was able to go home; I rode with him in the cab to make sure he got back okay, and I followed up later.

Imagine if I had taken the common personal training approach. I could have killed the poor guy.

This is not a commentary on the personal training industry. For the most part, trainers ask about medical histories, ailments, and other conditions. Of course, you always should consult a physician before embarking on any training regimen, including the one in this book.

What I'm trying to underscore here is that when people whose basic framework—the hips, shoulders, and midsection—has become locked down by an everyday sedentary lifestyle try to amp it up a few times a week, the results can do a lot more harm than good.

The bottom line is that if we don't first strengthen and stabilize the core region, we will inflict serious harm upon ourselves. At the very least, we'll get a lot less out of our workouts.

We wouldn't build a house without first pouring the foundation. We all know that a house built on sand will wash away. I cringe when I see people sit at a desk all day and then head to the gym to do some serious resistance training or, worse, go outside for a run without first addressing their core stability.

Whether you realize it or not, your body is full of imbalances. Let's say you spend long hours hunched over a computer or steering wheel. Then after work you play tennis. Ideally, you're employing all the wonderful muscles of the hips and shoulders to generate power in the tennis stroke.

More likely, those hips and shoulders are tight and locked down from sitting and hunching. The body is a phenomenal compensator, and you'll swing more from your forearm, producing tennis elbow.

Perhaps you twisted a right ankle years ago. Whether you realized it or not, this has triggered a series of events throughout your body's kinetic chain, producing tightness and a lack of flexibility in the hips that could produce knee and back pain.

All this is why we're going to focus on strengthening and stabilizing your core (your hips, shoulders, and midsection) using nothing but body weight for resistance. Don't worry if you're someone who has been throwing iron around for years. This will provide more than enough challenge.

WHY THIS BOOK?

Too many people come up with convenient excuses not to develop a strong physique that can empower them to create the life of their dreams.

Perhaps you think you don't have enough money. That's a good reason. I've worked at big-time gyms, and they're expensive to join. It's even more expensive to hire a trainer. It also can be pricey to eat right.

What if I told you that you've already made your only necessary purchase in the form of this book?

Perhaps you think you don't have enough time. That too is a good reason. After all, it takes time to drive to that expensive gym, work out for an hour alone or with that expensive trainer, shower, and drive home. That's a 2-hour process, or even longer depending on your commute.

What if I told you that you needed just 20 minutes to get a thorough, effective workout that would give you not only tremendous strength and stability in your hips, midsection, and shoulders but also a huge cardiovascular impact?

Perhaps you think you don't have enough space, especially if you're opting to forgo the gym in favor of training at home.

What if I told you that you could get a thorough workout in any 4×4-foot space? It could be in your living room, part of a bedroom, or even a cramped hotel room. I live in New York City, which has more than a few cramped living spaces, and I've yet to find a location where

FIT TIP

Ignore the fat-burning zone. It's a myth that you have to work out for 20 minutes before you begin burning fat. The thinking once was that you needed to exercise in a range between 60 and 80 percent of your maximum heart rate. Your body uses more energy with intervals of high intensities. Just look at the physique of a sprinter. Short, intense intervals will burn more calories and fat in half the time.

I can't carve out 16 square feet for Cardio Core 4×4.

Perhaps you think you must buy a lot of equipment or join that expensive gym that provides it. That too is understandable. The fitness industry has done an effective job of convincing us that we need the latest steel gadgets, weights, and pulleys to transform our bodies.

What if I told you the only gym equipment you need is found in the mirror? That's right. Your body can be your gym, providing ample resistance for dozens of exercises. There are elements of Cardio Core 4×4 that will remind you of Pilates, yoga, boxing, martial arts, wrestling—even break dancing.

Any one of those is a potent workout. By blending them together into a nonstop, integrated strength-and-cardio package, you have the most efficient and effective workout imaginable.

There's another excuse I hear: "This must be easy for your celebrity clients. They can afford you, along with chefs, massage therapists, assistants, and everyone else to keep them on task throughout their day."

You know what? You're right—to a point. Many celebrities have generated the resources that allow them to trade money for time. Most of us trade time for money. But having spent so much time around celebrities, I can tell you that other than being recognized constantly, there's not that much difference between their lives and ours.

No matter what your situation—working or not working, with or without kids, in or out of a relationship, wealthy or just getting by—your demands equal those of a celebrity. You are the

FIT TIP

Standing on one leg when you're brushing your teeth works deep core muscles. It's a perfect short workout, creating a degree of instability that works the smaller muscles essential for core strength. Now you'll have a great smile and a flatter midsection.

rock star of your world, and there's a lot of responsibility that goes with that.

3-D Fitness

How does it work? Imagine for a moment that your body is a table. If one leg of the table is uneven, it's going to wobble and not provide a stable surface. You'll have to place a piece of cardboard underneath to even things out.

The same is true of the alignment of your automobile. If the car is out of alignment, the tires will not wear evenly. Like your body, the car will compensate. Unlike the table, the problems in your car or body likely won't be evident until there's major damage. At that point, there's no easy, inexpensive solution like a piece of cardboard. Either you or the vehicle is looking at major repairs.

To avoid these types of imbalances, we're going to train the body across all three planes of motion. Straight down through the nose, dividing the body into right and left sides, is the *sagittal* plane, which involves flexing and extending movements. Now imagine cutting the body at the waist to produce a top and a bottom. This is the *transverse* plane, which references rotational movements. If you divided the body into front and back sides, you'd have the *frontal* plane.

It's important to train in all three planes because we live linear lives sitting at desks all day hunched over computers. That produces a lot of tension in the hips and shoulders, which is why people end up with back problems, exacerbated by work at the gym. Traditional workouts operate in only one or two planes of motion. We'll work in all three to support our joints and undergo "prehab"—movement that will strengthen us and protect us from injuries that require rehabilitation, or "rehab."

We want to have perfect balance, stability, and symmetry around the hips and shoulders, the key core components of the four limbs. This is why I call this program Cardio Core 4×4. A good chunk of this workout is done on all fours, and it can be done in as little as a 4×4-foot (16-square-foot) space.

If you've ever owned or driven a four-wheel-drive vehicle, you know the power that comes from having all four wheels receiving torque from the engine simultaneously. That gives the driver tremendous confidence, knowing it's possible to navigate through snow or mud without getting stuck.

Shouldn't our bodies be the same way? Like a car's wheels, the limbs are just along for the ride. We want to create a powerful engine (the core region) that delivers torque through the shoulders, hips, and midsection to power the four limbs.

The cardio component of the program is integrated into the workout itself. Most programs break up cardio and resistance training. Cardio is done separately, sometimes on different days; sometimes it's even optional. Here we do all movements in a continuous session that provides an incredible cardio workout.

By wrapping this up into one integrated system, we accomplish two things that I find are especially appealing to "celebrities" from all walks of life. We create a body with a strong foundation that's lean, powerful, resistant to injury, *and* aesthetically pleasing.

We also manage to accomplish this in just 20 minutes a day. That's all. That's 20 minutes for everything, no additional time for cardio work. It's built into the program.

This will be a tough 20 minutes, though we'll start slowly to build the foundation. As you progress, you'll be able to pack more repetitions and more advanced variations into the same 20 minutes. You can continue to progress indefinitely.

All you must commit to is a program of 20 exercises performed in 20 minutes a day, 4 days a week. That's all. It's a 40-day program to transform your body and perhaps your life.

Why 40 days? It's in keeping with the 4×4

theme, of course, but it's a time frame long linked to making change, going back to biblical times. I'm by no means inserting religion into this equation, though I hope whatever your faith (or no faith), you apply a spiritual element to the process.

We'll train for 20 minutes on Mondays, Tuesdays, Thursdays, and Fridays. Perhaps you're wondering if this is enough. After all, many programs ask for an hour a day, 5 or 6 days a week, for 12 weeks. Heck, most of my colleagues in the personal training profession expect an hourlong commitment from the clients 3 days a week.

That's great if you can sustain such discipline. Most people cannot. Not only that, the 12-week program conditions you to put a time frame on things. There's a tendency to take before-and-after photos and drift back to your previous ways, as if getting in the best shape of your life (for a brief period) were something to cross off a bucket list.

Studies suggest that it takes 30 days to install new habits, which is a cornerstone of many addiction and recovery programs. When people of the Christian faith successfully give up something for Lent, a period of 40 days, they discover they no longer want it. Even if what they gave up was not something especially harmful, they find they prefer life without it.

Several years ago, my coauthor, Pete Williams, gave up television for Lent. Pete didn't watch much TV anyway, but the process of not viewing a minute of television for 40 days changed his life. He felt more focused, less distracted, and as if he had more time on his hands. Now he rarely watches television.

Giving up TV would be a bigger sacrifice for many people. But the reason Pete was able to do so was because it was not much of a stretch. That's why it should not be much of an adjustment to adopt a mere 20-minute training program, 4 days of the week.

If I asked you to give me an hour a day, 6 days a week, for 12 weeks, that would be asking a lot. Maybe you'd get through it, though probably not, and if you did, you'd drop out the moment the 12-week period ended, because it would seem like crossing a finish line.

Cardio Core 4×4 is excuse-proof.

Let's say you're a businessperson who is on the road constantly like George Clooney in the movie *Up in the Air*. Through the magic of Hollywood, George's character managed to find convenient swimming pools wherever he went, but many road warriors struggle to fit in workouts between a brutal schedule of meetings, demanding clients, late dinners, and early wake-up calls.

With Cardio Core 4×4, you need only 20 minutes. No matter how tight your accommodations, you can make it work. I've stayed in some of the world's smallest hotel rooms, and I've yet to find one without a 4×4-foot space. Were it ever the case, a carpeted hallway would suffice. Even on nights when all you want to do is walk in the room and collapse in bed, you can take 20 minutes.

Let's say you're a stay-at-home parent unable to get to the gym or even outside for a short run on a consistent basis. Your life is a whirlwind of meal preparations, chauffeuring, doctor appointments, and perhaps diaper changes. You might not have room in your home for gym equipment and might not want the potential hazards anyway. But you can carve out 20 minutes and 16 square feet for yourself.

Let's say you're a young professional living with roommates in a small apartment and cannot afford a gym membership. Your life is about building a career, running in social circles, and perhaps navigating a new city. The idea of committing to anything else on a weekly or daily basis is unlikely. But you too can find 20 minutes and a 4×4-foot space to call your own.

FIT TIPS JUST FOR YOU

This book includes a nutritional component, but it will not be a traditional breakdown of protein, carbohydrates, and fats. You don't have to memorize any numbers or tables, and I'm not going to provide comprehensive grocery lists, discussions of high-fructose corn syrup and the glycemic index, or a lot of chapter and verse on what to eat and when.

I've found that nutritional information, like food itself, is best consumed in small bites. That's why for the last few years, I've created Fit Tips, little nuggets of information (mostly nutritional in nature) that help you eat better. Fit Tips started as insider info I sent to clients and friends via e-mail. That's still the case, though now I share it with thousands of friends on Facebook and Twitter.

These Fit Tips are generated from a wealth of experience. I'm a certified strength and conditioning specialist (CSCS), an accreditation awarded by the National Strength and Conditioning Association and considered the most prestigious certification in the industry. To obtain CSCS status, you must undergo extensive training in biomechanics, physiology, and nutrition.

I have 15 years of experience preparing meals for professional athletes. I've developed nutritional plans for athletes in boxing, baseball, football, mixed martial arts, polo, and other sports. By developing nutritional programs for people whose performance can be largely determined by how they fuel their bodies, I've come to understand how anyone can benefit from nutrition and avoid many of the common pitfalls.

Writing a Fit Tip or a Fit Food tip is the first thing I do in the morning, and I find these pointers resonate with readers. My wife rolls her eyes whenever friends or people I meet quote some Fit Tip back to me, but that's how memorable they are.

Here's an example: Ice cream after workouts? No wonder Fit Tips and Fit Foods are so popular. Since Fit Tips can pertain to other aspects of fitness and high-performance living, we'll sprinkle them throughout the book.

Think of Fit Tips and Fit Food as those celebrity secrets the magazines are always touting. It really has nothing to do with being a celebrity, of course. It's just a matter of finding methods to make the most of your time and maximize your energy so you can dominate your own celebrity world.

> **FIT FOOD**
>
> Eat ice cream after your workout. Yes, it's true. Having a *small* bowl of ice cream, up to 2 hours after your workout, will help trigger a surge of insulin better than most other postworkout foods. Also, ice cream will put a damper on postworkout protein breakdown.

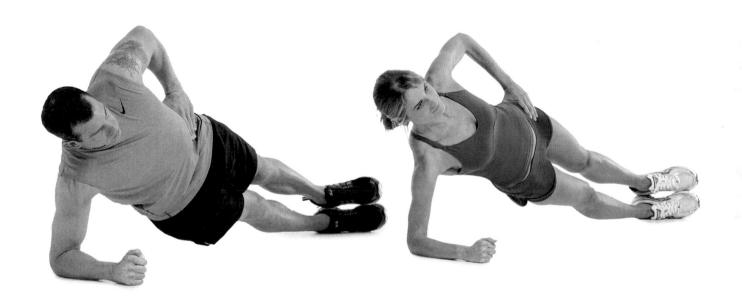

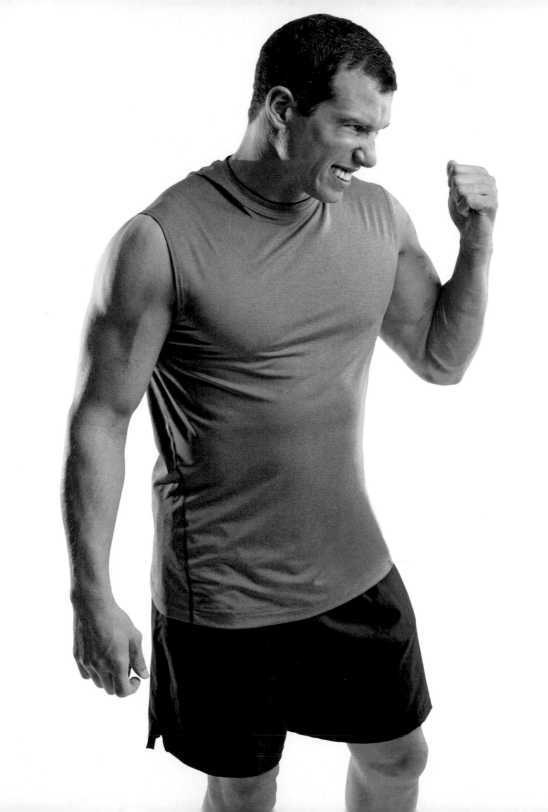

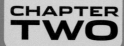

THE FIRST PILLAR OF SUCCESS

· ·

WE MIGHT NOT BE CELEBRITIES, but we have celebrity-like obligations professionally and personally, hectic schedules that demand that we be on the top of our game at all times. Like celebrities, we have little time to commit to training.

This book will show you that there's more to training than pursuing a bikini beach body or replicating a celebrity's quick-fix program to get ready for a movie or photo shoot. While Cardio Core 4×4 *will* produce mirror-pleasing results, it also will motivate you to create a lean, strong physique that gives you the energy and stamina to achieve your most ambitious goals.

Look, who doesn't want to look like the celebrity on the cover of *Us Weekly*? But if you're going to train to look better, why not train in a manner that also allows you to perform better both in the short term and down the road?

The 4×4 theme resonates throughout the book, including the four-part organizational structure of spiritual, emotional, nutritional, and physical. We won't spend nearly as much time on the first two as on the physical and nutritional, but they're still key parts of what I call the "four pillars of success."

The first pillar of success is *spiritual*. This part of the program is not based on religion and what you believe or don't believe, though if you have religious beliefs, they no doubt function as a pillar of strength upon which you can build.

But when I talk about spirituality, I'm referring to the notion that what lies inside affects what happens on the outside. It's about how your belief systems dictate how you're growing on the inside.

Take the word *try*. In fact, take it and leave it. People say, "I'm going to *try* my best" or "I'm going to *try* to make it." That's not a confident approach, is it?

"Trying" should refer only to the process of experimenting with new foods. If you say you're going to *do* your best or that you're *going* to make it, you're more likely to do so. You've made a commitment to others but, more important, to yourself.

FIT TIP

Here's a quick tip that will add years to your life. Ladies, learn men's ability to not sweat the small stuff and to face adversity with aplomb and sense of humor. Guys, take a cue from women and deal with health concerns as soon as they arise, rather than waiting until they escalate into serious conditions.

You don't fail if you get up to the plate. That's trying, to be sure, but it's also taking your best swing. You're doing your best. Anyone who finishes last in a marathon or triathlon is a success because he or she finished.

My track coaches at the University of Arkansas, conditioned as they were to winning one national championship after another, would say second place is the first loser.

Everyday life, however, is based on little victories, performing well in order to fulfill professional and family responsibilities. Still, it's a plan of action. You don't wake up in the morning and say, "I'm going to try to get my work done and perhaps provide for my family today."

There are plenty of people who look great on the outside but inside are very weak. You need to implement a strong spirit within in order to shine on the outside.

We have a self-confidence problem in this country. People are scared of change, wondering what happens if they fail. I'm referred to as a celebrity trainer, but I don't think of myself as someone who trains celebrities. Rather, I train *celebrations*.

Celebrate the little victories in life. If you train for 5 minutes, that's 5 minutes more than you did previously. If you eat one healthy meal, you're one ahead of where you were yesterday.

Deep down, people don't want to be Brad Pitt or Jennifer Lopez. They want to be the best versions of themselves. Become your own celebrity of sorts. Your mind-set is what positions you for success.

If I sound like a sports psychologist, it's because I've worked with a few of them over the years. Years ago, I worked with one whom I didn't agree with at first.

"I want to be the best," I told him.

He nodded. "Just think in terms of being the best you can be."

I didn't like that response. It sounded like what your mom might say to cheer you up after you came home as a kid after a tough loss. You know the spiel: "As long as you tried your best, you're a winner."

It wasn't until I reached my early thirties that I understood what the sports psych guy meant. Being the best you can be *is* being the best, because once you accept who you are as a person, you accept the notion that the greatest success is being the best you can be.

That's spiritual wellness, and, no, it's not just maturity, coming to grips with reality, or the adult version of Mom's rationalization. It's maximizing what you have.

Eighteen inches is what separates the heart from the brain, yet a lot of times the two organs don't work as one. The heart is what's driving us, and sometimes the mind doesn't believe in it. The spirit is what unites them together and gives you confidence.

My late father once told me that 5 percent of the people in this world make things happen. Fifteen percent watch what's happening, and the other 80 percent have no idea what's happening.

I've shared that philosophy with everyone I train, from celebrities to groups taking my Cardio Core 4×4 classes. These days, I'm entrenched in the 5 percent category, but it took me a long time to get here.

You need all of it—the heart, brain, and spirit working together—to become one of those "5 Percenters." Successful people accept who they are, recognizing their strengths, weaknesses, and faults and working to become better people.

That's how you achieve greatness. I made a decision a long time ago that I had to stop fighting the person in the mirror, quit battling myself mentally and physically. I accepted who I was (and am)—that I didn't have the God-given ability to be a professional athlete. I had 13 surgeries, and I know that each one of the scars I wear has gotten me to where I am now.

When we reach the physical part of this program—the third pillar of success—we'll talk about training from an anterior versus a posterior standpoint. Your anterior refers largely to your chest and biceps, the so-called beach muscles that men in particular spend a disproportionate amount of time training.

Your posterior refers to the group of muscles that runs from your lower back down behind your legs. This group includes the lower back, glutes, hamstrings, and calves. We train with a 2-to-1 ratio of posterior to anterior because it's far more important to have fully functioning glutes and lower back from a performance and health standpoint than the big beach muscles that look great but contribute little.

We want to be posterior rather than anterior people. Just as an athlete trains the posterior, we want to have a strong spiritual base that's like the roots of a tree. If you follow a certain religious faith, you think of that as your strength already. If you have a strong trunk and roots, a hurricane can come and rip off all your branches—family, finances, career—but the trunk still will be intact. It will be possible to rebuild everything else.

It's like what a young Tina Turner said during her divorce hearing when she extricated herself from a miserable marriage to Ike Turner: "You take everything I've made in the last 16 years. I'll take my future."

Talk about a strong spirit. Adversity is one of the best gifts I've ever received. If I had never encountered adversity, I never would have known how good I *could* have it.

People have no idea about the power of a strong spirit. Whenever I teach a class or talk to groups, I pull out the biggest, strongest-looking guy and tell him to put his arm out straight.

"Now," I'll say, "I want you to say, 'I will try my best,' and resist me."

"I will try my best," the guy says, and I have no trouble pushing his arm down.

"Now say, 'I will *do* my best,'" I suggest.

Inevitably, I can't push the arm down. This is not cheap theatrics or my letting up on the pressure. It's an example of the power of the spirit.

Try and *can't* are such limiting words. I have another drill I use with elite athletes. I measure their vertical leap, which for some can be 36 or 37 inches. Then I'll ask them if they can jump any higher.

"I can't," they'll say.

That's when I pull out a $100 bill, place it 6 inches higher, and tell them if they can grab it, they can have it.

I lose a Benjamin every time. Obviously, this would not work if I placed the money 2 feet higher, but when you give yourself a goal, you give the body a map. When you give the body a map, you have direction. When you see the end product, there's 100 percent certainty that you will obtain it.

If you look at my academic track record growing up, I had no business attending a top-flight college like William & Mary. I had a learning disability and was often put in classes for "special" kids.

When I decided to leave the University of Arkansas and transfer to the College of William & Mary, I called Sam Sadler, the school's longtime vice president of student affairs. I had not yet been admitted and figured I needed all the help I could get. Even though I had thrived academically at Arkansas, I still wielded a transcript with 580 SAT scores.

"Mr. Sadler," I said, "my name is Jay Cardiello, and I want to attend your school in the fall. If you admit me, I promise you I'll go on to become one of the school's greatest alumni."

William & Mary, of course, is the nation's second-oldest college and the alma mater of three US presidents, including Thomas Jefferson, as well as 16 signers of the Declaration of Independence.

Looking back, it was a brash approach, but Sam at least was willing to play along. "Well," he said, "I don't make those decisions."

Sam retired from William & Mary several years ago, but we stay in touch. The school might not be including my name on the list of its most prominent alumni yet, but at least I've justified my admission by becoming the best I can be.

What does being the best you can be mean? It means using your entire arsenal of gifts and talents at full capacity with a tireless work ethic to create the best possible product.

There's a tendency to look at our limitations rather than our strengths. You reflect on your background, lack of education, experience, or finances and think, *Surely there are people more qualified than I am.*

Yet the people who are most successful usually are not the most talented. Talk to pro athletes about their upbringing, and they'll mention people they played with who were far more talented but for any number of reasons did not leverage and maximize the opportunities to capitalize on those talents. The New York City playgrounds are full of legends, guys who were far better than some of the NBA's biggest stars but never made it.

We're a nation of people who stand around watercoolers complaining about our jobs and lots in life. Isn't it funny how 5 years later those same people are still standing there complaining while others have moved on to bigger things? People who complain the most never leave—unless they're shown the door.

Everyone has an excuse for why they can't thrive as opposed to having a plan and putting it into action. When people talk about why they deserve a promotion or opportunity, they point to their skills and experience. But did they have a plan?

A year before I wrote this book, I told my wife that within the next year I was going to land a DVD and/or a book deal or I would start looking for another line of work. It was the same ultimatum I gave myself when I left my job in radio sales for ESPN and vowed to become a top full-time trainer within the following year.

The key was that I had a plan of action and a deadline. We never want to ask ourselves years later the "what if?" question. It's easy to get comfortable and think you have things pretty good, but if you're not constantly pushing for growth, you'll fall behind. What's the old saying about experience? Do

FIT FOOD

"Beet up" your next workout. Did you know that drinking beet juice can increase stamina by up to 16 percent? Your body converts the nitrates in beets into nitric oxide, which dilates blood vessels, increasing bloodflow to muscles. Beet juice also helps your muscles produce energy more efficiently, making exercise less exhausting.

you have 20 years of experience or just 1 year repeated 19 times?

We need to have an action plan in place, and it can be something as simple as a to-do list. To-do lists are great for building momentum and tracking progress. To get the ball rolling, put some things on your daily list you know you'll get done, like eating, taking a shower, or working out. At the end of the day, at least you'll know you made some progress.

Back in the late 1990s, when I was working for the Tampa Bay Buccaneers, I was walking around the University of Tampa when I found a piece of paper on the ground. Some girl had dropped her to-do list. It included action items such as "finish term paper" but also "do makeup" and "do hair."

At that moment, I knew I wasn't alone in this strategy.

Admittedly, we want to accomplish bigger things, even on a daily basis, but this shows the power of goals, lists, and deadlines. It also shows the importance of making incremental progress every single day.

We want to make progress toward all of our goals every single day. No matter how busy and stressful a day you've had, consider it a success if as you place your head on your pillow you can answer in the affirmative to this question:

"Have I advanced toward achieving my goals?"

Maybe you've budged just an inch, but that's okay. I've dealt with a number of athletes going through excruciating rehabilitations, a process I know all too well. They've undergone major knee or arm surgeries, and on many days it feels like they're never going to return. But I always ask them at the start of each day if they feel 1 percent further along than they did 24 hours earlier. Even the biggest pessimists concede that they've progressed at least that far.

Through the miracle of compound interest, a 1 percent return every day adds up quickly. Any investor would take 1 percent a month. That's why daily, weekly, and monthly progress toward goals is so important.

Having a plan and being prepared gives you loads of confidence.

I did not get involved in track until my last 3 months in high school. Later, at Arkansas, I had no business trying to compete with all these perennial all-Americans. But even though they had more talent and experience, I was in such great condition that I was keeping up with them in conditioning drills and exceeding them in the weight room. That gave me the confidence to stand on the runway with them for the long jump. And even though I didn't jump as far as they did, I felt like I belonged.

GOAL WORKSHEET

Right now, I want you to set four big goals for yourself to accomplish in the next 6 months. They can relate to your professional or family life. They can be fitness, financial, or hobby related. Whatever they are, make them significant. Write them down here or on a separate piece of paper.

GOAL ONE _____

_____

GOAL TWO _____

_____

GOAL THREE _____

_____

GOAL FOUR _____

_____

Now set one big, ambitious goal for the next 3 years. It can be something that seems unattainable at the moment. Perhaps it's a more advanced accomplishment that builds on one of the previous four goals. Whatever it is, make it something significant.

BIG 3-YEAR GOAL _____

_____

Perhaps all this sounds a little touchy-feely. You might be thinking, *C'mon, Jay. I'm ready to tackle Cardio Core 4×4 already. I don't need a checkup from the neck up.*

No? I find it interesting that athletic coaches are always saying success is 95 percent mental and 5 percent physical, but they spend 95 percent of their time on the physical part.

If people say they've undertaken a new fitness regimen, you applaud their efforts. But if people say they've started to see a counselor, you ask what's wrong.

We should commend that decision as well. After all, they've made a decision to get better internally.

A few years ago, a client helped me create a system I've used both personally and with others. Gary needed reconstructive hip surgery, but before the procedure he wanted to be able to walk without pain for his wedding. That was my primary task, getting him better physically. We also wanted to improve his life overall. He was deep in debt, which was a concern, but the bigger issue was that there was a lot of negativity with his relationships and overall emotional state.

We took a piece of poster board and drew the equivalent of a dartboard. Next we took 30 index cards and placed the names of key people in Gary's life on each card. For people who were positive influences in Gary's life, we placed a green plus sign. The negative folks received a red minus.

Gary got his own card, which was placed in the bull's-eye of the dartboard. We drew two rings around the bull's-eye. The people Gary was spending the most time with were placed on the ring closest to Gary. The ones receiving little of Gary's time were on the outer circle.

Not surprisingly, Gary's card was virtually surrounded by red minuses. The people he liked and cared about most, the green pluses, were on the outer circle, light-years away. His fiancée, the woman for whom he was working so hard to overcome hip pain so that he could walk down the aisle, was off in the distance.

Think of the emotional stress that causes. Admittedly, it can be difficult to rid yourself of some negative people. It might take a job change to get away from a lousy boss or an insufferable co-worker. Leaving a bad marriage or relationship can be even tougher. Still, it can be done. Other negative people—friends, acquaintances, business relationships, etc.— usually are easier to leave.

Over the next 3 months, Gary flipped the rings on his dartboard. He brought the green pluses closer and pushed the red minuses to the outer rings or off the board. From a physical standpoint, we hit Cardio Core 4×4 and strengthened his posterior chain. The hip held up for the wedding, and after exchanging vows, he *carried* his new wife down the aisle.

This dartboard exercise isn't exclusive to people. Use it to see where your time is going or to measure the quality of food you're eating.

It's amazing what you can accomplish when you change yourself from a spiritual standpoint. Again, it has little to do with religion, though if you are a person of faith, put that to work. The power of goal setting or flipping the positives and minuses in your life can drive your success.

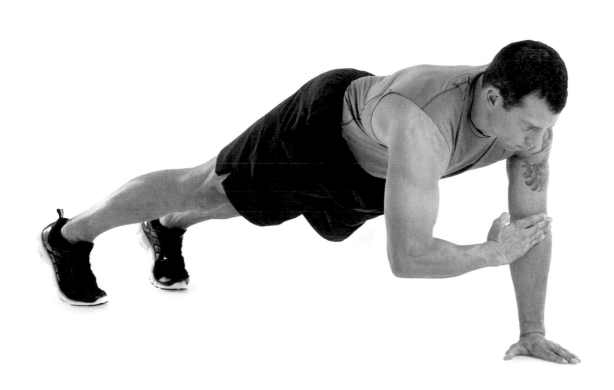

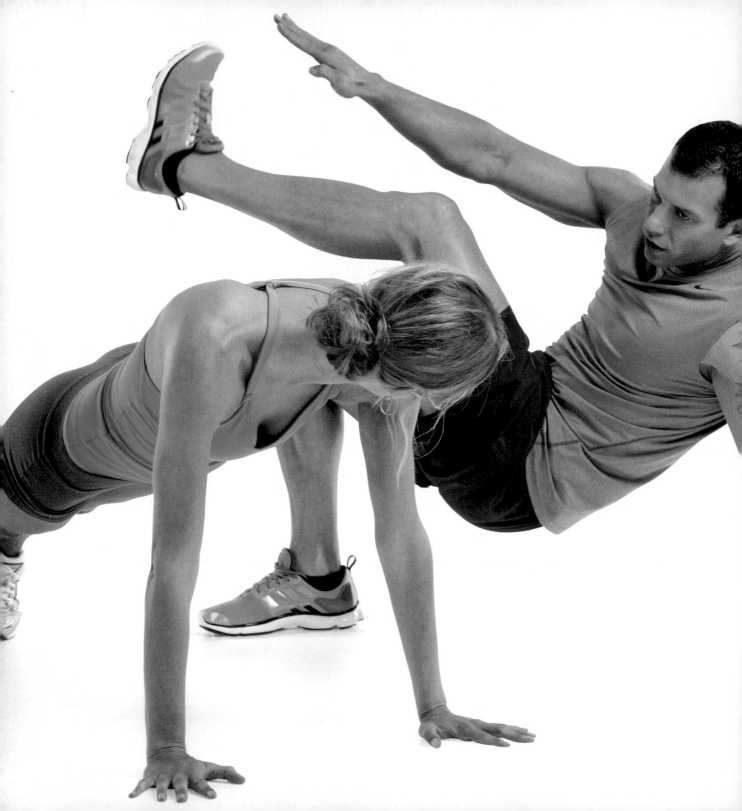

THE SECOND PILLAR OF SUCCESS

EMOTIONS GOVERN OUR ACTIONS to a greater degree than many of us realize. That's why the second pillar of success is emotional. This might sound similar to spiritual, but it's not. With the spiritual realm, we're putting ourselves in position for success with a new mind-set. We still need to get a handle on our emotions and channel them in the right direction.

When we talk about the spiritual aspect of this program, we're talking about what lies within: your core values and what makes you who you are. The emotional pillar is how you deal with external pressures. That's a fine line, perhaps, and one aspect can definitely overlap with the other, but look at it this way: The spiritual pillar is how you handle your internal life; the emotional pillar is you how deal with the external world.

I have a client who is prone to gaining weight. I asked him one day what he'd had to eat, and he replied, "Tofu and cottage cheese."

"So how are you gaining weight?"

"Well," he said, "I did have a cookie."

Two days later he admitted he had not been truthful. In fact, he routinely was eating doughnuts.

"That's great," I said.

He looked at me, puzzled.

"That's right," I said. "Now you're putting yourself in position for success, because you've told me the issue, and now we're going to work at it. When we know you're going to be in a meeting when your energy is down and you need a pick-me-up, we're going to pack sugar-free doughnuts and fruit."

The first step on the path to looking and feeling great is being honest with yourself. You can't change a habit or a behavior until you acknowledge it. Being emotionally honest with yourself and facing facts that might not be the most pleasant or attractive is the tough work you need to do to get to the place where you feel good about yourself inside and out. Your mind-set—and the emotional pillar is a huge part of this—is one of the most important factors in whether you're going to succeed or fail in your quest for fitness. I can teach you how to perform the exercises, but to achieve lasting change, you have to do the hard work of being emotionally honest yourself.

Whenever I meet with clients, I recognize

that they want to change. That's why they come to me. Even if the client is a celebrity just looking to get in shape for a movie role or concert tour, the person is in a heightened emotional state.

We need to channel this feeling into confidence. It grows as we build momentum with each training session, traveling further away from that lull in our lives.

No matter whom I work with, I stress the importance of conceiving, believing, and achieving. I'm not the first to string those words together, but I've found they're especially relevant when it comes to training.

If you can conceive of goals, whether it's losing 3 pounds or meeting a personal or professional challenge, you're well on your way. Next you have to believe in them, and finally you can achieve them.

When you train the physical, the emotional and spiritual fall into place. This isn't just about endorphin rushes and positive energy, though that no doubt helps. Instead, it's about confidence and empowerment and what you will be able to accomplish with this lean, energetic physique.

When I began working with 50 Cent, he weighed 238 pounds and had 19 percent body fat. He knew he had to make a change, and he did. In 6 months, he transformed his body

(199 pounds, 5.6 percent body fat) and used it to meet the physical demands of his schedule and accomplish great things.

Back when I coached at William & Mary, I dealt with an athlete who was going through a terrible time. She was having boyfriend, family, and academic problems and also dealing with an eating disorder. I'd get calls in the middle of the night; it seemed like she was always on the verge of leaving school.

It reached a point where she was beating herself up so much emotionally that I marched her into the women's locker room—thankfully nobody was in there—put her in front of a mirror, and asked her to repeat to herself all the horrible things she was saying about herself to others. It was only a few moments before she began breaking down. That was a good thing, because she hadn't realized how she was projecting herself to the outside world.

When you put that mirror in front of yourself and say all those things you've been saying internally, you don't believe them. In fact, you get ticked off. The reason actors recite lines in front of a mirror is because it helps them get into character. It's tough to say things with conviction in real life if you don't believe them.

And deep down, like that athlete at William & Mary, none of us believe bad things about ourselves.

FOUR WAYS TO DE-STRESS IMMEDIATELY

Working out is a great way to relieve stress. So is taking a bath or making love. Sometimes, however, you have neither the time nor the opportunity for those methods. When that's the case, try these quick de-stressing techniques.

- **Say "cheese."** It sounds, well, cheesy, but it's true. Research shows that a fake smile activates the pleasure center in your brain, which can make you feel calmer and happier immediately.

- **Chew on your stress.** Next time you feel stressed, chew on a stick of gum to defuse tension. While under moderate stress, gum chewers had salivary cortisol levels that were 12 percent lower than nonchewers'. There is a link between high cortisol levels and storage of body fat, particularly visceral abdominal body fat. However, it is the stress that will stimulate your appetite and lead to overeating.

- **Put a dot on your phone.** Stress is one of the leading causes of illness, and the phone is one of life's biggest stress inducers. To avoid phone stress, place a yellow dot on your phone. This will be your secret reminder to take a deep breath before you answer a call. Not only will you feel better, you'll sound more confident.

- **Tug on your ears.** Grab the lobes of your ears and begin moving them slowly in circles in opposite directions (10 to 12 circles should do the trick). This motion can help move the tentorium membrane in your head, which has been shown to relieve stress.

If you can conceive it, you'll believe it and definitely be in position to achieve it. The more times we say it, the more we believe it. The more it's conceived, the more it's achieved. My role is to lay the framework of a foundation. After all, when a hurricane rips down a house, the foundation is still there. It's the same process here. If you suffer a horrible injury, your foundation—emotional, spiritual, physical, and nutritional—still will be strong.

It's possible to transfer our emotions. We do this all the time. I used to marvel at how actors can summon a full range of emotional states with seemingly little effort. They can produce tears, get violently angry, or show love and affection to people they really don't know—fellow actors. There's an art to this, obviously, and actors hone their craft over many years of practice.

At the same time, any of us can transfer our

emotions without much effort. Heck, sometimes it's hard *not* to walk around angry if we keep thinking of a certain person. It can be difficult not to cry if we talk about a deceased loved one or not to laugh at a memory of someone who always made us smile.

The next time you find yourself feeling a negative emotion—anger, hurt, frustration, regret, stress, or pain—take a deep breath and focus on your heart. Replace that negative energy with a positive picture. It could be your child's laughter, a recent vacation, or any pleasant memory.

There's a reason children and others with quick tempers are told to count to 10. If you spend 10 seconds doing this, you can change your emotional state more effectively.

Back in high school, we had a meet against our archrival high school. This was before my father died, and I always looked forward to seeing him in the stands, easy to spot in his New York Yankees cap. He was the guy I most wanted to please, and I drew inspiration just seeing him there. But because Dad worked in a series of blue-collar jobs, he could not always make my midafternoon meets, and this was one of those days.

I was competing in the long jump, and the kid on the other team was putting on a show of macho arrogance. He wasn't talking trash, just sort of preening and glaring and backing it up with some long leaps.

This stuff usually didn't get to me, but for some reason that day it did. Because I couldn't look to the stands and see the calming face of my dad, I fouled on my first two jumps, with my foot landing beyond the starting line. Usually I had the other problem, jumping well before the line.

I was an emotional wreck. Fortunately, my English teacher, Joseph McBride, recognized it. He had become my mentor, a wonderful man who recognized that I did not belong in special education classes and was capable of much more than just enlisting in the army, as the guidance counselor had recommended.

Mr. McBride grabbed me by both shoulders and asked what was wrong.

"I can't jump today," I said, eyes welling up.

"Why not?"

"My dad isn't here."

Mr. McBride exhaled, looked me in the eyes, and said, "Jay, today I'm your father."

I had just one jump left, but that's all I needed. I projected a Yankees cap onto Mr. McBride as I ran down the runway, jumped over the sandpit, and landed a foot beyond my opponent's best jump.

When I got up, Mr. McBride was there to greet me, in tears. I hugged him and said, "I love you, Dad."

We see this all the time in sports, when an athlete inevitably will give a strong performance just days, sometimes hours, after losing a loved one. When you can emotionally project someone into your reality or pull from the power of the relationship, you're tapping into something special.

Don't forget to turn this equation around. You want to be that person whom others will look to when they need an emotional boost, whether you're physically present or not.

That's why following Cardio Core 4×4 is so important. Each of us plays some combination of important roles: friend, parent, child, significant other, work colleague, teacher, coach, or mentor. There's perhaps no more rewarding experience in life than to give of your time and talents to others.

But if you haven't taken care of yourself from a physical standpoint, you're not going to have the energy and drive to give of yourself to others. That's why I cringe whenever I hear people say they don't have time to train or eat properly because they're too busy with work or family commitments.

That's a noble sentiment, but sooner or later your body is going to break down, and then you won't be able to handle those work or family commitments. Maybe it won't happen in the form of injury or illness, but you'll be walking around like a zombie, struggling to make it through the day.

By devoting just 20 minutes a day, 4 days a week, along with following proper nutrition, you'll be more productive, thus creating more time to share of yourself with others.

Celebrities get accused of being self-centered and thinking of nobody but themselves. Having worked with a number of them, I've found that to be an unfair characterization. It's true that many of them need to look a certain way on camera or on the playing field. But what drives them is the knowledge that they will perform better by training and that they'll ultimately have more time for the people who matter most.

That's a powerful connection, and it will go a long way in terms of shoring up that second pillar of success.

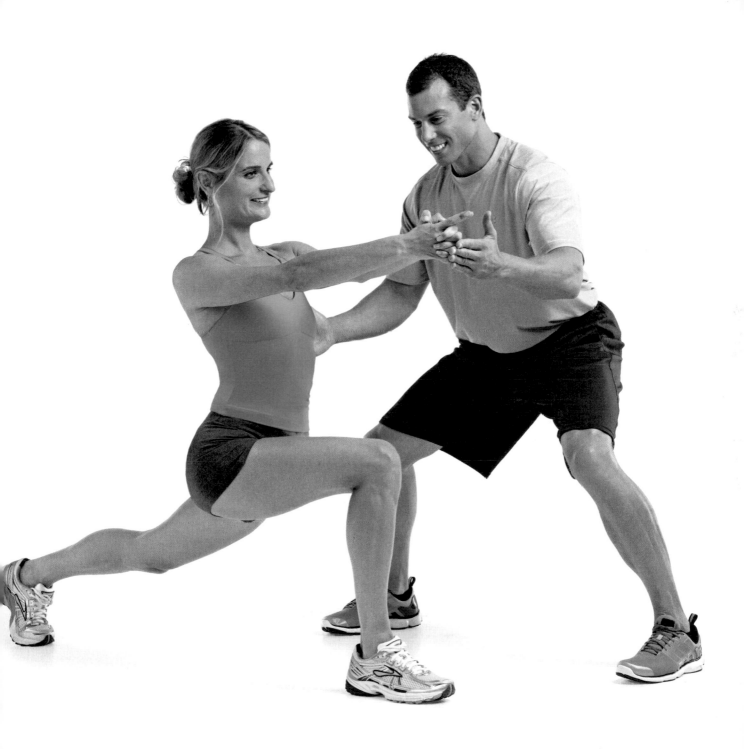

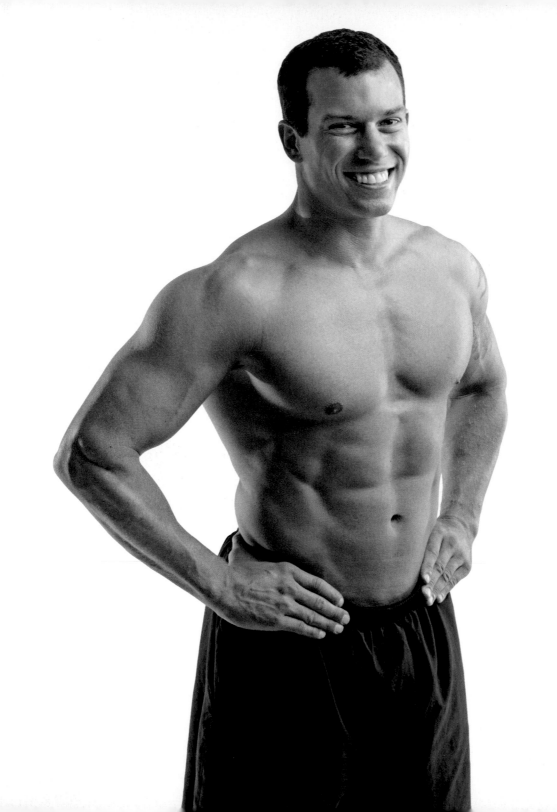

THE THIRD PILLAR OF SUCCESS

. . . .

THINGS HAVE CHANGED. Think back to when you were a kid. We ate from smaller plates with smaller portions. Sizes were smaller in general. It wasn't so long ago that a small drink meant a Dixie cup. Now a small drink is 20 ounces, and you can get a 64-ounce Big Gulp.

As kids, we ate well-portioned lunches and went out to recess. After school, we had a snack and rushed outside to play all afternoon before it got dark. These days, kids are overscheduled and no longer play on their own. Instead of thinking of physical activities as just something they did, kids now think only in terms of organized sports. Whatever happened to disorganized sports like pickup basketball and street football? Or just riding your bike all afternoon from one informal outdoor gathering to another?

FIT FOOD

Bake with applesauce. Next time you're baking, replace oil with applesauce. Two tablespoons of oil is about 200 calories, but 4 tablespoons of applesauce is only 40 calories. (Recipes typically call for twice as much applesauce as oil.) You'll be saving 160 calories without sacrificing flavor.

We need to get back to how we ate and moved then. This notion of "regression to progression" is a cornerstone of this program, and it especially applies to nutrition. The ages of 5 to 8 are the prime development years for motor skills. We never thought of "training" at that age. Our daily lives were nonstop movement.

As adults, we've formalized play into boring, repetitive movements in the gym. The same is true with nutrition. If we just ate our peas and broccoli like Mom said, we wouldn't be so nutritionally deprived that we'd have to pound coffee just to get through the day and constantly be on the prowl for the next fad diet to deal with the fat we've packed on because of our modern lifestyles.

If you follow Cardio Core 4×4, you'll get in tremendous shape while making gains in stability, flexibility, and mobility. You'll make yourself resistant to injury and slow the process of aging. But if you maintain a poor diet, you'll sabotage those results. Eating well will give you the energy you need to get through your day and burn off what would otherwise be excess calories.

We need to get back to the basics with nutrition. I'm not going to present comprehensive meal plans and philosophies. We've made things too complicated, building elaborate strategies and rule after rule to deal with the simple task of fueling our bodies for success.

Instead, I want to provide you with some simple strategies for eating for a high-performance, high-stress lifestyle. We'll take a trip to the grocery store, examine beverage options, and even look at how everyday food items can be used to cure ailments.

You've probably gathered by now that Fit Tips and Fit Foods are simple strategies that people can employ to eat better, and they resonate more than some 90-page section of a fitness book.

That's because nutritional information, like meals themselves, should be small, easy to digest, and yet nourishing. The common denominator for all of them is that they show you how to make better choices for food to improve your health, body, energy levels, and even cleaning strategies.

Rather than boring you with a hundred pages of facts and plans and rules that will go in one ear and out the other, I'm going to share with you the Big Seven. I've boiled the essentials of nutrition down into seven simple big-picture rules:

THE BIG SEVEN

EAT EARLY, OFTEN, AND LATE People who skip breakfast are more likely to be overweight. Here's why. Our bodies are craving nutrition after fasting all night. You may have noticed that *breakfast* breaks down into two words: *break* and *fast*. When you wake up, you want to rev your metabolism. Think of eating as adding wood to a hot fire. To keep the fire burning steadily, don't think in terms of three (large) square meals a day; instead, eat three smaller meals and two or three snacks, such as low-fat yogurt, a handful of almonds, an apple with peanut butter, or a low-cal protein shake. Have one of those snacks within 30 minutes of the end of your workout—the sooner the better—to help refuel your muscles. Eating before bed is not necessarily a bad thing. A healthy snack before bedtime will provide fuel for your recovering body and might ensure a good night's rest.

PLAN, PLAN, PLAN You don't have to plan a four-course menu for every day of the week in order to plan ahead. Instead, cook a lot of lean protein and veggies at once and portion the food into one-serving containers that can last for several days. Try stocking your backpack, purse, office desk drawer, and car with healthy snacks such as nuts, fruit, and energy bars. This way, you're always prepared to eat

FIT FOOD

Despite what many consumers seem to think, a food's "organic" designation does not mean that it is a lower-calorie choice. A recent study found that people assumed cookies labeled organic were 40 percent lower in calories than regular cookies.

healthy. There's nothing worse than eating bad food—and paying dearly for it—just because you had no other options. Planning saves time and money and keeps you on track with your fitness goals.

CARBS ARE NOT THE ENEMY Low-carb diets continue to be popular even though most everyone knows carbs are your essential fuel for daily life. It's true that if you eat too many carbs, they will be stored as fat, but the key is to strike a balance and focus on fiber-rich carbs that come from fruits and vegetables and avoid the processed carbs that come from breads, pastas, sugar, and baked goods.

FIT FOOD

Never eat from the original container. How many times have you dipped into a pint of ice cream or a bag of potato chips, only to find yourself staring at the bottom of the container or bag 15 minutes later? To save on calories and prevent overeating, try using a tea or coffee cup when serving ice cream and store small amounts of chips in resealable plastic bags.

KEEP PROTEIN LEAN Protein builds and maintains muscle. Avoid fatty protein and opt for lean protein sources such as chicken, fish, lean red meat, eggs, and dairy. There's a tendency to think that you can't have too much protein, but excess protein can be stored as fat. It also wreaks havoc on the kidneys and is one of the leading causes of kidney stones. So both the quality and quantity of your protein should be lean. To determine your recommended daily protein allowance, multiply your weight in pounds by 0.36, or your weight in kilograms by 0.8.

Keep in mind that your body expends calories to digest the food. Protein causes this inner fire to burn the hottest. Animal proteins increase thermogenesis more than vegetable proteins, so the best calorie-burning foods are lean meats. Eat some protein at each meal, building your dinner around a deck-of-cards-size portion of protein. That way you're burning the most calories through digestion at the end of the day, when the metabolism is slower.

FAT IS GOOD Fat can make you fat, but good fats are essential for cellular repair of the joints, mental clarity, and fighting inflammation. To slash body fat, you might need to eat more good fats. Research has found that people who up their fat intake to 40 percent while lowering carbs to 30 percent of their daily calories burn more blubber. Your muscles become better at converting fat to energy. The key is to go with healthy fats like fish, olive oil, and unsalted nuts.

DRINK WATER After all these years, we still have not come up with a healthier beverage than water, which regulates appetite and keeps our bodies hydrated and energized. You should drink a minimum of half your body weight in ounces of water a day. So if you weigh 180 pounds, you should be drinking 90 ounces—more if you live in a hot climate and train regularly.

SLEEP IT OFF Your body repairs itself while at rest. Good nutrition and adequate sleep go hand in hand. Sleeping less than 6 hours or more than 8 hours a night can cause you to gain weight and wreaks havoc on the body. Why do you crave sugar and carbs when you're having trouble sleeping? Leptin, a hormone that tells your brain that you're full, drops by 18 percent when you're tired, while levels of ghrelin, which makes you crave comfort food, increase by 28 percent. Lack of sleep raises levels of the stress hormone cortisol, making your appetite surge. So get 6 to 8 hours of sleep and avoid this vicious cycle.

FIT TIP

Slow down at the table. It takes the brain 10 minutes to register what you're eating, which is why consuming salad or tofu or simply dipping a small piece of whole grain bread in vinegar can stop you from overeating later in the meal. Plus, you are 84 percent more likely to be overweight if you eat quickly, according to an article in the *British Medical Journal*. Dutch researchers have determined that people who chew food for at least 9 seconds eat much less than those who chew for an average of 3 seconds.

FIT TIP

Here are some of my favorite tips to keep in mind when it comes to nutrition:

• Did you know that you're six times less likely to be overweight if you step on the scale at least once a week? Try weighing in on Friday and Monday mornings. Since most weight is gained on the weekends, this is a simple and effective way to keep yourself in check.

• Here's a simple and effective formula to figure out how many calories you should consume per day: Weight x 11 = your total daily calories. (This does not pertain to serious athletes, who need more calories.)

• Confuse your stomach and watch it shrink. The next time you're setting the family dinner table, try using 6-inch saucer-size plates instead of typical plates 12 inches in diameter. It might feel a bit like you're sitting at the kids' table, but studies show that people who ate food off saucers believed they were eating an average of 18 percent more calories than they really were—thus cutting down on overall calorie intake.

GROCERY SHOPPING

The next time you're grocery shopping, take a look down at the contents of various carts. Then look up at the people pushing them.

Isn't it funny how the appearance of the person pushing the cart is a direct reflection of the foods inside?

You are what you eat, after all.

It's no secret that the key to healthy eating is to keep your refrigerator and pantry stocked with nutrient-rich, high-performance foods. When you're hungry, you're going to eat whatever you can find, no matter how disciplined you are with nutrition. If the only options are pizza, chocolate, and soda, you're going to consume pizza, chocolate, and soda.

The key, of course, is to be an educated shopper. That's not always easy when food marketers throw around misleading terms like *low fat* and *all natural*.

We'll get to food labels in a moment. First, here are some supermarket strategies. When you enter a supermarket, think in terms of staying along the perimeter. That's where you'll find fresh produce, lean meats, and dairy products. The middle aisles are the danger zones, chock-full of processed foods designed to last on the shelf, and thus your waistline, a long time.

Most everything that makes crumbs can be found in the middle aisles. If you avoid these foods—cookies, crackers, snack foods, doughnuts, most cereals, and bread—you'll eat healthier *and* have a cleaner house.

A healthy nutrition program consists mostly of lean proteins, fruits, vegetables, whole wheat pastas, and water. What do they have in common? They don't produce crumbs.

FIT TIP

Use them or lose them: As you age, lost muscle is likely to be replaced by fat, according to a study reported in the *Journal of the American College of Nutrition*. That's problematic, because a pound of fat takes up 18 percent more space in your body than a pound of muscle does. Recent research suggests that eating spinach helps by increasing protein synthesis, which is a cornerstone of muscle growth.

Do all your grocery shopping for the week at once, perhaps on a Sunday, when you're not so rushed. Then again, though the weekend might be the most convenient time to shop, the best day to visit the store is Wednesday. Studies show that only 11 percent of people shop for groceries on hump day, and only 4 percent of people shop on Wednesdays after 9:00 p.m. You might have to track down someone to fetch fresh stuff from the back room, but what else do they have to do at that hour? You'll get in and out of the store quickly, saving time.

You never should go grocery shopping hungry, since you're more likely to eat unhealthy samples or just break open something and pay for it on the way out. If you're not making one large weekly trip, consider using a carrying basket. Supermarkets increased the size of pushcarts by 40 percent in the last 5 years, knowing that you're more likely to fill them.

Leave the kids at home when you go shopping, since kids increase your chances of choosing unhealthy foods and sampling snacks before checkout.

Once you're home, grill enough lean meat or fish and prepare enough vegetables for several meals over the course of the week.

Now let's take a spin around the market. There are pros and cons to shopping at a local grocery store versus a Whole Foods or a Costco. The important thing is to develop a routine that gets you in and out of the store quickly. This goes hand in hand with the advantages of habitual eating.

Let's take a look at labels. When consumers see the words *low fat* or *fat free* on a label, they often assume that the food won't make them fat. In reality, such terms, along with "no added fat," usually mean more sugar. Simple white refined sugar is the very stuff that converts to fat once in the body. Avoid anything that lists sugar as one of the first ingredients.

You can ignore fat altogether when it comes to bread. There's not enough in a slice

FIT TIP

How to shop for groceries: (1) Create a list before you go to the market. (2) Shop on a full stomach and in a good mood. (3) Unless you're stocking up, use a carry basket to tote purchases. These three strategies will keep your wallet fat and your waistline lean.

to make a real difference. Instead, focus on the amount of fiber per slice, low sugar content, and fewer ingredients. Whole grain should be the first ingredient. With whole grain, nothing nutritious is stripped away. That means you're eating natural fiber, not inulin and polydextrose, which are used to artificially boost fiber. Each slice should have at least 2 grams of fiber.

My choice? Arnold Grains & More Double Oat Hearty Oatmeal bread, with 110 calories, 5 grams of protein, and 3 grams of fiber per slice.

For breakfast, you can't go wrong with oatmeal, which is loaded with fiber. The fiber decreases your appetite by making you feel full so you can go for extended periods of time without eating while keeping your energy levels high.

Oatmeal will give you a lasting blast of energy that helps you work out longer and more intensely. It's better to eat steel-cut or old-fashioned oats and not the flavored oatmeal packets that contain a lot of sugar.

If you opt for a different cereal, consider that the average American consumes more than 160 bowls of cereal a year. Picking the right box could mean knocking 15 pounds off your waistline and infusing your diet with massive doses of vital nutrients. One of the best choices is Fiber One Original (60 calories, 1 gram of fat, 14 grams of fiber, and no sugars).

Can you eat eggs regularly and not get fat? Absolutely. Research shows that the dietary culprit in heart disease is saturated fat; eggs are low in saturated fat.

Eggs are relatively low in calories—75 calories if hardcooked and 110 calories if scrambled in 1 teaspoon of oil. They also have essential nutrients and antioxidants. The American Heart Association says that an egg a day is fine, but use light vegetable oil to cook the eggs.

Contrary to popular belief, there is no nutritional difference between a brown and a white egg. That's because brown eggs are laid by hens with red earlobes while white eggs are laid by hens with white earlobes. Who knew?

Yogurt can be a great breakfast option as well

as an effective midmorning or midafternoon snack. Unfortunately, many yogurts are loaded with sugar. Choose yogurt without fruit to save on calories and add your own fresh fruit. Go for yogurt with at least 20 grams of protein (i.e., Greek yogurt). Choose brands with 10 grams or less of fat per container, as some have up to 30.

It's tough to go wrong in the produce aisle.

I'm a big fan of most anything green—spinach, broccoli, asparagus, avocados, green beans—and I load up on apples and berries.

You can't overestimate the importance of eating fruits and vegetables. Your body burns 16 percent more calories after you eat a meal that's mostly fruits and vegetables than if you ate a meal without any produce.

Fruits and vegetables high in vitamin C (such as oranges, lemons, pineapples, grapefruit, apples, limes, tomatoes, broccoli, cabbage, celery, carrots, and watermelon) also boost your body's ability to burn fat. Adding them into your daily regimen will pay dividends in more ways than one.

You'll be hard-pressed to find a better food than tomatoes. Most are red, and that's a good thing, since red tomatoes are packed with more of the antioxidant lycopene. A diet rich in lycopene can decrease your risk of bladder, lung, prostate, skin, and stomach cancers.

When it comes to ground meat, don't agonize over whether beef, turkey, or chicken is healthiest. For ground beef, look for 90 percent–plus lean on the label, which equates to less than 10 grams of fat per 3.5-ounce serving. Just a few percentage points lower can make a big difference. Eighty-five percent lean beef packs a whopping 18 grams of fat—the same as a McDonald's Quarter Pounder.

As far as white meat versus dark meat, the difference is that dark meat is made up of mostly slow-twitch muscle fibers, used for slow, continuous activities. White meat is made up of fast-twitch muscle fibers, used for sudden bursts of activity. Fast-twitch muscles don't need the stored fat that slow-twitch muscles do. So white meat has less than half the fat of dark meat.

No discussion of nutrition is complete without mentioning salt, the most popular condiment. According to the US Department of Health and Human Services, Americans consume more than 3,400 milligrams of salt per day. That's well above the recommended daily allowance of 2,300 milligrams of sodium—1,500 if you fall into high-risk categories, which includes everyone age 51 and older and people with high blood pressure, diabetes, or kidney disease.

That daily limit of 2,300 milligrams is equivalent to just 1 teaspoon. Avoid adding table salt to food and be sure to examine product labels for salt content.

Try to be a habitual (good) eater. A lot of people eat oatmeal for breakfast every day of the week. This might sound boring to you, but there's nothing like a bowl of fiber-rich oats to get you going in the morning. When you don't have to think about what you're having for breakfast, you save time and energy.

The Hall of Fame baseball player, Wade Boggs, ate grilled chicken most every day of his career. He even wrote a cookbook of chicken recipes.

FIT FOOD

You'll lose weight faster if you eat fruits and veggies raw. Farmers feed pigs steamed or cooked vegetables to fatten them up because they know raw veggies will slim down the pigs. If you prefer your veggies hot, flash boiling is one of the fastest and healthiest ways to cook them. Just bring a pot of water to a rolling boil, add the veggies, count to 10, and then drain them. This softens them a bit but preserves much of their vitamins and minerals.

By choosing to eat grilled chicken—a quality lean protein, by the way—Boggs didn't have to spend much time worrying about food every day. That's because he didn't view every meal as a rich sensory experience but as a way to fuel his body for optimum performance.

Everyone enjoys treating the tastebuds and spending long sit-down meals with family and friends. But we should look at those occasions as exceptions to be savored. Most of the time, healthy habitual eating is the way to go.

A lot of people eat poorly out of habit. They continue to eat sugary cereals or fast food into adulthood because, well, that's what they've always eaten.

When you can draw the connection between a food and how it makes you *feel*, and not just how it tastes, that's a powerful discovery, and I believe it will be powerful enough to help you form new habits.

YOU ARE WHAT YOU . . . DRINK

We tend to focus too much on what we eat and not nearly enough on what we drink. People often mistake hunger for thirst, which is not surprising since you're not going to feel satiated when you're thirsty.

How much should you drink? You've no doubt heard the advice to consume eight glasses of water a day. That's not a bad starting point, but it's still not enough. You ought to be drinking enough to produce 2 liters of urine a day. That's right, enough to fill a 2-liter bottle. That means you'll need to drink 3 to 3.5 liters a day.

There are countless benefits to drinking more water. You'll have more energy and healthier skin and hair, and your kidneys will love you. Most kidney stones are caused at least in part by not drinking enough water. That alone should be adequate motivation. Many women who have given birth and had kidney stones claim the stones were more painful!

Caffeinated beverages don't count toward your daily 3.5 liters. In fact, if you drink enough water and follow a proper diet, you won't have to use caffeine.

That's right. It wasn't that long ago when the only people who drank coffee were people over 50, the type you'd see in TV commercials for Folgers and Maxwell House. Starbucks has done a wonderful job of convincing us that everyone over the age of 10 needs their products just to get through the day.

Here's the great thing about caffeine, though. When you stop using it, it becomes that much more effective. Non–caffeine users know the power of a jolt of caffeine when they rush into a meeting following a red-eye flight. But it was never meant as daily fuel.

FIT FOOD

Fruit is doused with pesticides prior to harvest to ensure blemish-free skin. By the time it arrives in the produce department, most fruit can be coated with up to nine different pesticides. So choose only fruit with the USDA organic sticker. Also, fruit has a natural wax coating that holds pesticides, so wash each piece with a sponge or scrub brush and a dab of dishwashing detergent to eliminate more than half of the residues.

That's what water was meant for. It doesn't matter what kind of water you drink. People tend to obsess about bottled water, but chances are what comes out of your tap is highly purified. A generation ago nobody drank bottled water. (Quick: What's Evian spelled backward? Naive.)

It's not just water, however. The liquids you drink play a major role in determining your health. Let's examine them one at a time.

MILK

For some reason, milk isn't as popular as it was a generation ago, when kids routinely drank milk with every meal. That would not be such a bad thing if today's kids replaced milk with water, but more often than not they've substituted soda and juice.

Milk has all sorts of benefits, starting with its calcium content. Men who add calcium to their diets lose up to 70 percent more weight and up to 64 percent more fat than men who have a poor calcium intake. Aim for 1,000 milligrams of calcium a day from low-fat milk, yogurt, or a supplement.

Drinking low-fat or fat-free milk is a smart move if you're looking to cut calories. When it comes to building muscle, though, whole milk might be a better choice. Scientists at the University of Texas medical branch in Galveston found that drinking whole milk after lifting weights boosted muscle protein synthesis—an indicator of muscle growth—2.8 times more than drinking fat-free milk did.

Milk also helps when you've consumed something fatty. Make up for this diet mishap by drinking an 8-ounce glass of milk. The calcium in milk will help metabolize fat more efficiently by speeding up the time it takes to get rid of fat as waste.

Contrary to popular belief, warm milk is more likely to keep you awake than put you to sleep. That's because the protein in milk actually will reduce the brain's serotonin levels, delaying sleep. Try cherry juice instead. Cherries are loaded with carbohydrates that will boost your brain's production of serotonin and induce sleepiness.

Perhaps the easiest way to add milk to your diet is to splash a couple of ounces on oatmeal for breakfast. And if you consider that many postworkout recovery drinks consist of little more than chocolate-flavored whey protein (a by-product of cheese manufacturing), you might as well go with a glass of chocolate milk.

SODA AND ENERGY DRINKS

There's no upside to drinking soda. Admittedly, I'll have a Diet Coke with pizza occasionally, but soda should not be an everyday

FIT FOOD

Need a one-word answer for fighting fat? *Vinegar.* This acidic liquid contains acetic acid, which can activate genes that produce enzymes to help break fat down. In simplistic terms, add a tablespoon or two to your favorite salad and begin your war on fat.

beverage, and until recently it was not. A generation ago, soda was viewed as a treat. Kids tended to have it only after sporting events or perhaps at birthday parties.

Adults, meanwhile, drink soda like water. Diet soda has fewer calories, but that does not mean it's good for you. Did you know that your risk of becoming overweight soars 41 percent with each daily can of *diet* soda you consume? Artificial sweeteners such as high-fructose corn syrup (HFCS) are many times sweeter than sugar and act as a potent stimulus for turning any sweet tooth into a fang.

Sodas, iced teas, and other sweetened beverages are the biggest sources of HFCS—accounting for about two-thirds of our intake. Research from the University of California at San Francisco indicates that fructose can trick our brains into craving more food, even when we're full. It works by impeding the body's ability to use leptin, the "satiation hormone" that tells us when we've had enough to eat.

The average American drinks up to 60 gallons of soda a year, which wreaks havoc on the pancreas. Drinking just two sodas a week increases your risk of pancreatic cancer by 87 percent over people who don't drink soda. That's because the sugar in soda spikes insulin levels, and repeated bouts of insulin spikes promote cancer in pancreatic cells.

FIT TIP

Got sunburn? Use milk to reduce the pain associated with a nasty sunburn by soaking a clean washcloth in cold milk and draping it over the burned area for up to 10 minutes. Repeat each hour for the first 6 hours. The lactic acid in the milk will help ease inflammation, while the coolness will help short-circuit the swelling.

As for energy drinks, it's scary to consider the sugar, stimulants, and other stuff that goes into them. I worry about any category where certain brands have been banned in some countries—and a few in this country. Anyone relying on energy drinks needs to implement some dietary changes immediately. Those afternoon energy slumps are a sign of poor adrenal function, inefficient metabolism of carbs and sugars, as well as consumption of nutrient-depleted foods. Reduce sugar, caffeine, and dairy foods at lunch and opt for foods such as brown rice, yams, kidney beans, pinto beans, or sunflower seeds to avoid the crash and the need for caffeine.

Bottom line: You can lose 14 pounds a year simply by switching from soda to water, since the typical soda is 140 calories, which translates into more than 50,000 calories a year.

COFFEE

Coffee consumption has grown exponentially in the past decade, rising proportionately with the obesity epidemic. There's not necessarily a direct correlation, though all those sugary, creamy drinks have contributed.

Instead, coffee consumption is more a symptom of people having poor diets that do not provide them with adequate energy. Sure, a lack of sleep contributes, but if people consumed more lean meats, fiber-rich vegetables, and healthy fats, they would not need constant short-term energy boosts with caffeine.

By following Cardio Core 4×4 nutritional program, you should be able to wean yourself off caffeine. Until then, try swapping your 2:00 p.m. coffee for green tea. Not only is green tea better for you, it also might prevent colds. Canadian researchers added green tea to lab samples of the adenovirus, one of the bugs responsible for colds, and found that it stopped the virus from replicating. All the credit goes to EGCG, a chemical compound found in green tea. Start pumping green tea into your body at the first sign of a cold and help stop the advance of the adenovirus.

If you still need a morning pick-me-up, eat an apple instead of drinking a cup of coffee. An apple can energize you naturally in the same way that coffee will and is a healthier alternative.

Ginseng tea also is a great substitute for coffee.

FIT TIP

Cola contains a lot of phosphoric acid, which destroys your insides as it produces that cool soft drink fizz sound. Did you know that some police squad cars carry a 2-liter bottle of soda to remove bloodstains after an accident? It's also effective for cleaning toilets. Just pour a can in the bowl, let it sit for 10 minutes, and flush. It also gets rid of rust. Is this what you want to put in your body?

A cup just before leaving for work can get you energized and ready to start your day, and it's cheaper and healthier for you than coffee. Hot tea of any sort can slash your risk of kidney cancer by 15 percent, according to a review in the *International Journal of Cancer*. Try pu-erh tea, which is purported to be better than green or black tea at preventing DNA damage.

Once you wean yourself from caffeine, it becomes a powerful weapon for those days when an infant kept you up all night.

Caffeine also is a proven training aid, though here again energy drinks do not provide the boost you might think. During one study, 17 fit adults drank up to two cans of a popular energy drink an hour before a sprint workout but didn't experience a performance boost. You're better off with a banana, a carb gel, or even dark chocolate.

JUICE

The great thing about eating a piece of fruit is all the fiber you get in addition to the nutrients in the juice. Unfortunately, you negate most of that nutritional value by simply consuming the sugar-rich juice.

If you eat an apple or orange, that fiber is going to satiate you. A glass of juice will spike your insulin levels and make you hungry. One compromise is to consume juice rich in pulp, but why not just eat the fruit?

If you must drink juice, dilute it 50 percent with water. That changes a 16-ounce bottle of cranberry/grape from 275 calories to 138, and you won't notice the difference.

When it comes to misleading marketing, nobody does it better than smoothie shops. It's true that there's some nutrient value to these beverages. Unfortunately, even a medium-size fruit-and-yogurt smoothie packs at least 60 grams of sugar. The fruit purees used in the smoothies are mixed with liberal doses of sugar or high-fructose corn syrup. Sure, it has juice. But linking your average smoothie to a piece of fruit is like comparing a bowl of Rice Krispies to a Rice Krispies treat.

WATER WITH LEMON (JUICE)

Unlike other juices, there's no sugar in pure lemon juice. If drinking plain water isn't appealing to you, make your own lemonade by drinking an ounce or two of H_2O out of a bottle and topping off the bottle with lemon juice.

Lemon peels contain pectin, a soluble fiber that has been shown to help with weight loss while also helping you to feel fuller. The combination of lemon juice and drinking adequate water also is one of the best ways to

FIT FOOD

Researchers at the University of Alabama fed rats 200 milligrams of vitamin C twice a day and found that it nearly stopped the secretion of stress hormones. If it relaxes a rat, it can work for you. Another study found that people who consume 500 milligrams of vitamin C daily burn 39 percent more fat during exercise than those who have less than 100 milligrams a day. Low levels of vitamin C might impede your body's ability to use fat as energy. Oranges are a terrific source of vitamin C, but did you know kiwifruit and peppers actually pack more of this vital nutrient?

ward off kidney stones.

Speaking of lemon, take a cue from the Greeks, who used lemon during ancient times to kill bacteria. Now they add it to everything. It's an excellent source of vitamin C and has fewer calories than other citrus fruit. I recommend whipping up the ultimate free-radical-fighting salad dressing or meat marinade with lemon juice, olive oil, oregano, and garlic.

A word of caution on lemons: In a 2007 study from the *Journal of Environmental Health*, nearly 70 percent of the lemon wedges smashed onto restaurant glasses contained disease-causing microbes. Researchers ordered drinks at 21 different restaurants, securing 76 lemons. Testing revealed 25 different microorganisms lingering on the lemons, including *E. coli* and fecal bacteria. Solution? Ask for lemon juice in a separate glass.

Most people don't drink enough water, and it's mainly because of the out-of-sight-out-of-mind mentality. If you keep water bottles on your desk, in your car, and alongside you in the gym and even while relaxing, you'll drink more water and lose weight.

Take a water bottle when shopping. You'll avoid those random hunger pangs that often are just thirst disguised as hunger. Your brain just does a lousy job differentiating between the two. Thirst can masquerade as hunger, which is one reason dieters should do their best to stay hydrated.

Water also fuels your body's fat burners. Metabolism rises 24 percent in the 90 minutes after drinking a bottle of chilled water. That's because of the energy your body requires to warm the water during digestion. One study found that athletes who drank cold water trained 23 percent longer than those who downed lukewarm water.

Drink water as soon as you wake in the

morning. Studies show that drinking 20 ounces of water before breakfast can boost your metabolism by 10 percent—meaning you'll burn 10 percent more calories than if you didn't drink up.

ALCOHOL

One of the toughest things for people to do when they embark on a healthy lifestyle change is to give up alcohol—or at least curtail it. I'm not going to suggest that you give up your favorite spirits, but what you'll likely discover is that the harder you work on your body, the less likely you'll want alcohol.

You might find that alcohol just drops out of your schedule, especially if you train after work instead of going to happy hour. If you get up an hour earlier to train, you'll go to bed an hour earlier, cutting into what previously might have been nightcap time.

If you picked up this book, chances are you're so busy that you need a quick training solution for your hectic schedule. Alcohol probably isn't a big part of your life.

I'm not passing judgment. Most of us like to indulge occasionally, especially during the holidays. A glass of wine is one of life's simple pleasures.

One way to cut down on your alcohol is to "choose your sin wisely." If you're going to indulge in alcohol, don't indulge in fattening food and vice versa. Pick your vice and stick with it—and try to keep it in moderation. If you do choose to imbibe, try to drink one glass of water in between the alcoholic stuff. That

FIT TIP

With billions of water bottles produced each year, it's important to be environmentally conscious. Use plastic water bottles with numbers 2, 4, or 5 in the triangle. Number 1 plastic bottles are safe to use but not meant to be reused. Bottles numbered 3, 6, or 7 can leak toxins into the water. These toxins can cause breast cancer in women or prostate cancer in men. Never store your bottle in your car or direct sunlight, which can release these toxins at a faster rate.

will slow you down *and* keep you hydrated for the next day.

Several studies have extolled the health benefits of drinking *one* glass of red wine per day. To reduce your risk of cancer, drink red wine from Chile. Chilean Cabernet Sauvignon is 38 percent higher than French wine in antioxidants that plunder free radicals that cause cancer (called flavanols).

When it comes to liquor, try to make the best choice possible. While, gin and tonic, for instance, is regarded as a lighter cocktail, it actually packs 210 calories and 22 grams of sugar. That's because tonic water has more than 20 grams of sugar per 8-ounce serving, making it nothing more than a glorified 7Up. Champagne is just as bubbly but contains only one-fourth of the sugar. Not only that, you look classier holding a champagne flute, right?

If you want to cut down on calories during the holiday season, stay away from eggnog. Its primary ingredients are milk, cream, and eggs, providing a gut-busting 350 calories, 19 grams of fat, and 22 grams of sugar. And that's before you add alcohol.

Should you overindulge, forget all those hangover pills you find in the checkout aisle. Instead, try a roast beef sandwich on whole grain bread. The protein in the beef helps your liver process the alcohol, while whole grain bread is loaded with vitamin B, which your body needs. Add some baby spinach (for vitamin A) and hummus to help with the morning-after anxiety. Then have a side of asparagus with your sandwich. When researchers exposed a group of human liver cells to asparagus extract, it suppressed free radicals and more than doubled the activity of two enzymes that metabolize alcohol. Translation: Asparagus can sober you up faster.

EATING OUT

A generation ago, eating out was a relatively unusual experience. Families gathered around the dinner table, kids and adults took their lunches to school and work, and people were more likely to eat breakfast at home.

Today? All bets are off. With both parents working in many households, meals are grabbed on the go. Whether it's at a restaurant, cafeteria, fast-food establishment, or one of the many "fast-casual" takeout places that have sprung up to feed our fast-paced, on-the-go lifestyles, it can be a challenge to eat healthy on the go.

Unfortunately, many people rely on sugar and caffeine to get through their hectic days. This causes the blood sugar to spike, giving you a temporary burst of energy. Soon you crash and need to repeat the process, creating a vicious cycle.

As with the rest of this fitness program, you can employ some simple strategies to improve your health and performance.

Did you know, for instance, that diners underestimate their caloric intake by up to 93 percent when eating out? Every time you eat at a restaurant, you're probably consuming twice as much as you think. Order a box with your entrée and put half of it away before digging into your meal.

Don't assume that a sit-down restaurant is healthier than a fast-food eatery. One menu analysis of 24 national chains revealed that the average entrée at a sit-down restaurant con-tains 867 calories, compared with 522 calories in the average fast-food entrée.

That's probably due to the "free" handouts at sit-down restaurants. But just because it's free doesn't mean it comes without a cost. Munch on bread or breadsticks and you will consume 300-plus calories before your meal arrives. That basket of chips at a Mexican eatery comes with a price tag of 500 calories, which easily can double the impact of an entrée. Not so free now, is it?

Then there's the "house salad," which sounds like it should be healthy, right?

Unfortunately, the iceberg lettuce it's served on offers little nutritional value. Two tablespoons of dressing can add more than 200 calories and 12 grams of fat. Instead, try seaweed salad. It's one of nature's strongest multivitamins.

The average salad dressing serving has approximately 300 calories, which means your salad could have as many calories as a cheese-burger. When ordering salad, keep the dressing on the side and dip your fork in it before spearing a piece of lettuce. You'll add taste without excess calories.

Order right away instead of opting for appe-tizers, which usually offer few healthy options. If you can't wait for the entrée, order vegetable or noodle soup. The fiber causes food to go through your digestive system faster, and water helps dissolve the fat. Tomato soup has the same effect. You'll eat less during the meal, and you will feel full longer.

FIT FOOD

It's tough to eat healthy at the movies. Consider, ahem, sneaking your own fruit or healthy snack into the theater. If you purchase popcorn, don't add salt—there's plenty already—and stay away from the butter pump, which can triple the calories of popcorn. Don't be surprised if you sleep better if you eat popcorn at a late movie. The carbs will induce your body to create serotonin, a neurochemical that makes you feel relaxed. Skipping the butter will slow the process of boosting those feel-good chemicals and will slow digestion in general.

Think of the menu as a starting point. Any restaurant—even fast-food joints—will tailor to your needs. So ask and save on the calories. Take a BLT: Ask for mustard instead of mayo, take off a slice of bacon, and you've cut more than 300 calories.

It's simple, really. Request whole grain bread for your sandwich at Panera Bread and ask for your pasta with whole wheat noodles at Macaroni Grill. When ordering at Chipotle Mexican Grill or Moe's Southwest Grill, get your burrito in a bowl and hold the tortilla. When you eat at a "fern bar" restaurant such as Applebee's, Ruby Tuesday, Chili's, or TGI Friday's, just ignore the menu and order grilled fish or chicken with vegetables.

The term "mystery meat" applies to restaurants and not just school cafeterias. Don't assume, for instance, that a turkey burger is a better option than beef. Restaurant turkey burgers often are made with a mix of light and dark meats, so the calorie count is similar to that of ground sirloin (200 calories for 4 ounces). But lean beef is rich in B vitamins and iron, nutrients often missing from women's diets.

Then there's "prime," which sounds like a positive term when it comes to beef. Actually, it's the USDA designation that means a piece of beef is sufficiently marbled—strewn with intramuscular fat. Only 3 percent of beef processed in the United States receives this rating, and most goes to restaurants. If your steak is prime, count on it packing 50 percent more calories.

Perhaps you like sushi? Stay away from the California roll, which contains some healthy ingredients but still is a nutritional lightweight. That's because most rolls are made with white rice and imitation crab, which are high in sugar. Both ingredients spike your blood sugar levels, leaving you hungry within a few hours. Opt instead for a vegetable roll with brown rice and raw fish.

Choose the veggie roll over the spicy tuna roll as well. In the sushi world, spicy means a spoonful of mayo spiked with an Asian chili sauce. The calorie counts can climb higher than 300, depending on how heavy a hand the sushi chef has with the spicy stuff. Either way, you're better off satisfying your need for heat with a touch of wasabi.

Pizza is a tempting choice for lunch, especially when you live in the pizza capital of the world (New York), like I do. The key, as always, is to make the best choice—and when it comes to pizza, that's thin crust. It has one-third fewer calories than a thick-crust slice. Order your pizza with double tomato sauce and light cheese. Men who eat a lot of tomato products lower their risk of prostate cancer, and the reduced-fat cheese can save up to 20 grams of fat per pie. And, yes, blotting the cheese with a napkin will cut down even more on the fat.

FIT TIP

Headed to a party? Wear fitted clothes and you will be more likely to avoid unhealthy eating. People generally feel better in fitted than loose clothing, which translates into less eating. Also, avoid seated conversations. People who stand during gatherings eat and drink less while burning more calories than their seated counterparts.

Bottom line with nutrition: By following some simple strategies and planning ahead, you can eat healthier and tastier and save money along the way.

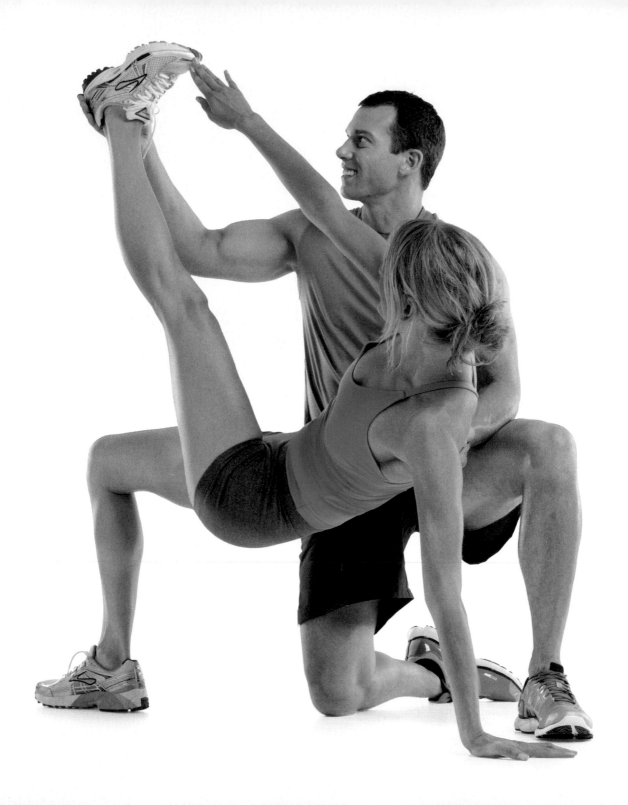

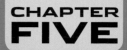

THE FOURTH PILLAR OF SUCCESS

Now that we've defined how to get our spiritual, emotional, and nutritional houses in order, it's time to turn to the *physical*.

When we look at professional athletes, we see people who train to perform well and to avoid injuries. So why don't the rest of us train that way? Most people train for aesthetics and thus do not create bodies resistant to injury and long-term deterioration.

Over the years, several of my clients have recovered from automobile accidents faster than doctors expected because they had developed tremendous core strength. I've also noticed people in gyms where I've worked suffer major hip and knee injuries that could have been minimized, if not prevented, had they focused their training on building a solid foundation rather than just looking good in a mirror.

The great thing is that you can do both. Why put forth all that effort to look good if you haven't created a powerful, injury-resistant physique along the way? As we age, the core becomes especially important. The reason so many seniors end up suffering terrible falls and needing hip replacements is because they did not establish the strength and stability around these joints that would have enabled them to avoid the falls.

Don't be that person in the gym whose house is built on sand. Build a strong foundation.

Believe me, I know. Outside the time spent training clients, I don't spend more than half an hour a day in the gym, and I'm able to maintain 6 percent body fat. When I do need to engage in some serious aesthetics training for photo shoots and videos, my strong foundation makes it simple.

That's because if you build this strong

FIT TIP

By following this program, you can cancel your gym membership. But in case you want to keep it, remember that January is the best month to negotiate gym fees and discounts and Sunday is the best day of the week to join. Salespeople are more likely to cut a deal and add perks like free training sessions and no initiation fees when you join on Sunday than on any other day of the week. And anytime you see balloons outside gym doors, you know it's a buyer's market.

foundation first, you'll reach your weight-loss and aesthetics goals much faster.

Why is it, then, that so much emphasis is placed on creating a bikini body, losing 30 pounds in 30 days, or building a massive muscle-bound physique?

The answers can be found in the recent history of fitness. In the 1970s, Arnold Schwarzenegger and his bodybuilding buddies taught us that spending long hours in the weight room to create big, showy muscles was the way to go. In 1977, Jim Fixx authored *The Complete Book of Running,* which started the first running boom. Americans everywhere took off running like so many Forrest Gumps, because it seemed like the thing to do.

In the 1980s, people like Jane Fonda and Kathy Smith turned us on to aerobics and body shaping. This paved the way in the 1990s for more specialized group fitness classes (remember "step aerobics"?). Thousands of young women, inspired by ESPN's coverage of figure modeling and fitness competitions, embarked on a hybrid training regimen that seemed like a cross between gymnastics and bodybuilding in order to compete in a muscular, breast-implanted version of Miss America pageants.

The 1990s also included a second running boom (thanks, Oprah!), and gym rats everywhere followed the lead of Major League

> # FIT TIP
> Think a postworkout sauna helps you recover faster? Not so! Forget about the steam room after a workout. A recent study tested athletes and found that a postworkout sauna actually impaired their performance and strength 2 days later. For optimum recovery, take a plunge in a cold whirlpool or hit a cold shower.

Baseball players, cyclists, and track stars, turning to pharmaceuticals of every variety to build the physiques of their choice.

At the turn of the 21st century, a number of pioneering "performance coaches" had seen enough, realizing that for all the time people were spending in the gym or pounding the pavement running, they were not becoming any fitter. In fact, they were exacerbating muscle imbalances through repetitive, joint-pounding running or weight lifting.

These coaches realized there was no point in "working body parts," as bodybuilders do, because the arms and legs are simply levers, not the core muscles of locomotion (hips, shoulders, midsection). Why do long, steady-state, joint-damaging running or aerobics classes when you would get a lot more out of some quick bursts of interval training?

Why train the body to look good in a mirror or figure competition when what we really need is a physique built for the stresses and challenges of everyday life and for functional movement that's resistant to injury and long-term deterioration?

Why spend long hours in a gym or outside running when we could accomplish so much more in a shorter, focused workout and get the same aesthetic look that others spend hours a day pursuing?

That's what the performance coaches who deal with elite athletes have stressed in recent years. They've borrowed from yoga, Pilates, track and field, and martial arts to train the body for everyday movement, creating strength, stability, and mobility around the shoulders, midsection, and hips.

My program is the culmination of the best learning of this new paradigm. Cardio Core 4×4 is the product of my backgrounds in track and martial arts. I developed it as a way to train elite athletes to excel in their respective sports without needing to camp out all day in the gym.

When you look at how we move, it all comes down to the shoulders, midsection, and hips, the three-dimensional, stabilizing rotational muscles known as the core. If we can strengthen and stabilize these muscles, we'll go a long way toward performing better and avoiding long-term deterioration.

This aha moment could not have come at a better time, as it coincided with the initial late-'90s Internet boom. Technology became a more prevalent part of our lives, mostly in a good way, but it caused us to spend more time sitting and hunched over computers.

As a result, our shoulders rounded forward

and our hips tightened up. Think of elderly people you know who have that hunched-over look or who walk with small, uneasy steps because their hips are so locked down they no longer can generate motion with their hips. Instead, they rely on their knees and as a result must endure costly and painful hip or knee replacements.

But at least baby boomers have lived mostly during the pretech era. What about all the Generation Xers and Millennials who have grown up slouched over computers, sitting in front of screens all day, far less active than their predecessors? What will happen when they start hitting their fifties and sixties?

Isn't the answer obvious? There will be an epidemic of hip, knee, and back problems. The real problem is a lack of core stability.

We're living longer, and if you believe the economic doomsayers, we will have to work longer than ever before. How will we live and work if we're in constant pain?

You might not think this applies to you. Perhaps you're a runner or a gym rat. But how is your flexibility? If you stand in profile in front of a mirror, is there a straight line from your ear to your toe? Or are you slightly hunched forward? Do you experience back problems?

Whether these issues are apparent or not, you must address them. People don't tend to think of their shoulders and hips as key areas to train. After all, they're not nearly as sexy as the biceps or triceps.

There's a tendency to think of the hands and arms as carrying the workload for the upper body. But it's really the shoulders that bear the weight. That's why we talk about *shouldering* a burden.

When it comes to upper-body movement, we want to think in terms of moving from the shoulder, not lifting with our arms and hands. The arms are just levers, along for the ride. The power comes from the shoulders, though few people realize it.

That's because the body is a phenomenal compensator. Let's say you spend all day in meetings or sitting at your desk. Then you rush out to play a game of tennis or hit the gym. Because your shoulders are tight, your body will compensate when you swing a racket by putting more stress on the elbow. This creates tennis elbow.

Imagine if you start throwing some weight around in the gym without first opening your shoulders from sitting in that hunched-over position all day. Having a less effective workout will be the least of your worries.

FIT TIP

Getting sick is your body's way of telling you that you need time off. Your body can get so caught up with repairing muscles that it won't have the energy to fight off a virus if you continue to train hard with a cold. So when a cold hits, take a day off from your workout.

You'll eventually end up with a shoulder injury, probably something involving the rotator cuff.

How do we prevent this? The easy way is to think constantly in terms of squeezing your shoulder blades together. You'll open up and strengthen the muscles around your shoulders throughout Cardio Core 4×4, but think of squeezing your shoulder blades together throughout the course of the day. If you can do that, you'll counteract the forces of gravity, to say nothing of the effects of being hunched over a computer or squeezed into an airline seat, looking to pull you forward.

If the shoulder is the control center of the upper body, the hip cuff controls the lower half. It affects the thighs, knees, and foot position.

Because of the hip's central location in the body, it has an impact on the upper body as well.

People with sore backs assume there must be something wrong with their lower lumbar regions. In reality, it's usually due to tight hips. Having tight hips forces you to move with your back or knees to make up for the immobility in your hips. It's like walking around with your hips welded to your pelvis instead of forming this wonderfully efficient and powerful ball-and-socket joint.

Think of how some elderly people walk. They're moving gingerly, from their knees, and as a result cannot stride very far.

As if this weren't bad enough, anyone with tight hips will have a flat, unattractive butt. Yep, all the work undertaken in the gym, especially by women, to create the proverbial buns of steel will be for nothing if we don't focus on the relationship between the hips and the gluteal muscles, which are the engines of all movement.

Think of what are perhaps the most famous glutes in the world—the ones on the backside of Jennifer Lopez. Yes, Jennifer can thank her parents to some degree, but that would not recognize the tremendous hip stability and mobility that she has worked hard to create over the years.

This has nothing to do with her dazzling

moves onstage, though it takes hip stability to pull those off. What Jennifer has managed to do better than 99 percent of people is to execute proper human movement from the hips, which results in a strong, powerful set of glutes. If she did not constantly do that—and train accordingly—she'd have a flat butt.

Well, maybe not a flat butt. But not one that has inspired songs and videos.

So how do you activate your glutes? Just squeeze them one at a time. Yes, this might seem odd at first, puckering your left butt cheek and then your right, but it's that simple. It's a good exercise to do when sitting at your desk, in the car, or on a plane or train, but it's especially important when walking.

If you can squeeze your glutes, you'll extend your legs farther. You'll walk with your chest over your knees and a straight line from ear to ankle. The pressure will be on your hips, where it's supposed to be, and not your knees. With each step, you'll be developing those glutes.

This is important to know for your own training and well-being, but it also comes in handy when you're caught admiring someone's butt in the gym or on the beach.

If you're called on it, you can say, "Sorry, but I was just admiring how fluid your movement is from your hips and glutes. Most of us have tight hips and a flat butt from sitting all day, but I couldn't help but notice how you've managed to keep your hips strong and stable, activating your glutes, and that's something you just don't see every day. If you don't mind my asking, what's your workout regimen?"

Not a bad conversation starter, no?

You cannot overstate the importance of moving properly from the hips. Whether

FIT TIP

Don't pop a pill after you work out. Researchers at the University of Arkansas for Medical Sciences found that ibuprofen (Advil, Motrin) and acetaminophen (Tylenol) were no more effective than a placebo in relieving postexercise muscle soreness. More important, they say the drugs may actually suppress muscle growth when taken after a workout.

you're walking, going up steps, or squatting to pick something up, you want to squeeze your glutes until your legs are extended.

If you find that your hips are tight and your glutes deactivated, don't worry. I've trained some prominent pro athletes and celebrities, and they've been in the same boat. Get excited because you've discovered a simple way to activate your glutes—squeeze those butt cheeks!—and some strategies to move from the hips as nature intended.

Now that we've addressed the hips and shoulders, it's time to focus on the core.

"Core training" has become a popular catchphrase over the past decade as some fitness magazines and trainers have used it as just another way to market and obsess over washboard abs.

In reality, the core has little to do with rocking an impressive six-pack. Granted, washboard abs *can* be a manifestation of a strong core, but not necessarily. You can have a strong core and more than the 8 percent body fat that's the minimum requirement to display washboard abs.

Show me bodybuilders with washboard abs and, more often than not, I'll show you people who have stressed their hips and backs through overdeveloped muscles—and their insides through pharmaceuticals. That six-pack often is just a temporary manifestation of draining the body of water prior to a bodybuilding or figure competition or a photo shoot.

True core stability is the link between hip and shoulder stability and consists of the muscles of your torso, primarily the abdominals and lower back. This includes muscle groups such as the transverse abdominis, rectus abdominis, lats, obliques, and many small stabilizing muscles between the vertebrae.

Unfortunately, I'm an expert in this area, having undergone 13 surgeries following my devastating track injury at the University of Arkansas. And while it's true that I have washboard abs, it has nothing to do with situps, crunches, or anything you'd consider abdominal exercises.

Think about it. Our sedentary society is causing us to hunch over. Our shoulders are rounded forward and our hips tightened. Most people are a half inch to an inch shorter than they really are because of this gradual phenomenon.

So why would you want to do exercises such as situps and crunches that curve your body even farther forward, exacerbating this problem? I spent more than a year of grueling rehabilitation to get my body back in alignment because it had been thrown out of whack so dramatically. I would never do something that puts strain on my back and hunches my shoulders forward—even if it was effective in producing washboard abs.

Here's the dirty little secret, though. Crunches, even if they weren't potentially harmful, are a terribly inefficient way to flatten your belly.

Researchers at the University of Virginia found that it takes 250,000 crunches to burn 1 pound of fat. That's 100 crunches a day for 7 years.

The best exercise for belly fat? Simply changing your eating habits by avoiding fast foods and sodas and working your abs on a multidimensional level, as you do in yoga, boxing, martial arts, and sprinting. Cardio Core 4×4 is inspired by all four disciplines. (If you insist on doing crunches, at least put your tongue on the roof of your mouth when doing a crunch. This will help align your head and reduce neck strain.)

Core strength, on the other hand, is created when you train your core muscles to become strong and stable, enabling them to work in tandem with your shoulders and hips.

This concerted movement between the shoulders, midsection, and hips is the key to all movement. It's what gives you power when you're swinging a golf club, baseball bat, or tennis racket. It's what enables you to reach to

FIT TIP

Did you know that the average person blinks approximately 17 times a minute? Staring at a computer screen can cause that rate to drop to around six, which can cause your eyes to dry out. To avoid dry eyes, turn away from the computer every 20 minutes to restore natural blinking, and use eye drops frequently throughout the day. Also, supplementing your diet with flaxseed is a great way to keep your eyes naturally moistened.

open a door or pick up a sack of groceries without wrenching your back.

Remember: The limbs are just along for the ride. Bodybuilders talk about working their arms on one day and legs on another. The body is not a collection of parts. It's one amazing operating system working together, or at least it should be.

My coauthor, Pete Williams, often made an analogy between core strength and a mannequin with no limbs. That mannequin, were it a real person, still could generate incredible strength and power from the hips, midsection, and core.

Pete's point was proven recently when he met a remarkable triple-amputee triathlete named Rajesh Durbal. Rajesh was born with a congenital deformity and has no legs and only a left hand. But Rajesh, with the help of prosthetic legs, is able to generate incredible power from his core, which propels him through Ironman triathlons consisting of a 2.4-mile swim, a 112-mile bike ride, and a full 26.2-mile marathon.

Rajesh has washboard abs, but it has nothing to do with crunches and situps. He's had to learn by necessity how to move from his hips, midsection, and shoulders.

We're all born with proper movement patterns. As we grow older, spending more time behind a desk, our bodies hunch over and compensate. We're able to move, sure, but we do so with too much strain on our knees, backs, and shoulders.

Rajesh never has had that luxury and has been forced to maintain the proper movement patterns just to get through daily life.

The rest of us need to rediscover those childhood movement patterns, what I call "regression to progression." If we can regress to how we moved as kids, we can progress by building a stronger and more stable platform, something that's become uncommon.

I spend a lot of time watching people move. I live in New York City, after all, the people-watching capital of the world, but it's more out of professional curiosity than anything else.

As I watch people blow by me on the sidewalks or in the subway, I take note of how their

FIT TIP

Stick to your workout goals by asking your spouse or significant other to start Cardio Core 4×4 with you. According to one study, nearly half of men who exercise alone quit their programs after 1 year, but two-thirds of those who exercise with their wife or girlfriend stick it out. Plus, both genders will benefit, since both men and women work 12 to 15 percent harder when training with a loved one.

bodies are aligned. It's easy to diagnose when someone is standing in profile. Few have the optimal position of a straight line from ear to heel. Their shoulders are rounded and forward, sliding away from the spine. The ears are significantly ahead of the shoulder, and, regardless of the person's age, there's a slight hunch forming in the back.

The scary thing is that most people don't realize it, since it's such a gradual process. If you looked at an elderly woman with osteoporosis—women tend to be more affected than men—you'd think, *There's no way I'd allow that to happen to me.* And yet that process already has started for many people.

There's a reason mothers and teachers are always telling children to sit up straight in their chairs. We don't want to end up in this position.

So how do we avoid it? Be cognizant of your posture. I like to wear clothes with lines and seams along the sides so I can check my alignment. If I'm standing with proper posture, my ears are in line with my shoulders, my hips are in line with my knees, and my knees with my ankles. If I'm seated, there should be a straight line between my ears and hips.

Keep in mind some of our previous techniques that you can do over the course of the day, such as squeezing your shoulder blades

FIT TIP

Brush away your cravings! The next time you finish a meal, be sure to brush your teeth. Reason: The toothpaste will take away the food taste in your mouth, which actually can cause you to yearn for more of the food you just ate, while the minty taste will reduce the likelihood of your reaching for something sweet.

together and squeezing your glutes. You also want to activate your transverse abdominis, which is the first muscle that's recruited every time you move. It's located beneath your rectus abdominis, also known as the six-pack muscle.

Perhaps you've been told to keep your tummy tight. This does not mean sucking in your gut and holding your breath. Instead, think in terms of pulling your belly button back from your belt buckle. This will keep your transverse abdominis activated, and after a while this posture will become second nature.

In fact, the easiest way to flatten your gut is by activating your transverse abdominis. Work your "TA" by pulling your belly button toward your spine and holding for 10 seconds while breathing normally. Repeat five times. You can do this while sitting at your desk, in the car stuck in traffic—anywhere.

People tend to think of working out as something they do in a fixed period of time. If they're not in the gym or out running, well, they're not working out. Take advantage of all the little windows of opportunity you have during the day. No matter how busy you are, you're going to be stuck in a meeting or on a never-ending conference call. Use that time to squeeze your glutes or activate your transverse abdominis.

Just as we're making the most of our 20-minute workouts, let's make the most of every minute we have over the course of the day. Every so often, I'll pass a bookstore in New York City where people are standing in line waiting to have a celebrity author sign their books. They're looking at a 20- to 30-minute wait, and you'd think they just might crack open the book they presumably have some interest in reading. Instead, they just stand in line impatiently, books tucked under their arms.

The great horror novelist Stephen King, who no doubt has witnessed this phenomenon, once wrote about how he reads so many books by "sipping" throughout the course of the day. He doesn't have hours to sit and "gulp" one chapter after another, but by taking a book wherever he goes, he knocks off a few pages here and there, whether it's standing in line for takeout food or even between innings at baseball games.

Let's apply that philosophy to our training, making the most of every opportunity we have during the day. For instance, stand on one leg when you're brushing your teeth and you'll provide a degree of instability that works the smaller muscles essential for core strength. You'll create a great smile and a flatter midsection at the same time.

This time management philosophy also

applies when it comes to activating your transverse abdominis, which helps coordinate all those abdominal and lower-back muscles every time you move. By keeping it activated, you'll be able to move properly and fortify yourself against injury and long-term deterioration.

Because of the importance of creating true core stability, you will not find any popular abdominal routines in Cardio Core 4×4. The last thing we want to do is contribute further to the hunching over of your body.

Instead, the exercises in this program will be in a 2-to-1 ratio in favor of the posterior chain over the anterior chain. The posterior chain refers to the muscles that run from your lower back down behind your butt. The posterior chain includes those ever-important glutes.

The anterior chain refers to the chest, abs, and quads. Those look good in a swimsuit, especially on guys, but such training runs contrary to what we're trying to accomplish.

Bodybuilders and figure models spend a lot of time working their chests. They even refer to "chest days," spending long hours on their pectorals, biceps, and triceps, the murderers' row of beach muscles. That might produce some showy muscles, but it does little to improve your shoulder and core stability.

Ab-specific training, as we've discussed, contributes to being hunched over. As for training the quads, there's some value to that, but it's more important to be hip and glute dominant in our movements than quad dominant.

When we talk about the anterior chain, we're referring to that front part of the body from quad to neck, but the emphasis is on the shoulder and midsection and *decreasing* anterior tilt.

Situps strengthen the abs, albeit inefficiently. They also pull the sternum toward the pelvis, creating lumbar flexion and ultimately a hunchback. By putting your hands on the back of your head and crunching forward, you're placing massive pressure on your lumbar spine.

I'm not a fan of situps, especially the endless parade of infomercial abdominal

FIT TIP

Take your phone calls standing up and you'll burn 50 percent more calories than sitting. Also, did you know that "good cholesterol" levels decrease by 20 percent and that there is a 7 percent increase in your risk of diabetes after a couple of hours of sitting?

machines promising to build you a wash-board quickly. Eighty percent of people don't have the strength in their lower lumbar regions to lift their legs and necks off the ground properly. We're placing so much strain on the back in everyday life, why exacerbate the problem?

Then there are the guys who spend a lot of time working on their anterior: the chest, biceps, and abs. They place a ton of pressure on the lumbar region, creating roundness in the back.

By following a 2-to-1 ratio when it comes to training the posterior versus the anterior, we're decreasing the chance of anterior tilt and increasing the chance of having a healthy spine.

Need more incentive? A Syracuse University study revealed that people burned more calories the day after they did lower-body resistance training than after they worked their upper bodies. The legs carry more mass than your upper body. Work more muscle, and your body uses more energy to repair and grow.

After my track accident and 13 surgeries, I came up with the idea of "prehab before you rehab." The idea is that if we can take preventive measures to prehabilitate our bodies, we'll likely avoid the horrific injuries that will require rehabilitation, or "rehab," later.

I didn't popularize the term *prehab*. That honor probably goes to Mark Verstegen, with whom my coauthor Pete Williams wrote some groundbreaking *Core Performance* books. But having undergone those 13 surgeries, I can appreciate the concept of prehab as much as anyone.

You might think you have nothing to

FIT TIP

The pushup is the all-American exercise. Too bad most people can't do one. So I put a test together to determine base levels of fitness. For men 45 and younger, doing 35 or more pushups equals fit, 20 to 34 is average, and less than 20 is out of shape. For women of the same age, we cut the number of reps by 40 percent. So to get a fit score, a woman needs to be able to do 14 pushups.

FIT TIP

Want to get a good workout in bed? No, not like that. The next time you have a minute, perform as many pushups as you can in 60 seconds on your bed. Since you'll be working on an unstable surface, the bed will force your body to work twice as hard as performing pushups on the floor. One set of these, and you'll call it a day.

worry about. After all, you're not competing in track and field. But think of all the everyday mishaps we encounter, whether it's slipping on a patch of ice, falling off a short ladder, or tripping in the dark. Such everyday moments, like my routine tumble on the track, can be devastating.

That's why we're going to focus on strengthening and stabilizing all these muscles around our hips, midsection, and shoulders. That's going to stabilize our joints to the point where we're less likely to take such a tumble. We do this by improving our proprioception, our system of pressure sensors in the muscles, tendons, and joints that provide the body with information to maintain balance.

I don't want anyone to undergo what I endured nearly 20 years ago. While that was a freak athletic accident, the reality is that our sedentary, technology-based culture has so locked down our bodies that routine falls can have life-altering consequences, and not just for elderly people.

So think of this 20-minutes-a-day, 4-days-a-week program as not only an investment in your short-term health and performance but also an insurance policy against future injury.

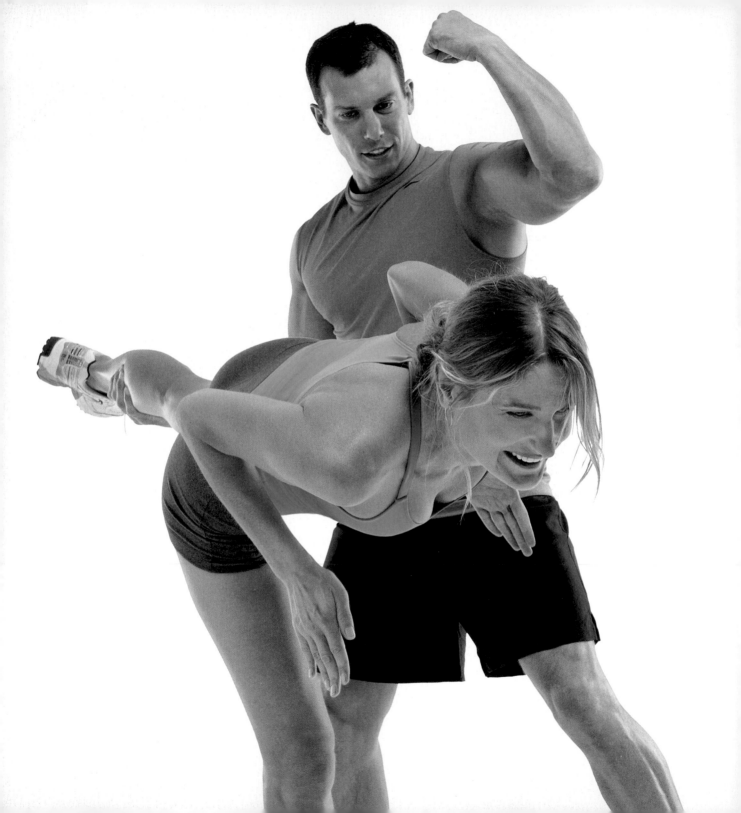

CHAPTER SIX

THE CARDIO CORE 4×4 WORKOUT

THIS SECTION INCLUDES CARDIO CORE 4×4 WORK-OUT, which you'll do for just 20 minutes a day, 4 days a week. On Mondays and Thursdays, you'll do a 4×2 version consisting of movements done standing. On Tuesdays and Fridays, you'll perform a 4x4 version in which your feet and hands start on the floor.

If you aren't able to do the workouts on the exact days I suggest, don't worry. As long as you sneak in four 20-minute workouts a week, you'll be golden.

There's also an optional Cardio Core series of exercises that you can perform on Wednesdays and/or during the weekend. Again, this is optional, but as you advance with your training, you might find that you're looking for something additional. Cardio Core is 10 exercises and can serve as active recovery.

There are roughly 50 exercises in the program. That might not sound like a lot, but if you consider that most of them have a version for each side of your body and some have multiple variations, it actually comes closer to 100. We might do only 20 in any given workout, but it will be a powerful 20-minute mix of movements.

At first, you may be able to do only a few repetitions of any given movement. That's okay. As you progress, you'll become more efficient and be able to do more repetitions and thus pack more into the same 20-minute workout. As you become more proficient with the movements, you'll inevitably become faster, again allowing more time for additional reps.

Have you ever practiced to give a speech? If so, you probably found that the more you practiced, the shorter your talk became. That's because you gradually became more comfortable with the talk and your material, using fewer words and perhaps speaking a little more quickly. The same phenomenon is at work here.

For each exercise, start at 10 and work up to 20 reps on each side, unless otherwise indicated. The exact number is up to you, depending on how far you have advanced.

Let's begin with the 4×2. When I teach this in the form of a group class, I play the opening notes of "We Will Rock You" by Queen. You need not play the familiar stomping, clapping beat, but it wouldn't hurt to get it into your head for inspiration.

One other tip before you get started: As you count reps of each exercise, count down (10, 9, 8) instead of up (1, 2, 3). You're more likely to achieve the reps you set out to perform, since you've subconsciously told yourself you'll do that many.

THE CARDIO CORE 4×2 WORKOUT

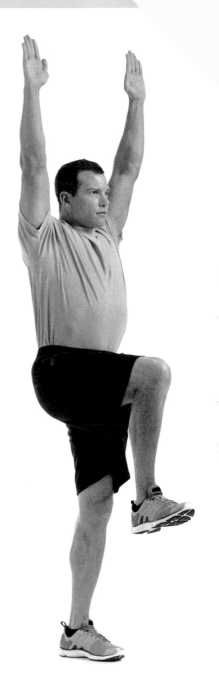

CARDIO CORE
4×2 WORKOUT
AT A GLANCE

2 times a week, 10–20 reps of each exercise Mondays and Thursdays (or whatever 2 days a week you choose)

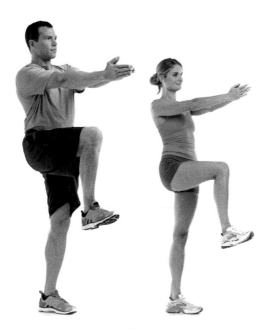

1. ROUNDUPS
(PAGE 80)

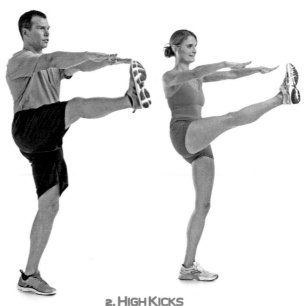

2. HIGH KICKS
(PAGE 82)

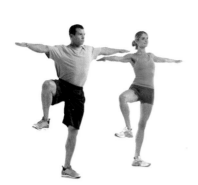

3. OVER THE FENCE
(PAGE 84)

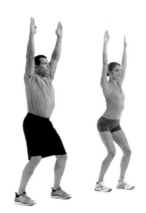

4. BALL AND SOCKETS
(PAGE 86)

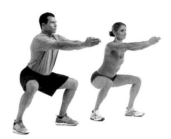

5. LUMBERJACKS
(PAGE 88)

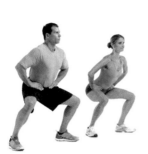

6. MADMAN SQUATS
(PAGE 90)

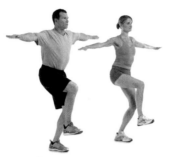

7a. SCARECROW MATRIX
Karate Kids
(PAGE 92)

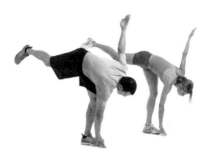

7b. SCARECROW MATRIX
Leaning Tower of Pisa
(PAGE 94)

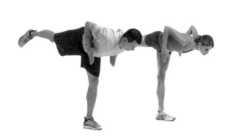

7c. SCARECROW MATRIX
Union Rows and Flying Eagles
(PAGE 96)

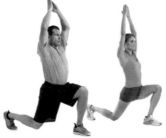

7d. SCARECROW MATRIX
Drop-In Lunges, Charlie's
Angels, and Tip Taps
(PAGE 98)

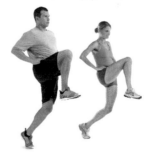

7e. SCARECROW MATRIX
Rocking the Cradle
(PAGE 102)

THE CARDIO CORE 4×4 WORKOUT 77

4x2 WORKOUT AT A GLANCE (Continued)

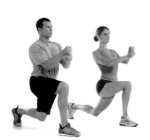

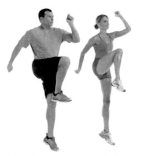

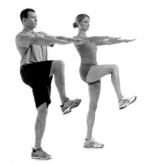

7f. SCARECROW MATRIX
Wimbledons
(PAGE 104)

7g. SCARECROW MATRIX
Kiss the Sky
(PAGE 106)

7h. SCARECROW MATRIX
Knee Drives
(PAGE 108)

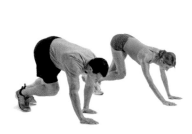

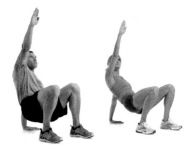

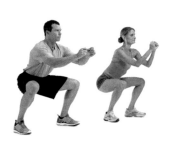

8. WALK OUTS
(PAGE 110)

9. GET UPS
(PAGE 112)

10. ROUND THE WORLD SQUATS
(PAGE 114)

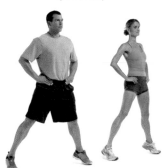

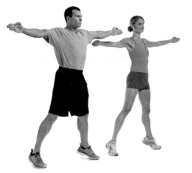

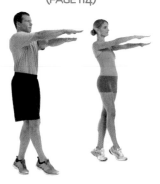

11. WIDE OUTS
(PAGE 116)

12. SEAL JUMPS
(PAGE 118)

13. CROSSOVERS
(PAGE 120)

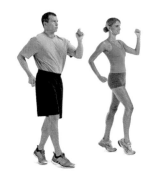

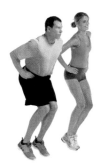

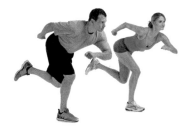

14. Sprinter Jacks
(PAGE 122)

15. Pogo Pops
(PAGE 124)

16. Speed Skaters
(PAGE 126)

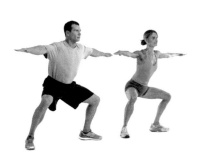

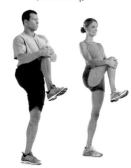

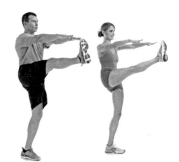

17. Squat Holds
(PAGE 128)

18. Alternating Knee Grabs
(PAGE 129)

19. High-Kick Toe-Ins
(PAGE 130)

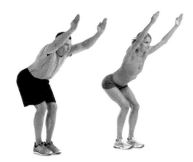

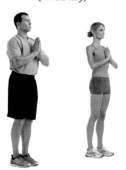

20a. Cooldown
Butt-Up Pose
(PAGE 132)

20b. Cooldown
Cardio Calmers
(PAGE 133)

1. ROUNDUPS

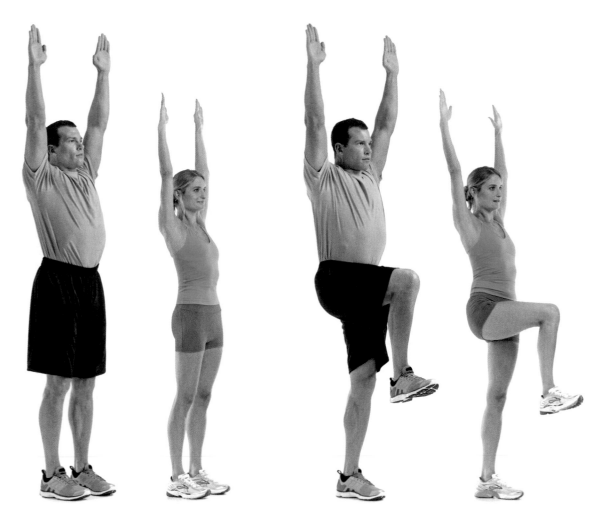

OBJECTIVE: To open up the shoulders as part of a dynamic warmup at the beginning of the workout.

STARTING POSITION: Stand erect with your legs shoulder-width apart and your arms extended straight up.

PROCEDURE: Lift your left leg and clap your hands together in front of you and then circle them out to the side. Repeat on the other side. Done in quick succession, this movement will simulate marching. Think of "We Will Rock You" playing in your head and clap every third beat.

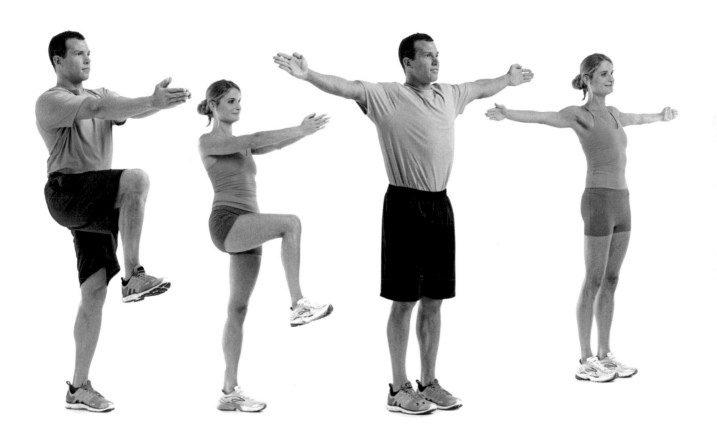

YOU SHOULD FEEL IT: In your shoulders and hip flexors.

2. HIGH KICKS

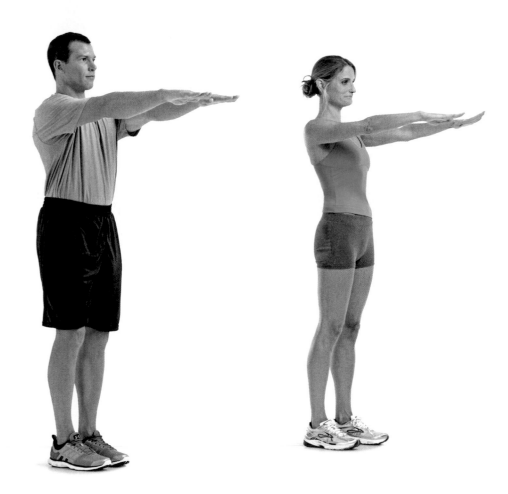

OBJECTIVE: To strengthen the hamstrings, improve hip flexibility, and stabilize the lower back.

STARTING POSITION: Standing with your arms extended in front of your body.

PROCEDURE: Perform alternating leg raises, keeping your legs as straight as you can. If you can touch your toes to your hands, terrific, but go as far as you can. Your feet should be dorsiflexed, which is to say the toe is pointed toward the shin. This is part of the warmup but also a movement to generate strength and mobility in the hamstrings and lower back.

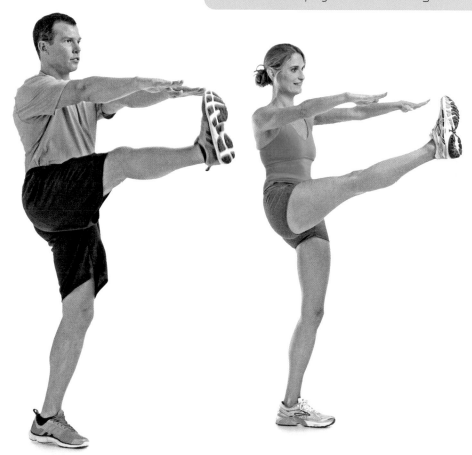

YOU SHOULD FEEL IT: In your hamstrings.

3. OVER THE FENCE

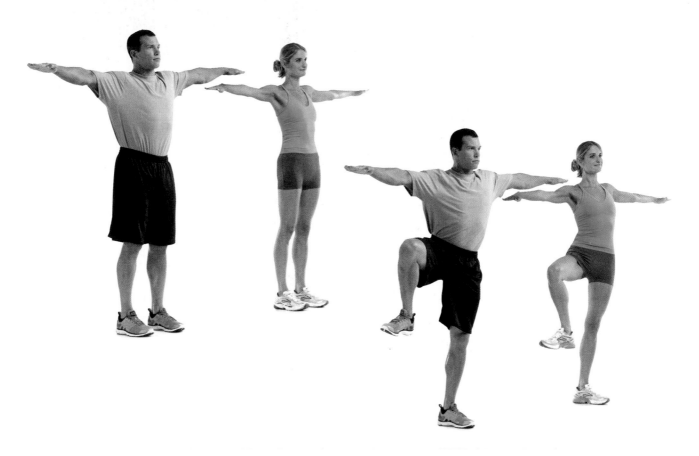

OBJECTIVE: To improve your abduction and adduction. Abductors are the outer-thigh muscles located on the sides of your hips and are important for lateral movement and stabilization. Adductors are the muscles located in your inner thighs that help pull your legs back toward your body and stabilize your hips and pelvis.

STARTING POSITION: Standing, your feet shoulder-width apart, with arms extended to the sides.

PROCEDURE: Imagine stepping laterally over a hurdle, one leg at a time. Stand tall, open up your right hip, and swing your right leg slightly back, as if over an imaginary hurdle. Repeat on the other side. Your leg should drag slightly and then whip over the fence quickly.

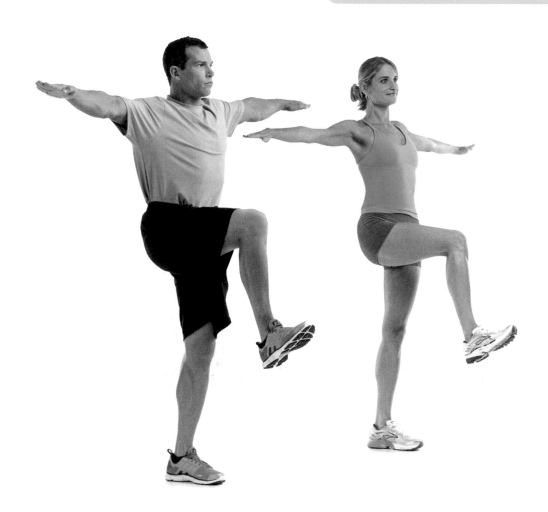

COACHING KEY: Stay as erect as possible and don't contort your body. Move from your hips.

YOU SHOULD FEEL IT: In your hips.

4. Ball and Sockets

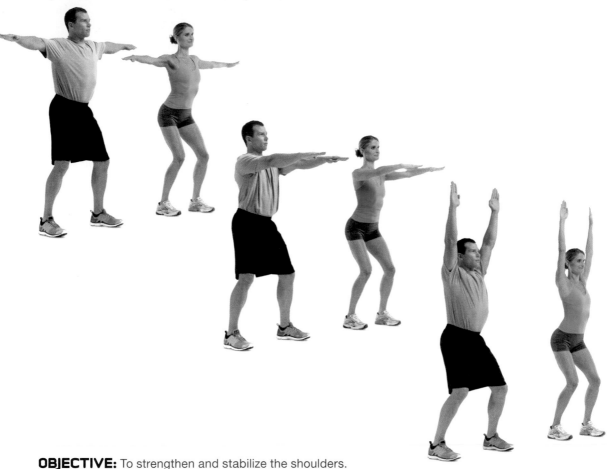

OBJECTIVE: To strengthen and stabilize the shoulders.

STARTING POSITION: Athletic stance with your legs shoulder-width apart and your arms extended to the side; squat down slightly.

PROCEDURE: Extend your arms to the sides and circle them forward for however many reps you have progressed to, and then perform the same number of reps backward. Next, extend your arms in front of you and do the same number of circles clockwise and counterclockwise. After that, reach your arms directly above you and circle the same number of times clockwise and counterclockwise. Finally, extend your arms to the sides. Bend your elbows so they form right angles and then press your forearms down as if you are closing a window. Repeat for the number of reps you have progressed to.

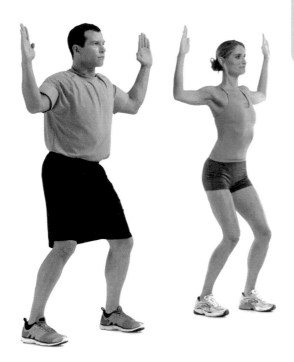

COACHING KEY: Don't think of this as swinging your arms. Instead, think of it as rotating from the shoulders. Your arms are moving, of course, but they're really just along for the ride.

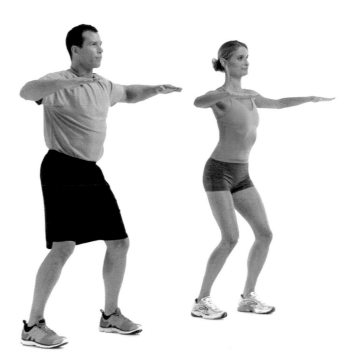

YOU SHOULD FEEL IT: In your shoulders and arms.

5. LUMBERJACKS

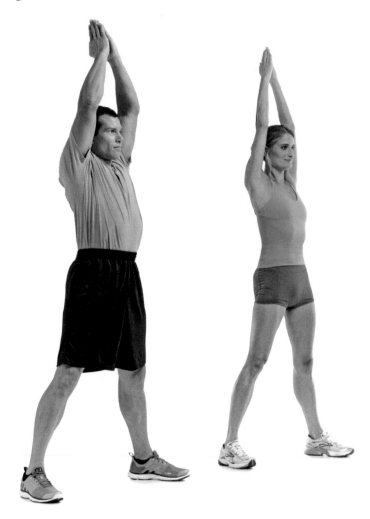

OBJECTIVE: To improve stability in the hip and core regions.

STARTING POSITION: Standing with your legs slightly wider than shoulder width and arms extended overhead.

PROCEDURE: As you squat, bring your hands from over your head down as if swinging an ax or sledgehammer. Keep your thighs parallel to the ground.

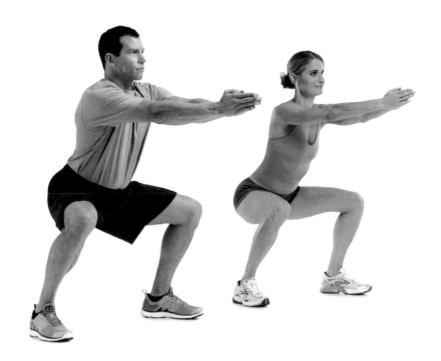

YOU SHOULD FEEL IT: All over, but especially in your hips.

6. MADMAN SQUATS

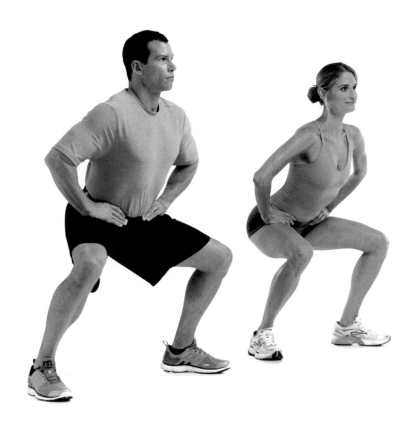

OBJECTIVE: To create stability and strength in everyday functional movements in which you're shifting weight.

STARTING POSITION: Squatting position, your legs slightly wider than shoulder-width apart. Good posture, back straight, hands on hips.

PROCEDURE: Lift your left leg toward the ceiling, while standing on your right leg. Your left leg will be bent. Come down to a squat. Switch legs.

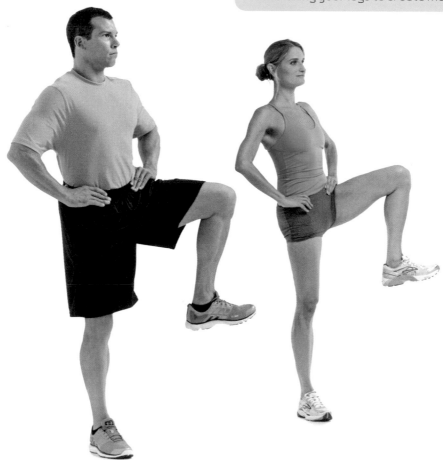

COACHING KEY: Think of this in terms of everyday movements such as pulling a lawn mower starter, standing in a subway car, or playing golf. If you feel it in your back, you're leaning too far forward. Step softly, no stomping. Do not bounce. Complete the squat. You're controlling your legs to create more stability.

YOU SHOULD FEEL IT: In your hips, hamstrings, and quads.

SCARECROW MATRIX

This is a series of seven exercises (*a* through *g*) from the "scarecrow position," which is standing tall, your arms extended to the sides. We'll do everything first with the left leg planted and the right leg in motion.

7a. SCARECROW MATRIX
Karate Kids

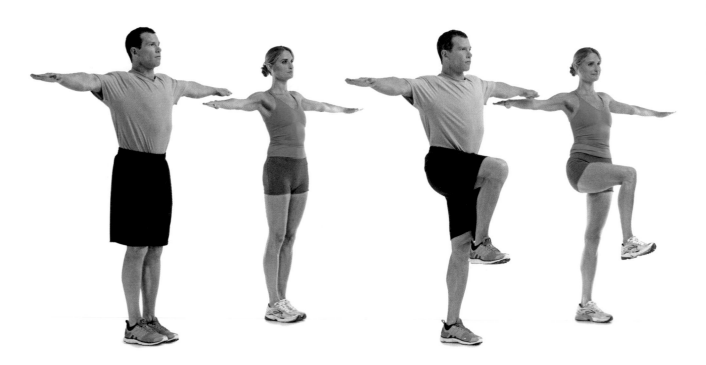

OBJECTIVE: To create hip stability and improve overall balance.

PROCEDURE: Bring your right leg up and down in a pumping motion. Raise the knee as high as possible while keeping the thigh parallel to the floor, placing yourself in a flamingo or Karate Kid position. When you lower the leg, don't let your right foot touch the ground, if possible, instead keeping it 3 inches in the air. Next we'll do the same movement but with a shorter lift. From there we raise the leg back to the Karate Kid position and do some one-legged squats.

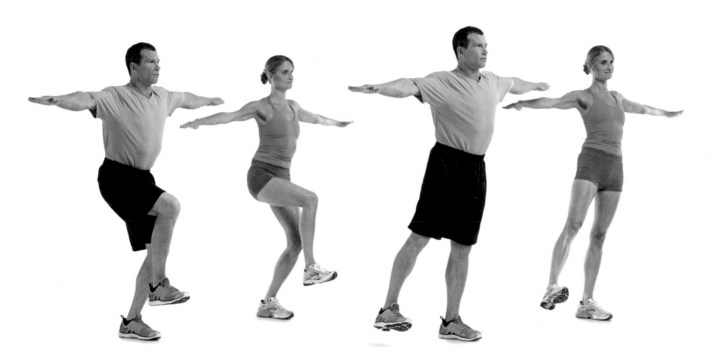

When you've completed the prescribed number of reps, drop your right foot to the ground and get back in the scarecrow position. Keeping your right leg straight and locked, swing it out to the right and then back under your body in a circular motion, first counterclockwise and then clockwise.

YOU SHOULD FEEL IT: In your lower back, hip flexors, quads, and hamstrings. With your hands out, you'll also feel it in your rear deltoids.

7b. SCARECROW MATRIX
Leaning Tower of Pisa

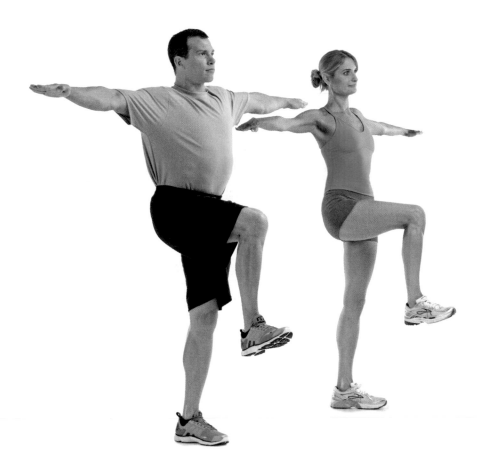

OBJECTIVE: To open up the body and create hip rotation, which is important for everyday movements. Think gardening or picking up kids. This exercise creates balance and stability in the lower lumbar region.

PROCEDURE: From the scarecrow position, extend your right leg backward, keeping it as straight as possible, while you rotate to touch your left toes with your right hand. Always keep your right foot off the ground.

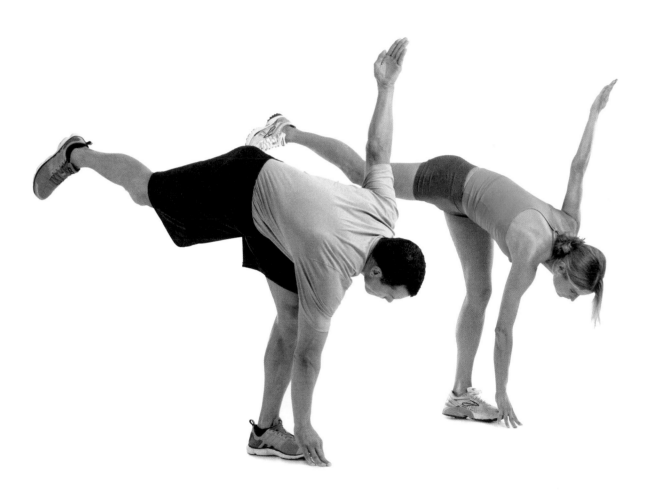

YOU SHOULD FEEL IT: All over.

7c. SCARECROW MATRIX
Union Rows and Flying Eagles

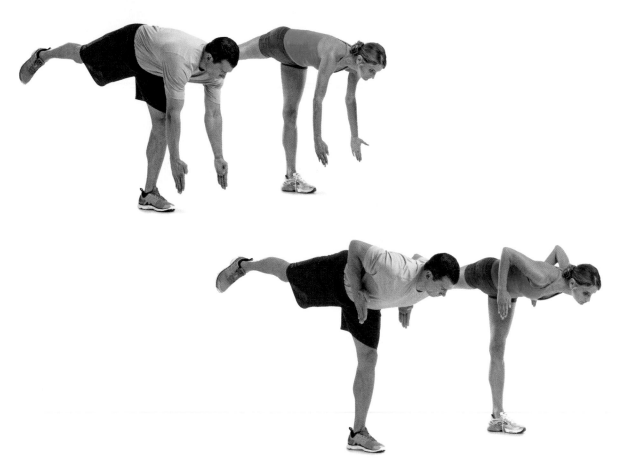

OBJECTIVE: To create stability in the shoulder and lower lumbar region.

PROCEDURE: *Union Rows:* With your left leg still planted on the ground, extend your right leg back and lean forward until your upper body is parallel to the ground, so your body forms a T. With your arms hanging down, simulate rowing with dumbbells, pulling your arms up with your elbows close to your body. Squeeze your shoulder blades together and release. *Flying Eagles:* While still in this T position, extend your arms to the sides. Release your arms toward the ground.

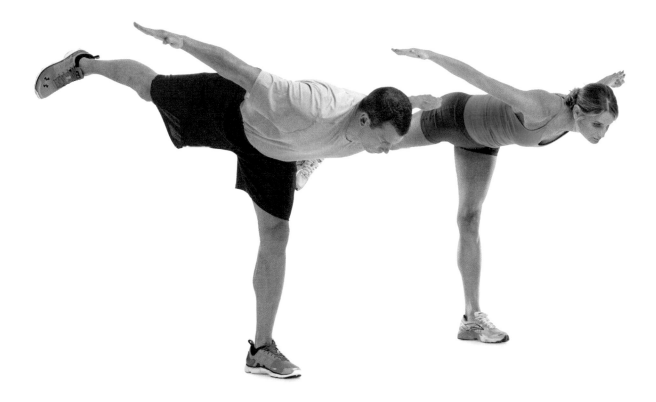

YOU SHOULD FEEL IT: In your glutes and the stabilizing leg.

7d. SCARECROW MATRIX
Drop-In Lunges, Charlie's Angels, and Tip Taps

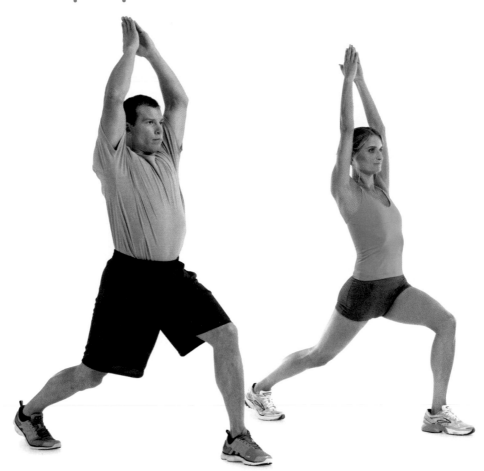

OBJECTIVE: To move from one strong, erect pillar.

PROCEDURE: From the Flying Eagle T position, step back with your right leg, keeping your left leg in front, until you're in a lunge position. Extend your arms over your head and move up and down from the hips. This will be a familiar pose if you've done yoga. We're calling it the Drop-In Lunge.

COACHING KEY: The front knee should not go forward. Move from your hip, which goes up and down. Don't think of it as a lunge but as an up-and-down movement from the hip.

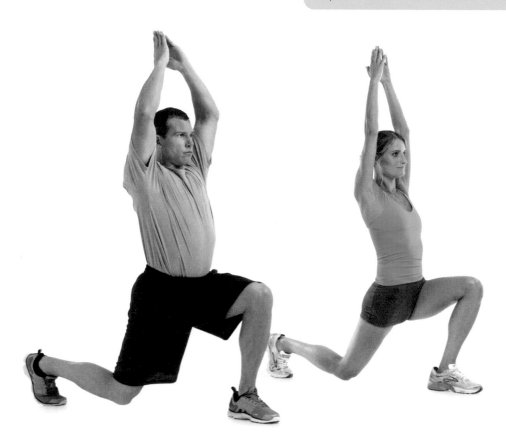

YOU SHOULD FEEL IT: Throughout your lower body, but especially your quads.

(continued)

7d. SCARECROW MATRIX
Drop-In Lunges, Charlie's Angels, and Tip Taps (Continued)

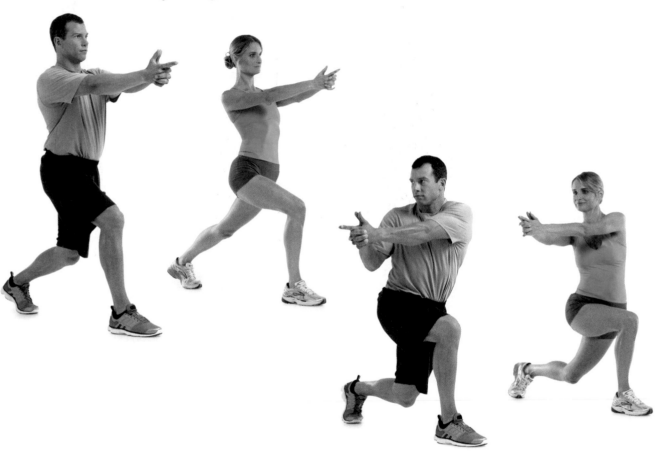

PROCEDURE (continued): From that lunge position, extend both hands forward and connect the fingers as if making a gun to assume the Charlie's Angels position. With your right foot forward, rotate as far as possible to the right side for the prescribed number of reps. From this lunge position, hop on your front (right) foot to the right side and then the left, tapping the ground with your front foot. These are Tip Taps. Repeat the Tip Taps with your right leg in back. Remember to stay in the stable, low lunge position, with your hips low. This is a fun but aggressive move that really works the glutes.

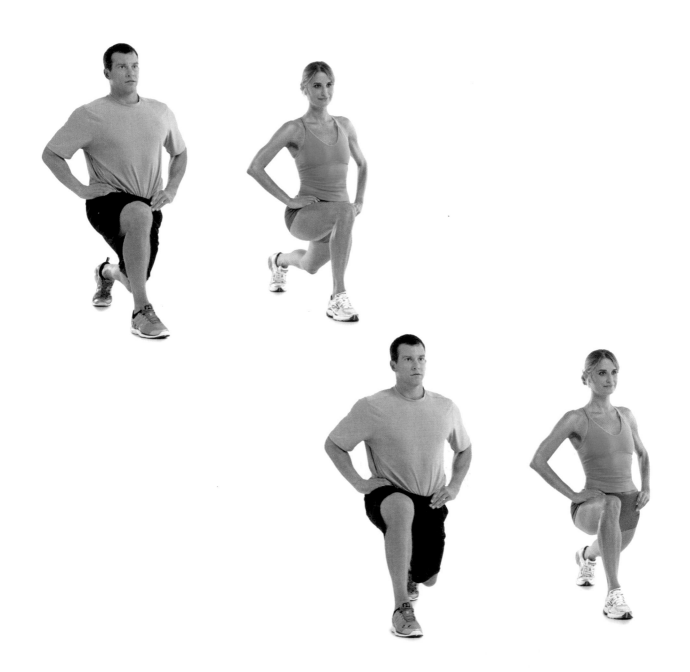

7e. SCARECROW MATRIX
Rocking the Cradle

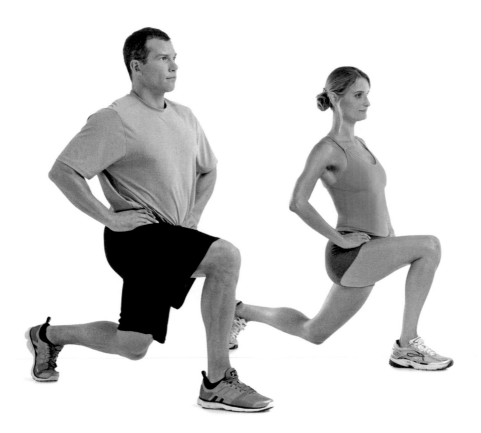

OBJECTIVE: To engage the body, especially the hip flexors, through a full range of movement.

PROCEDURE: From that same low lunge position, with your hands on your hips, rock back onto your left foot, bringing your front (right) leg up as high as possible. Your left leg provides support. Then rock back into the lunge position. The knee stays bent throughout the movement.

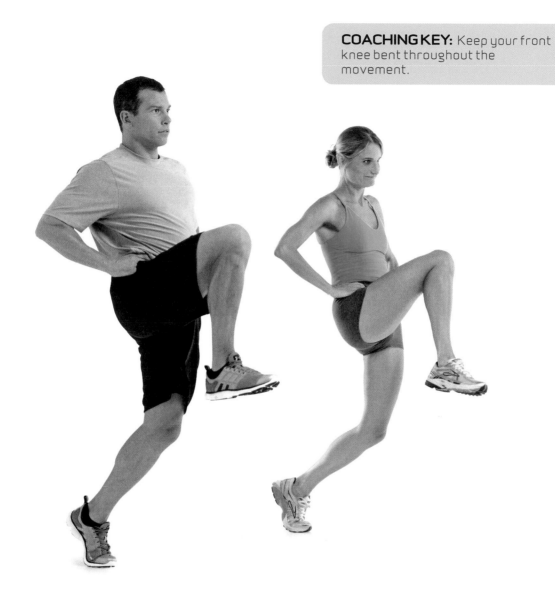

COACHING KEY: Keep your front knee bent throughout the movement.

YOU SHOULD FEEL IT: Throughout your lower body, but especially your hamstrings.

7f. SCARECROW MATRIX
Wimbledons

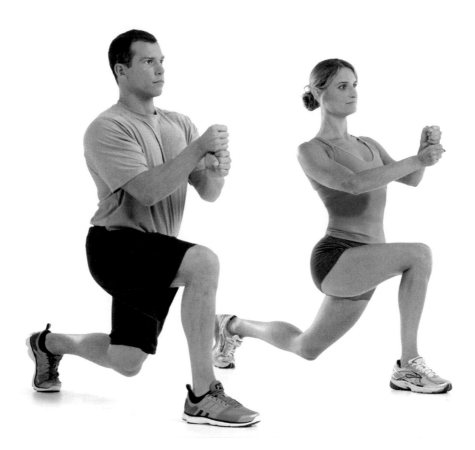

OBJECTIVE: To create balance and coordination in one point in space. Think of a boxer jumping rope in one place (as opposed to the rest of us moving all over the map).

PROCEDURE: Wimbledons mimic the tennis stroke. Staying in the low lunge position, with your right foot forward and your hands in front of you as if you are holding a tennis racket, jump with both legs 6 inches to the right and then to the left. Both legs leave the ground at the same time. This is a whole-body movement. Remain in that low lunge position. You're shifting back and forth, much like a tennis player. Picture yourself on hot coals where you don't want to spend any time on the ground. Imagine that the photos on these two pages show the people jumping 6 inches to the right and then 6 inches to the left.

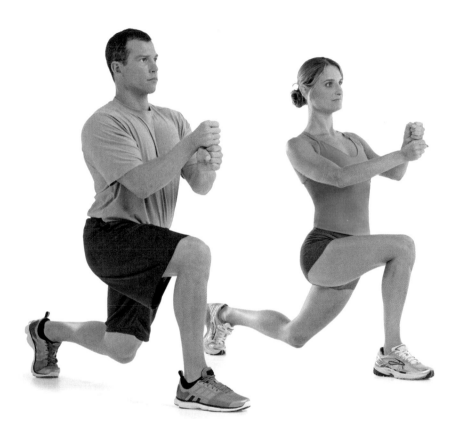

YOU SHOULD FEEL IT: Throughout your posterior chain, especially your calves and Achilles tendons, and also your lower back.

7g. SCARECROW MATRIX
Kiss the Sky

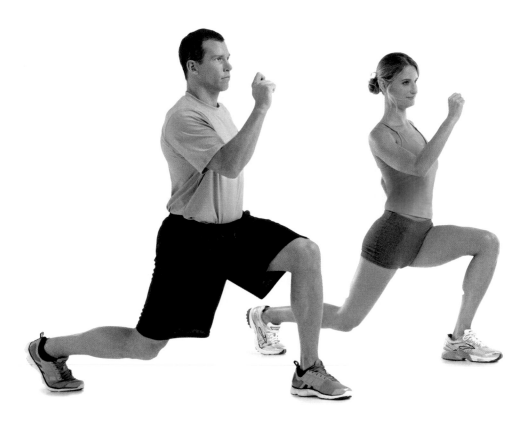

OBJECTIVE: To build strength in the core region.

PROCEDURE: From the low lunge position, with your right fist in front of you, drive up your right knee as high as possible, toward the hand in front of you. Return to the lunge position. From the lunge position, drive the knee backward.

COACHING KEY: Be sure to exhale thoroughly during this exercise. That will make all the difference.

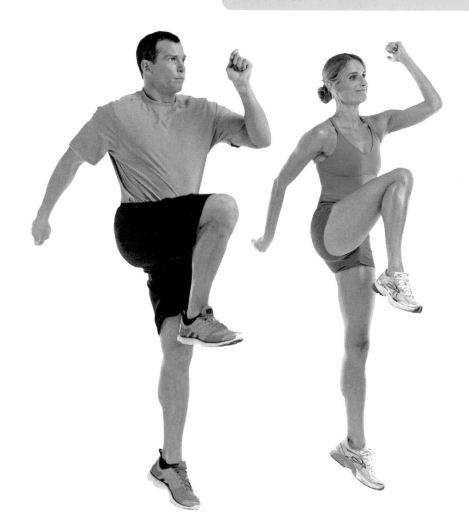

YOU SHOULD FEEL IT: In your abs and in the stabilizing leg.

(continued)

7h. SCARECROW MATRIX
Knee Drives

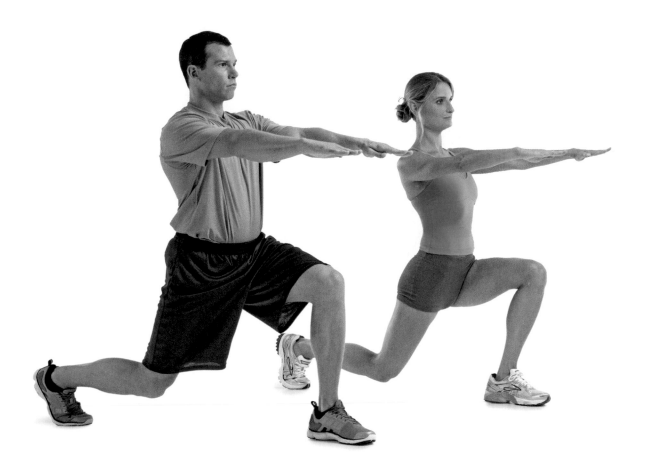

OBJECTIVE: To build strength in the core and hip region.

PROCEDURE: From the low lunge position, with both hands extended in front of you, drive the right knee as fast as possible to the mid line of the body. The left leg is planted; the right leg is doing all the work.

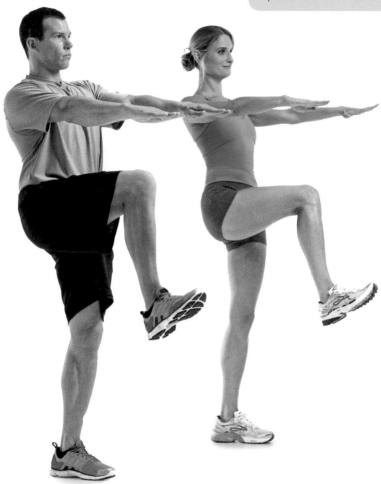

YOU SHOULD FEEL IT: In your abs and in your stabilizing leg.

Now that we've done all seven parts of the Scarecrow Matrix with the left leg planted and the right leg in motion, it's time to go back and reverse the legs.

8. WALK OUTS

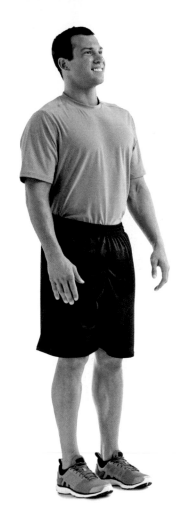
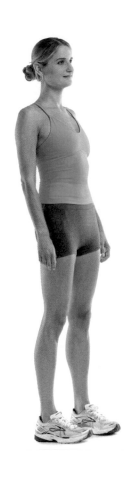

OBJECTIVE: To build stability in your shoulders and core while strengthening the lower lumbar region.

STARTING POSITION: Standing, with your feet shoulder-width apart and your hands at your sides.

PROCEDURE: Keeping your belly button drawn in, walk your hands out to a plank position. Now walk your hands back until you're in the original standing position.

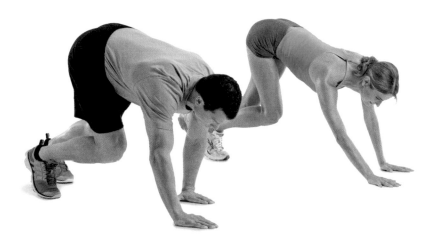

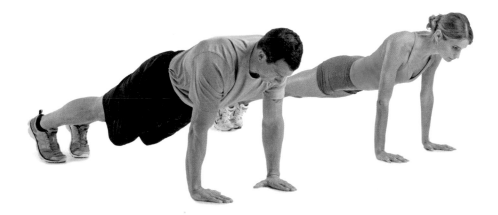

YOU SHOULD FEEL IT: In your shoulders and lower back.

9. Get Ups

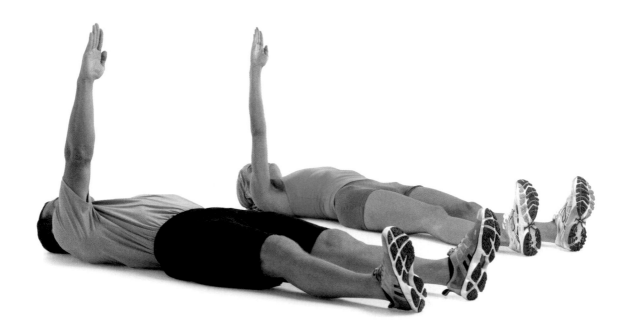

OBJECTIVE: To challenge your core. If you can get to the point where you can do this with no hands, you've developed some serious core strength.

STARTING POSITION: Lying on your back on the floor.

PROCEDURE: Raise your right hand in the air and stand using (at most) your left hand. If you have sufficient core strength, get up without the use of your arms. Do the prescribed number of reps with your right arm raised and then switch arms.

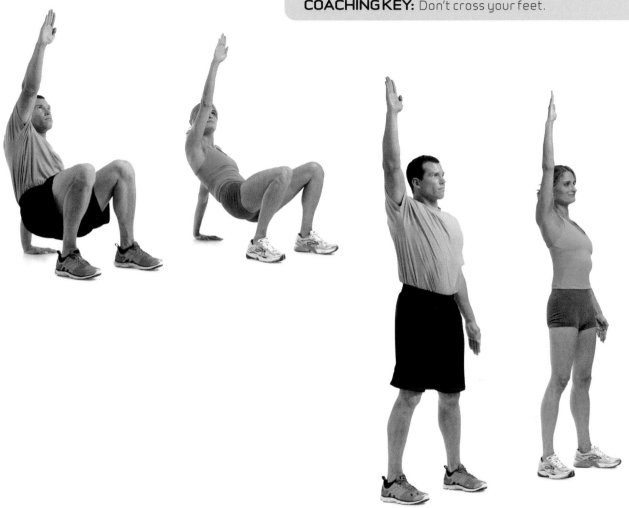

YOU SHOULD FEEL IT: All over, especially in the stabilizing shoulder.

10. ROUND THE WORLD SQUATS

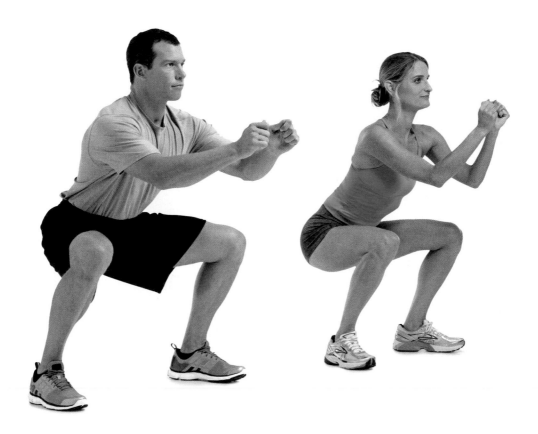

OBJECTIVE: To create hip stability and mobility.

STARTING POSITION: In a full squat, your feet shoulder-width apart and your arms in front of you.

PROCEDURE: Squat and jump 180 degrees to the left side. Imagine there's a video camera behind you and you want to face the camera. Squat while facing the camera and jump back the way you came. Squat again and jump to the right. Repeat this process for the prescribed number of reps.

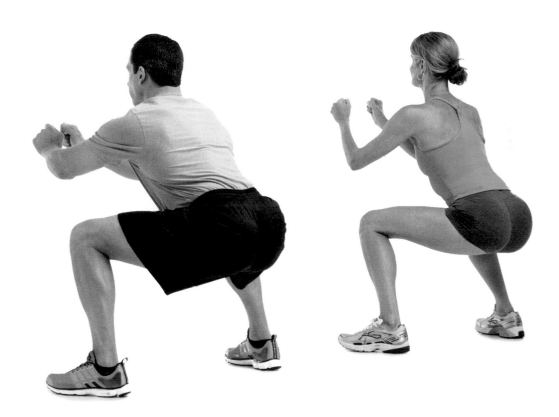

YOU SHOULD FEEL IT: In your hips, quads, and groin.

11. WIDE OUTS

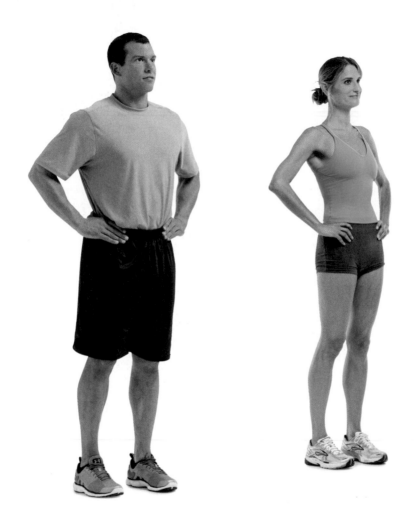

OBJECTIVE: Cardio conditioning, reaction time, and overall speed.

STARTING POSITION: Standing with your feet shoulder-width apart.

PROCEDURE: Perform a jumping jack with only your legs.

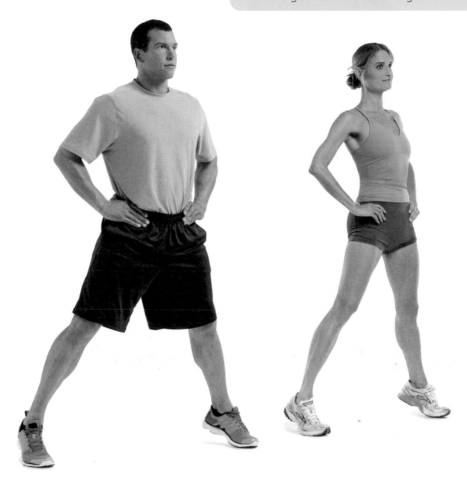

YOU SHOULD FEEL IT: In your hips.

12. Seal Jumps

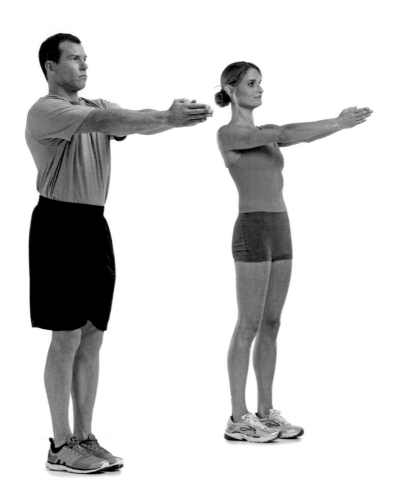

OBJECTIVE: To improve stability in the shoulders.

STARTING POSITION: Standing with your feet shoulder-width apart, your arms extended forward.

PROCEDURE: This is similar to a jumping jack, but instead of taking your hands overhead, clap your hands forward like a seal would. Jump your legs out to the side and land so that your feet and arms are extended to the sides, your body forming a star.

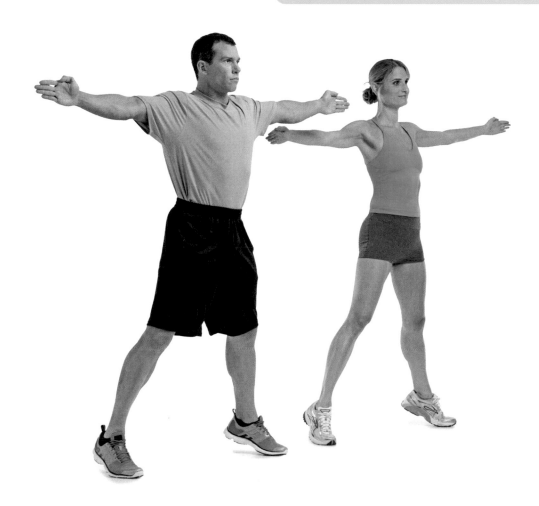

YOU SHOULD FEEL IT: In your shoulders and throughout your lumbar spine.

13. Crossovers

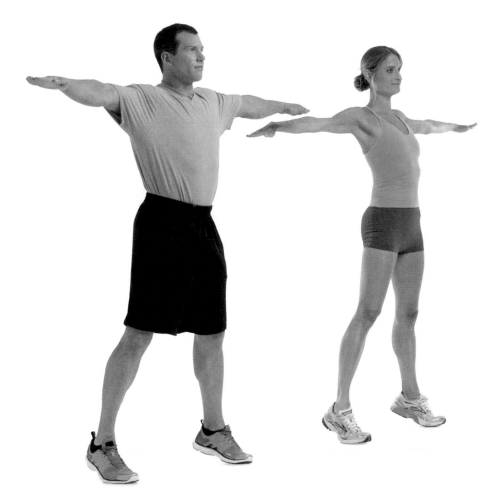

OBJECTIVE: To train your upper and lower body to work in unison.

STARTING POSITION: Standing with feet shoulder-width apart, arms extended out to the sides.

PROCEDURE: Cross your right leg and right hand over your left leg and left hand. Go back to the starting position (feet shoulder-width apart, arms extended out to sides). Now cross your right leg and right hand over your left leg and left hand. Don't get crossed up. If you're old enough to think that this resembles an early-1990s dance move, you've got the right idea.

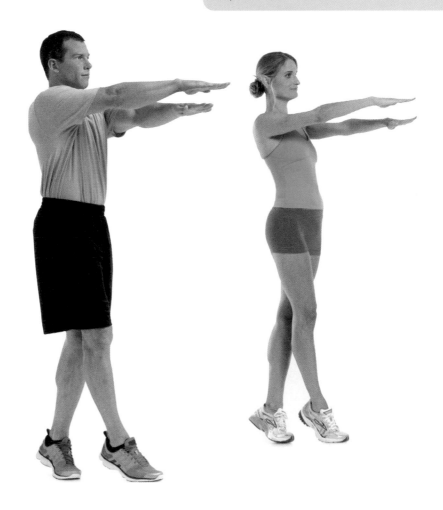

YOU SHOULD FEEL IT: In your hips.

14. SPRINTER JACKS

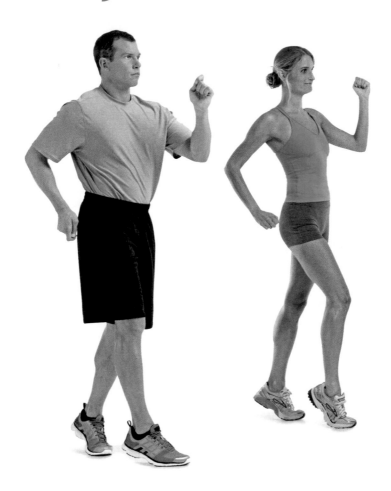

OBJECTIVE: To train your upper and lower body to work separately. This is called "disassociation," and it allows you to generate incredible power across three dimensions.

STARTING POSITION: Standing on the balls of your feet with your right foot 6 to 12 inches in front of the left.

PROCEDURE: This is a plyometric movement that mimics the motion of a sprinter. Drive the right arm and left leg forward as if sprinting, alternating with the left arm and right leg. This back-and-forth motion should be similar to training on an elliptical machine.

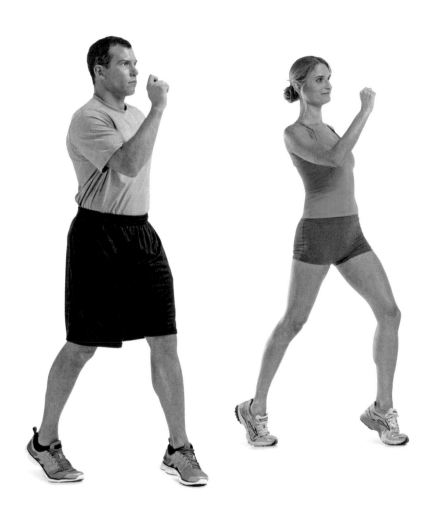

YOU SHOULD FEEL IT: In your hips and shoulders.

15. POGO POPS

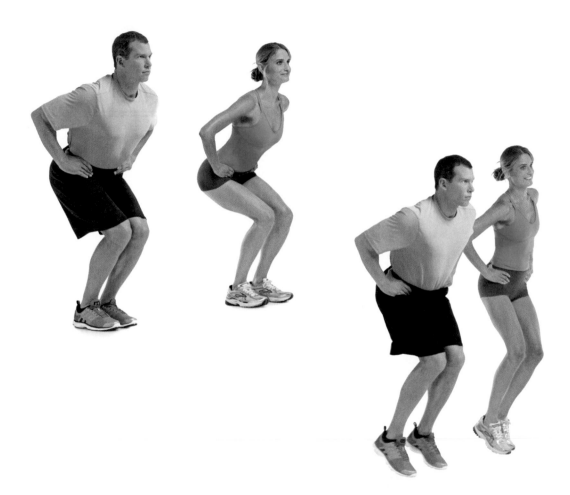

OBJECTIVE: To train your body to store and release energy powerfully, much like a pogo stick. The more efficiently we can store and release energy, the less effort it will take.

STARTING POSITION: Standing in a squatting position with your hands on your hips.

PROCEDURE: Keeping your feet together, jump from side to side as if over a line or an object no more than 6 inches high. Think of moving your body like a pogo stick—without the pogo stick.

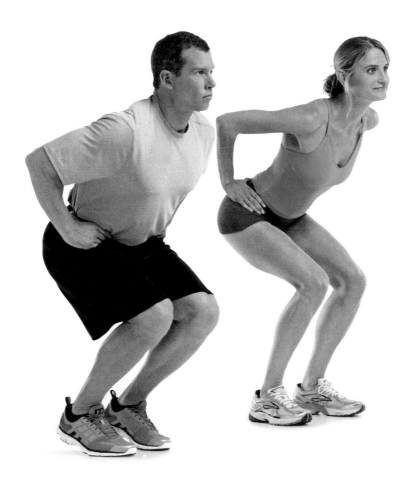

YOU SHOULD FEEL IT: Everywhere, but especially in your hips and legs.

16. SPEED SKATERS

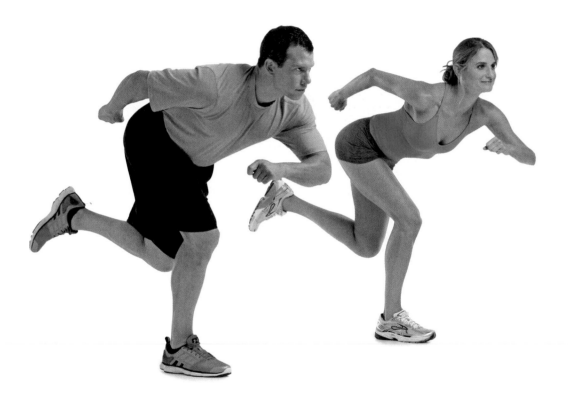

OBJECTIVE: To improve overall core stability.

STARTING POSITION: Standing on one leg, poised to jump laterally.

PROCEDURE: Leap as far as you can to one side, landing on the other foot as if you were ice-skating. Move your arms like a speed skater (or inline skater), swinging both arms. This should look like a skating movement without the blades.

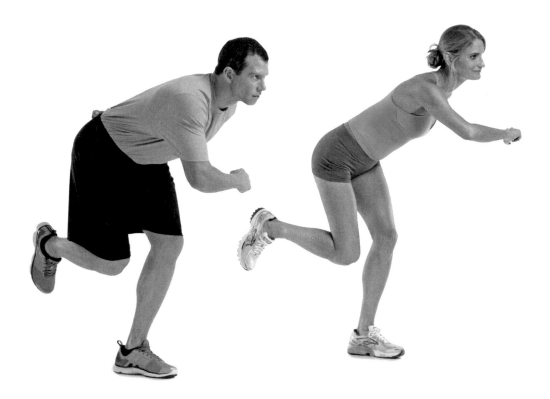

YOU SHOULD FEEL IT: In your lower body from your ankles to your hips.

17. SQUAT HOLDS

COACHING KEY: Think in terms of sitting with your hips back and down until your thighs are parallel to the ground. Your back should be erect and straight, not hunched.

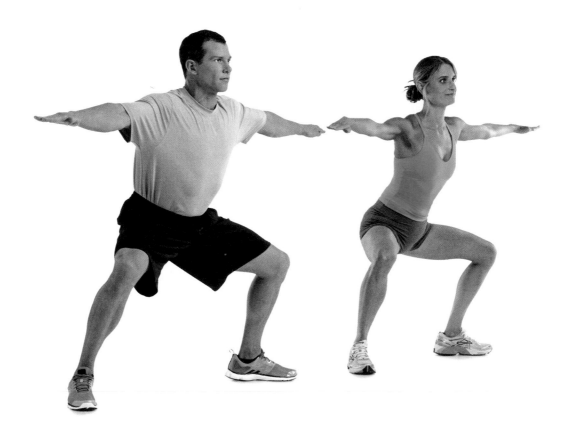

OBJECTIVE: Hip stability.

STARTING POSITION: Standing in a wide squat with your arms out to your side.

PROCEDURE: Hold the position for 10 to 30 seconds, depending on your ability, for the prescribed number of reps.

YOU SHOULD FEEL IT: In your hips and quads.

18. ALTERNATING KNEE GRABS

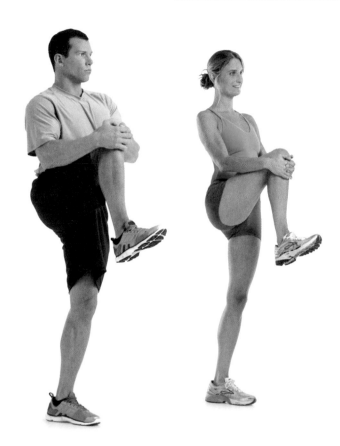

OBJECTIVE: To stretch the hips and hamstrings as we transition into the cooldown.

STARTING POSITION: Standing tall with your back straight and your arms at your sides.

PROCEDURE: Lift your right knee to your chest and grab below the knee with your hands. Pull the knee as close to your chest as you can. Squeeze your left glute (butt cheek) to help with stability. Return to the standing position and repeat on the other side. Alternate knees for the prescribed number of reps.

YOU SHOULD FEEL IT: In your hips and hamstrings.

19. HIGH-KICK TOE-INS

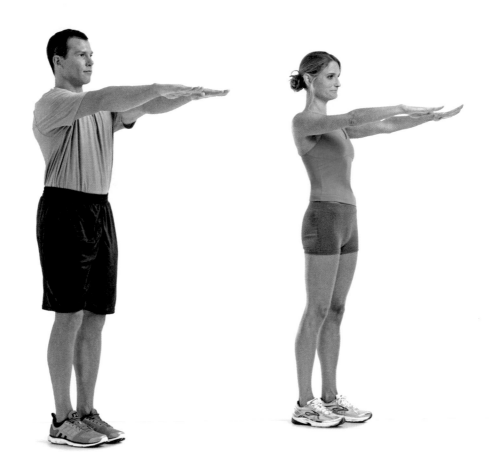

OBJECTIVE: To strengthen the hamstrings, improve hip flexibility, and stabilize the lower back.

STARTING POSITION: Standing with your arms extended in front of you.

PROCEDURE: Perform alternating leg raises. If you can touch your toes to your hands, terrific, but go as far as you can. Your feet should be dorsiflexed, which is to say the toes should point toward the shin. This is part of the cooldown but also a movement to generate strength and mobility in the hamstrings and lower back.

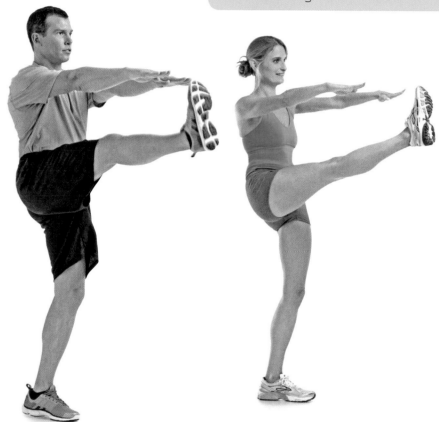

COACHING KEY: Make sure your toes are pulled toward you (dorsiflexed) to get a better stretch in your calf muscles because of the amount of bouncing and dynamic movement. Keep your chin up; don't round your neck and back and don't drop your hips. If you're having trouble with this, do it with your back against a wall. That keeps you from cheating.

YOU SHOULD FEEL IT: In your hamstrings.

20a. COOLDOWN
Butt-Up Pose

COACHING KEY: Move from the hips. Do not round your back.

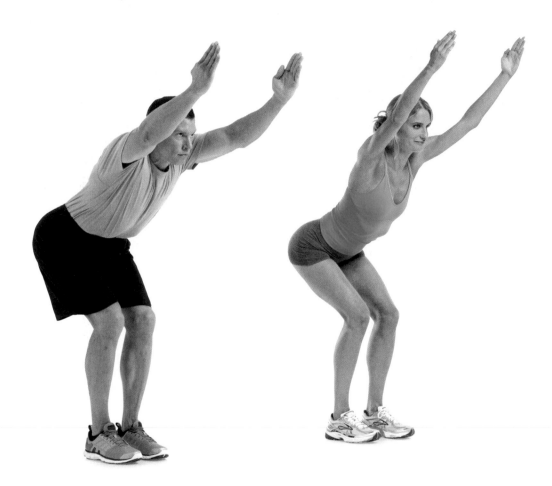

OBJECTIVE: A full-body stretch.

STARTING POSITION: Standing with knees slightly bent and arms extended in front.

PROCEDURE: As you reach forward, bend at the hips so that your butt extends back and up.

YOU SHOULD FEEL IT: All over, but especially in your hamstrings.

20b. COOLDOWN
Cardio Calmers

COACHING KEY: Bend from the hips. Don't forget to breathe.

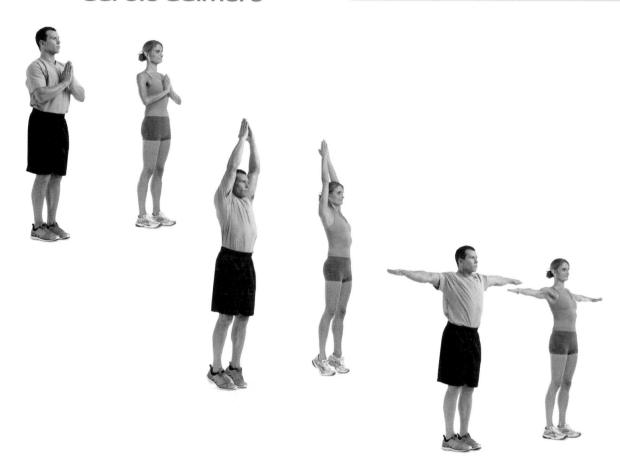

OBJECTIVE: A full-body stretch as part of the cooldown. Also to finish the 4×2 calm and relaxed.

STARTING POSITION: Standing with your hands together in prayer position. Exhale.

PROCEDURE: Inhale and keep your hands together as you reach overhead standing on your toes. Inhale and return to the standing position with your arms stretched out to the side. Perform four times.

YOU SHOULD FEEL IT: In your hamstrings.

Now that you've learned the 4×2 Standing Workout, it's time to take it to the floor. Athletes train on the court; most people's playing field is their desk. We need to train on a pre-hab basis to avoid injuries associated with the common modern lifestyle. 4×4 Cardio Core workout does just that.

As in the 4×2 workout, you should start with 10 reps on each side and work up to 20 as you get stronger unless otherwise indicated. Anytime you are on all fours, do your best to keep your core and glutes engaged and to keep your toes in a dorsiflexed position. This helps to strengthen your anterior muscles and helps you to stabilize your foot better whether you are running or wearing high heels.

THE CARDIO CORE 4X4 WORKOUT

THE CARDIO CORE
4×4 WORKOUT
AT A GLANCE

2 times a week, 10–20 reps of each exercise
Tuesdays and Fridays (or whatever 2 days a week you choose)

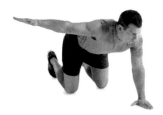

1. GEAR-UPS
(PAGE 140)

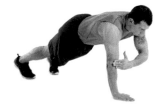

2. PUSHUP SERIES
(PAGE 142)

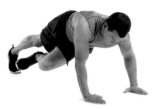

3. ACROSS THE BODY
(PAGE 146)

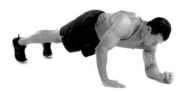

4. MOUNTAIN CLIMBERS
(PAGE 148)

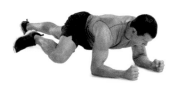

5. JACKKNIVES
(PAGE 150)

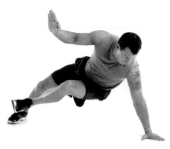

6. BREAK DANCERS
(PAGE 151)

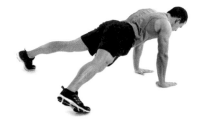

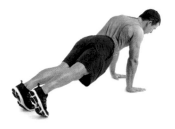

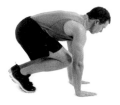

7. SCISSORS
(PAGE 152)

8. TOGETHER HOPS
(PAGE 153)

9. TUCK JUMPS
(PAGE 154)

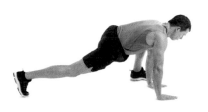

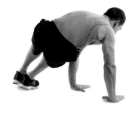

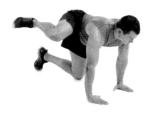

10. FORK JUMPS
(PAGE 155)

11. FORK AND KNIFE JUMPS
(PAGE 156)

12a. 4X4 MATRIX
Fire Hydrants
(PAGE 158)

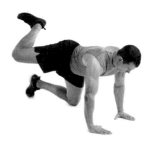

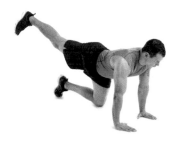

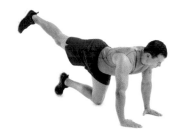

12b. 4X4 MATRIX
Forward/Backward Circles
(PAGE 160)

12c. 4X4 MATRIX
Leg-Ups
(PAGE 162)

12d. 4X4 MATRIX
Leg Circles (Internal/External)
(PAGE 164)

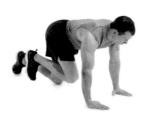

12e. 4X4 MATRIX
Pistons
(PAGE 166)

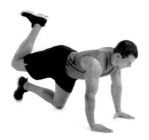

12f. 4X4 MATRIX
Curls
(PAGE 167)

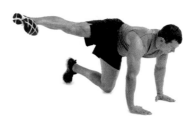

12g. 4X4 MATRIX
Sideout Lifts
(PAGE 168)

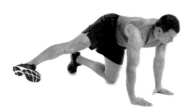

12h. 4X4 MATRIX
Sideout Circles
(PAGE 170)

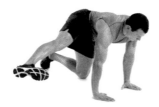

12i. 4X4 MATRIX
Windshield Wipers
(PAGE 172)

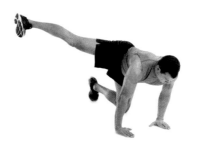

12j. 4X4 MATRIX
Karate Kids
(PAGE 173)

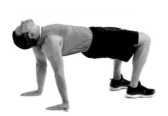

13a. REVERSE 4X4 MATRIX
Tabletops
(PAGE 174)

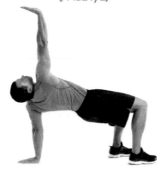

13b. REVERSE 4X4 MATRIX
Crab Trees
(PAGE 176)

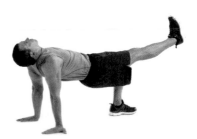

13c. REVERSE 4X4 MATRIX
Crab Legs
(PAGE 178)

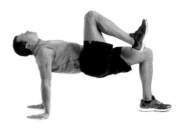

13d. REVERSE 4×4 MATRIX
Crab Claws
(PAGE 179)

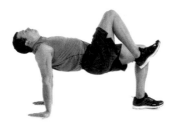

13e. REVERSE 4×4 MATRIX
Running Man
(PAGE 180)

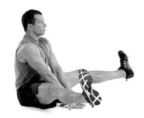

14. HIP LIFTS
(PAGE 181)

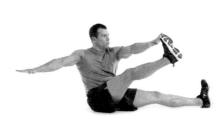

15. ALTERNATING HIP LIFTS
(PAGE 182)

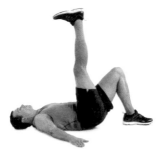

16a. ON-GROUND MATRIX
Leg-Ups
(PAGE 183)

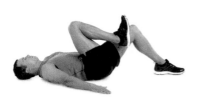

16b. ON-GROUND MATRIX
Reverse Pistons
(PAGE 184)

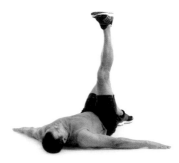

16c. ON-GROUND MATRIX
Tick-Tocks
(PAGE 185)

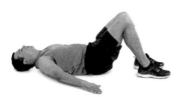

16d. ON-GROUND MATRIX
Pelvic Tilts
(PAGE 186)

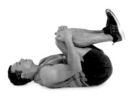

17. COOLDOWN
(PAGE 187)

1. GEAR-UPS

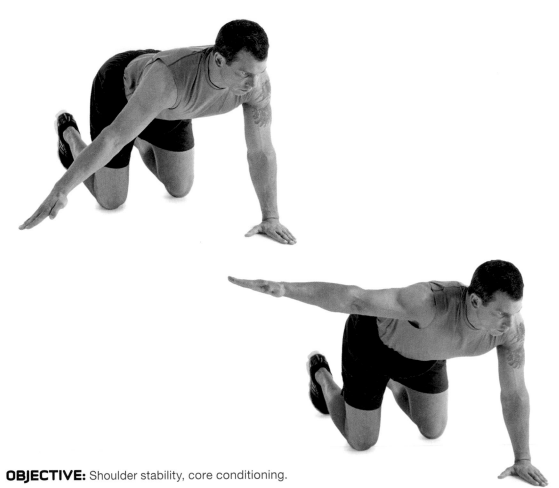

OBJECTIVE: Shoulder stability, core conditioning.

STARTING POSITION: On your hands and knees, 4×4 position.

PROCEDURE: Extend your right arm laterally (to your right) and do the prescribed number of reps, up and down. Your hand should come down to within an inch of the ground, without touching, and go no higher than perpendicular to your body. Next perform circles, clockwise and then counterclockwise. After that, take your right arm forward and repeat the process, up and down, clockwise and counterclockwise.

YOU SHOULD FEEL IT: In your shoulders, lower back, and core.

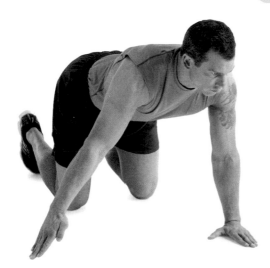

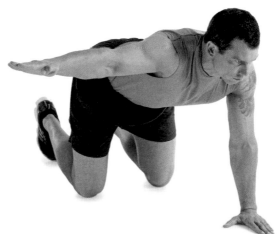

Repeat all these movements with your left arm.

2. PUSHUP SERIES

For the next series of exercises, we're going to depart from our 4×4 stance (hands and knees on the ground) and assume a pushup position, with your hands and feet on the ground. If you're unable to do a pushup, begin with your knees on the ground.

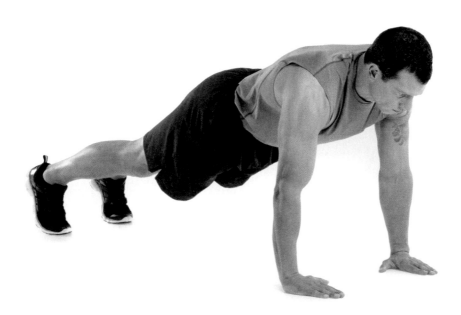

OBJECTIVE: Shoulder stabilization.

STARTING POSITION: On all fours, in the pushup position.

PROCEDURE: With your right hand, touch your left forearm on the inside of the elbow. Repeat on the other side and alternate. Next, touch your left shoulder with your right hand. Switch hands and alternate. Finally, use your right shoulder to raise your right arm from the elbow. Lower it and repeat on your right side, and then do the same number on the left side. The movement should resemble a dumbbell row.

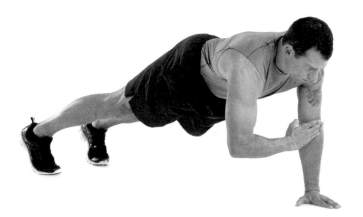

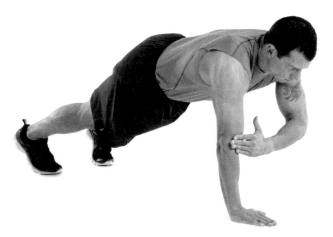

YOU SHOULD FEEL IT: In your shoulders.

(continued)

2. PUSHUP SERIES (Continued)

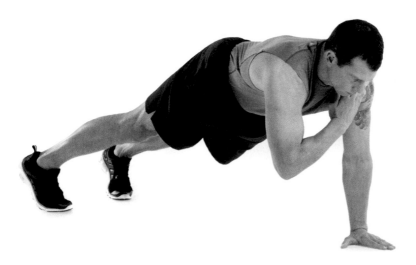

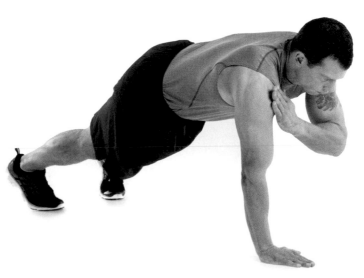

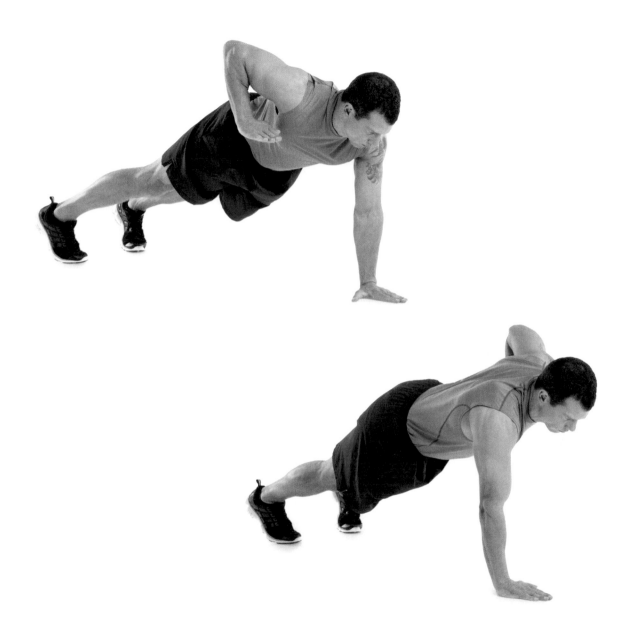

3. ACROSS THE BODY

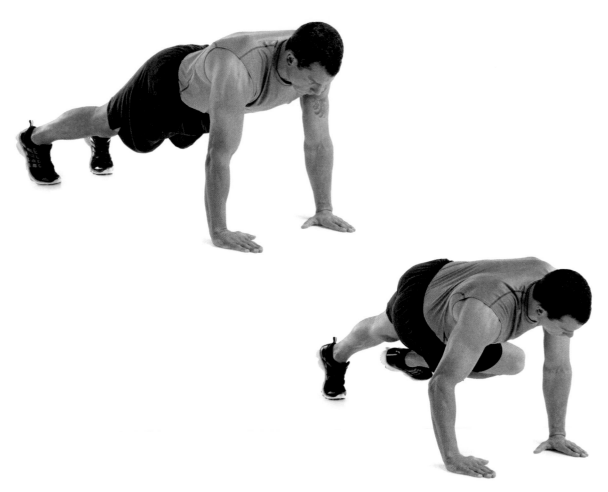

OBJECTIVE: Shoulder stability and hip mobility.

STARTING POSITION: Pushup position.

PROCEDURE: Bring your right knee across your belly button. Think of your knee as a thread and the space under your left arm as the needle hole and bring the knee across the midline of your body to thread the needle. Alternate knees. Think of driving your knee to the opposite elbow.

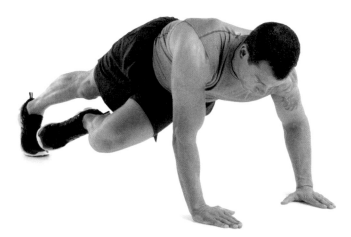

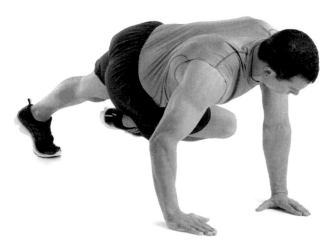

YOU SHOULD FEEL IT: In your hips and groin.

4. Mountain Climbers

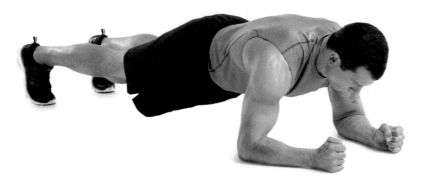

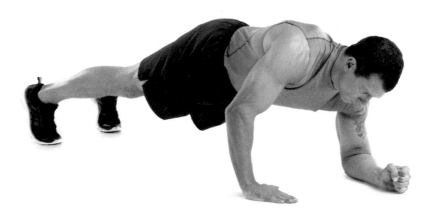

OBJECTIVE: Shoulder stability and strength.

STARTING POSITION: Plank position: facedown in a modified pushup position, with your forearms on the ground. Your elbows should be under your shoulders and bent 90 degrees.

PROCEDURE: Raise your right forearm and place your right hand on the ground. Do the same with your left forearm. You're now in pushup position. Return by moving your right arm back to plank position (forearm on the floor) and then your left arm. Repeat for the prescribed number of reps. This mimics a mountain climber's progression.

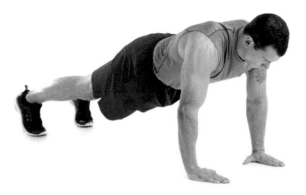

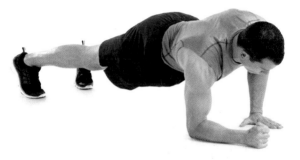

YOU SHOULD FEEL IT: In your shoulders and core region.

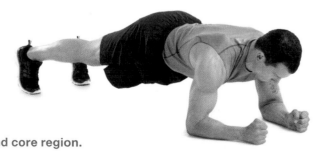

5. JACKKNIVES

COACHING KEY: Open your hips and groin as much as possible to get a good stretch.

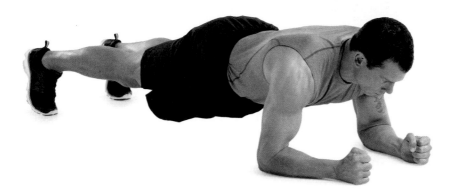

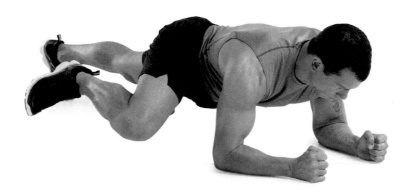

OBJECTIVE: Hip and shoulder mobility.

STARTING POSITION: Plank position: modified pushup position with your forearms on the ground.

PROCEDURE: Take your right knee to the right side so that it grazes your elbow, go back to the plank position. Do the prescribed number of reps on the right side, and then do the same with your left knee.

YOU SHOULD FEEL IT: In your hips and groin.

6. BREAK DANCERS

COACHING KEY: Focus on making your belly button face the floor and then the ceiling. Or think of it as your hips doing the same thing. Bend your elbow and knee to better stabilize your body.

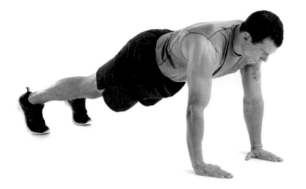

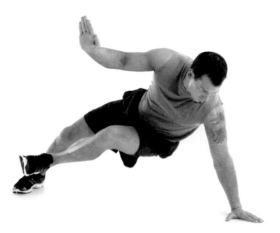

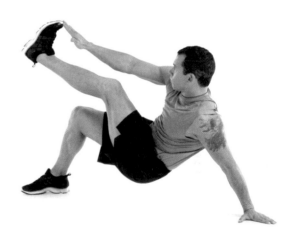

OBJECTIVE: Hip and shoulder stability.

STARTING POSITION: Pushup position.

PROCEDURE: Raise your right hand and left foot at same time, swinging your left hip and leg under your body toward your right hand so that you're basically rotating your belly button till it faces the ceiling. Try to touch your left foot (or left knee) with your right hand, and keep your left knee bent. Hold for a second and rotate back. Then swing your right hip and leg through and touch your right foot or knee with your left hand.

YOU SHOULD FEEL IT: All over. This is a full-body exercise.

7. SCISSORS

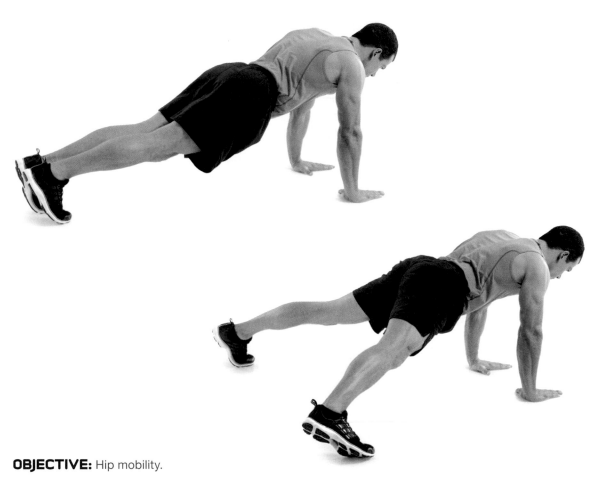

OBJECTIVE: Hip mobility.

STARTING POSITION: Pushup position.

PROCEDURE: Jump your feet out as wide as possible. Return to the starting position. This is the same movement we did standing in the 4×2. The reason we replicate this move and others from different angles is that the body has three planes of motion, and we want to work all three planes.

YOU SHOULD FEEL IT: In your hips and groin.

8. TOGETHER HOPS

COACHING KEY: Don't slouch. Keep your body tall with your shoulders back.

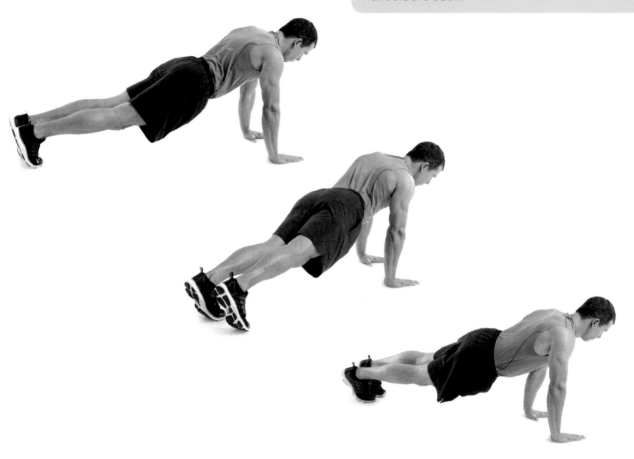

OBJECTIVE: Similar to the Pogo Pops in the 4×2, the goal here is to train the body to store and release energy powerfully, much like a pogo stick. The more efficiently we can store and release energy, the less effort it will take.

STARTING POSITION: Pushup position with your feet together.

PROCEDURE: Jump laterally as if you're going back and forth over a line on the ground.

YOU SHOULD FEEL IT: Everywhere, but especially in your hips and legs.

9. TUCK JUMPS

COACHING KEY: Keep your feet together.

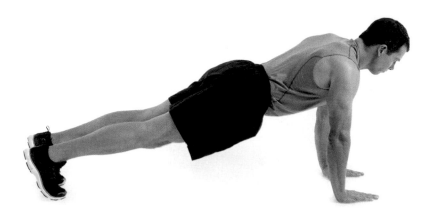

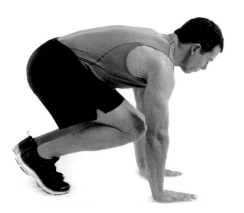

OBJECTIVE: As with Wide Outs, the goal is to develop the body's "elasticity," its ability to store and release energy powerfully.

STARTING POSITION: Pushup position.

PROCEDURE: Jump forward with both feet together. Your knees should come as far forward as possible. Return to the starting position.

YOU SHOULD FEEL IT: In your hips, legs, and calves.

10. FORK JUMPS

COACHING KEY: If you can't get your foot adjacent to your hand immediately, get it as far as possible.

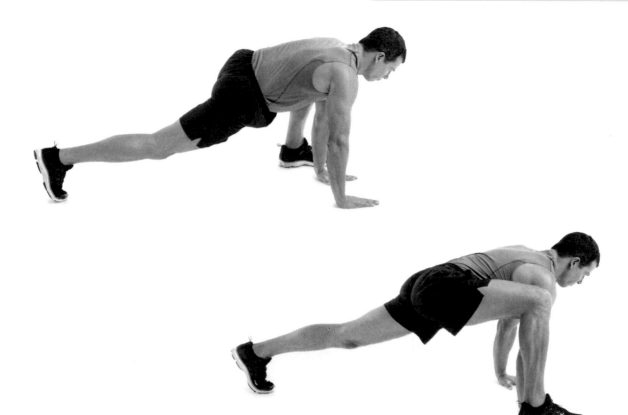

OBJECTIVE: Hip mobility and explosive power.

STARTING POSITION: From the pushup position, bring your right foot next to your right hand or as far up as possible.

PROCEDURE: Jump up with your left foot to your left hand as your right foot drops back for stability. Alternate for the prescribed number of reps.

YOU SHOULD FEEL IT: Everywhere. This is a full-body exercise.

11. FORK AND KNIFE JUMPS

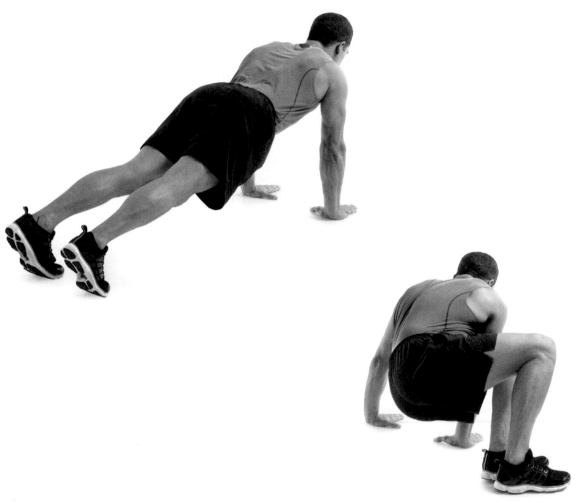

OBJECTIVE: Hip mobility and explosive power.

STARTING POSITION: Pushup position.

PROCEDURE: With your feet together, jump toward the right hand. Return to the starting position and jump to your left hand. This is different from Tuck Jumps in that you're moving at an angle.

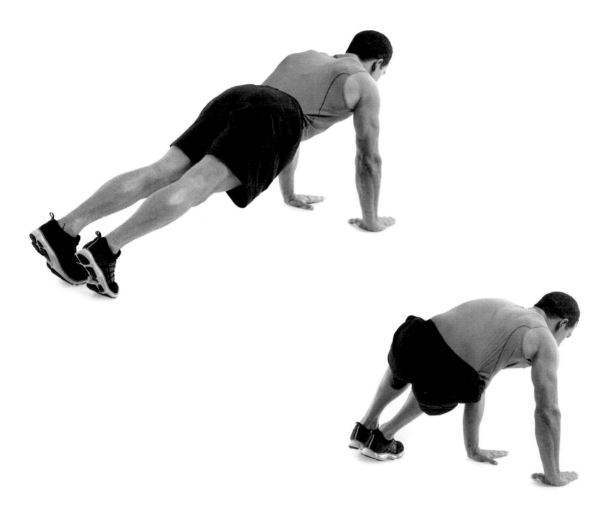

YOU SHOULD FEEL IT: Everywhere. This is a full-body exercise.

4×4 MATRIX

This is similar to the Scarecrow Matrix in the 4×2, where we performed a series of exercises to strengthen and stabilize the shoulders. That's the same philosophy here, only we're strengthening and stabilizing the hips. As we did with the Scarecrow Matrix, we will do the entire matrix on the right side first and then follow with the left side.

12a. 4×4 MATRIX
Fire Hydrants

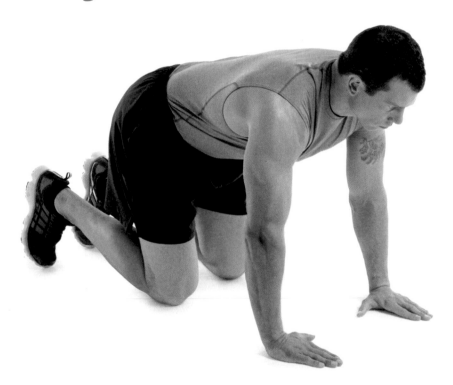

PROCEDURE: From your hands and knees (the 4×4 position), raise your right leg from the hip until the leg is parallel to the ground, mimicking a dog's movements, then lower it again. Do the prescribed number of reps.

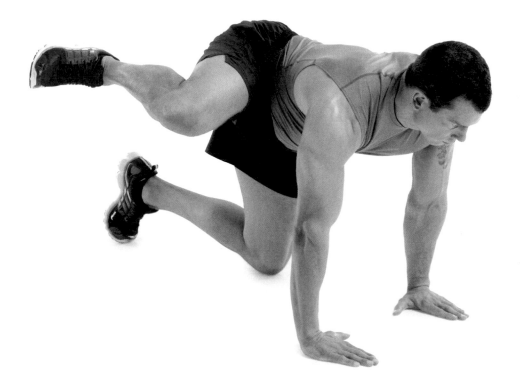

YOU SHOULD FEEL IT: In your groin, glutes, and shoulders.

12b. 4×4 MATRIX
Forward/Backward Circles

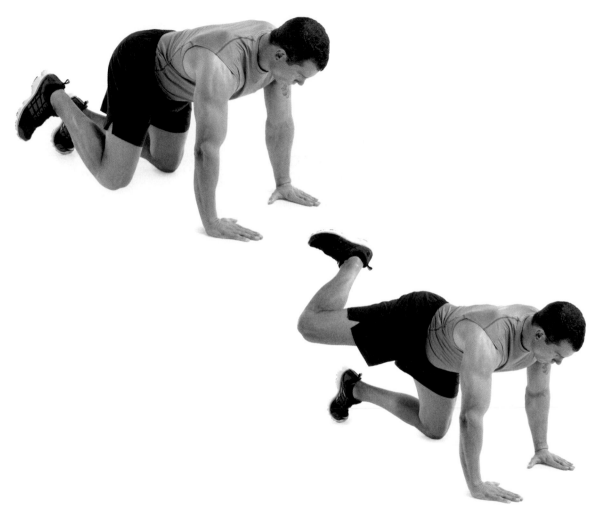

PROCEDURE: From the Fire Hydrant position, raise your right leg as if you're lifting it over a hurdle. Circle your leg from the hip joint. This is the same movement we did earlier with the 4×2 in Over the Fence, only from all fours.

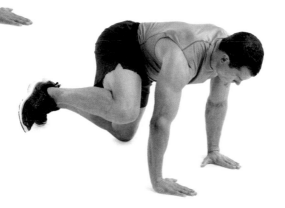

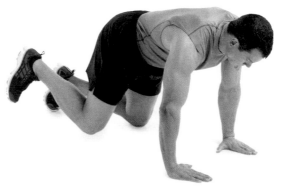

YOU SHOULD FEEL IT: In your groin, glutes, and shoulders.

12C. 4×4 MATRIX
Leg-Ups

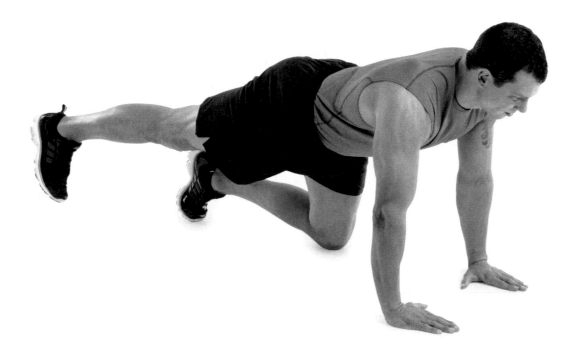

PROCEDURE: From the 4×4 position, extend your right leg back. Keeping the knee straight, lift the leg up and then lower it.

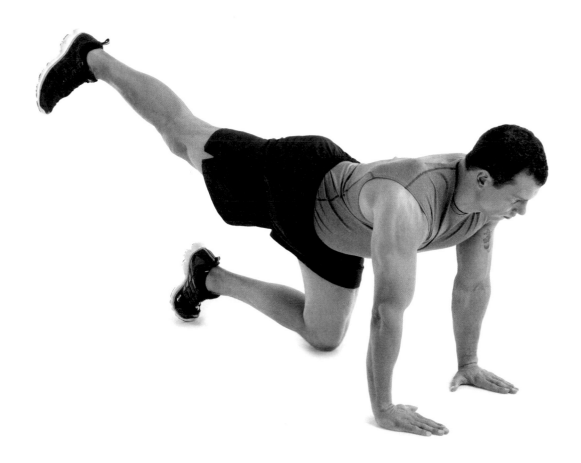

YOU SHOULD FEEL IT: In your glutes and lower lumbar region.

12d. 4×4 MATRIX
Leg Circles (Internal/External)

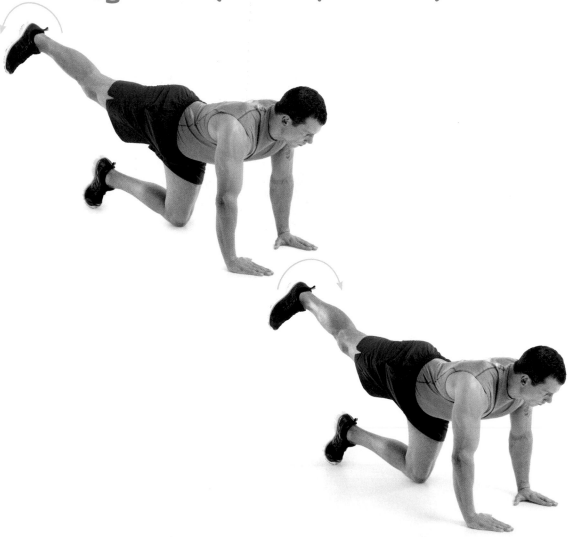

PROCEDURE: Picking up from the previous movement (Leg-Ups) with your right leg extended, make a circle with your leg counterclockwise and then clockwise.

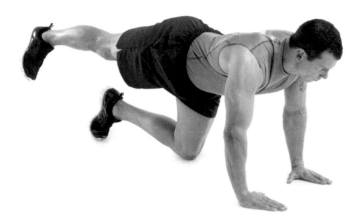

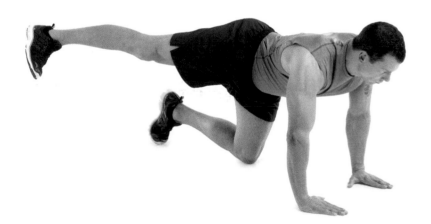

YOU SHOULD FEEL IT: In your hips, lower lumbar region, and glutes.

12e. 4x4 MATRIX
Pistons

COACHING KEY: Breathing is key here. Inhale as you bring the knee toward you and exhale as you kick. When you're kicking toward the ceiling, kick from the hip.

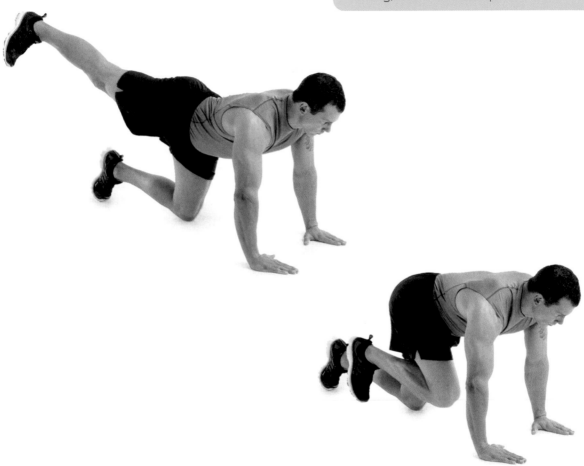

PROCEDURE: Beginning with your right leg extended, bring your right knee under your body and then kick the leg out straight, donkey-style.

YOU SHOULD FEEL IT: In your hips and core.

12f. 4×4 MATRIX
Curls

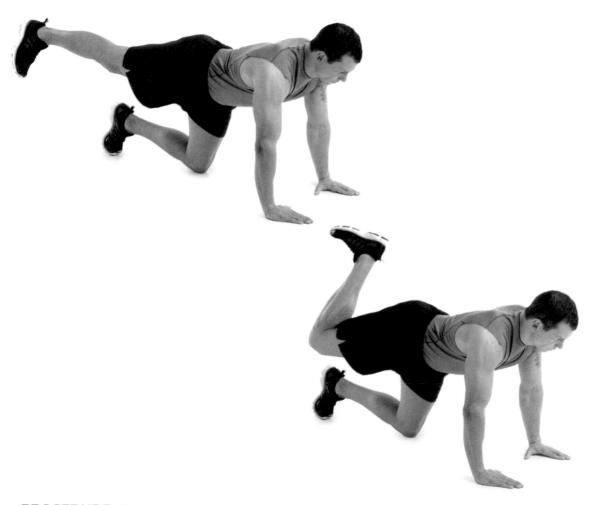

PROCEDURE: Here we're working the hamstrings but also the hip flexors, glutes, and lumbar spine. With your right leg extended back, bend your knee to curl your lower leg as if doing a biceps curl.

YOU SHOULD FEEL IT: In your glutes and hamstrings.

128. 4×4 MATRIX
Sideout Lifts

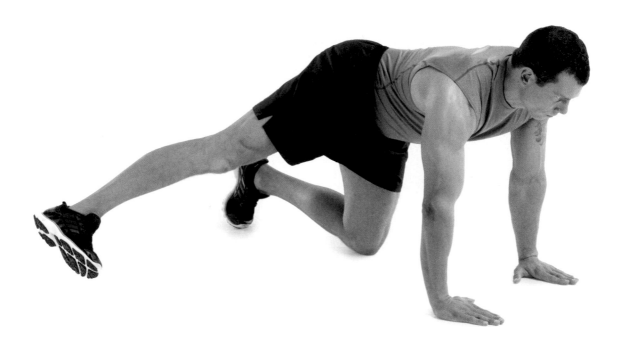

PROCEDURE: From the 4×4 position, bring your right leg out to the side until it's almost perpendicular to your body. Depending on your degree of flexibility, you'll be able to go between 20 and 90 degrees. Regardless of where you start—and don't worry if it's on the low end of the flexibility scale—lift your leg and lower it, isolating the outside part of the hip.

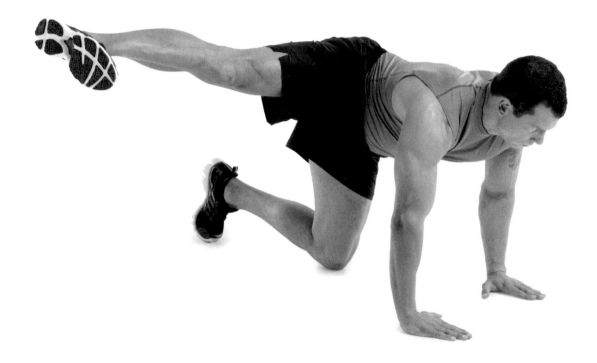

YOU SHOULD FEEL IT: In your iliotibial (IT) bands, the tough group of muscle fibers that run along the outside of the thigh, and in the side of your hip.

12h. 4×4 MATRIX
Sideout Circles

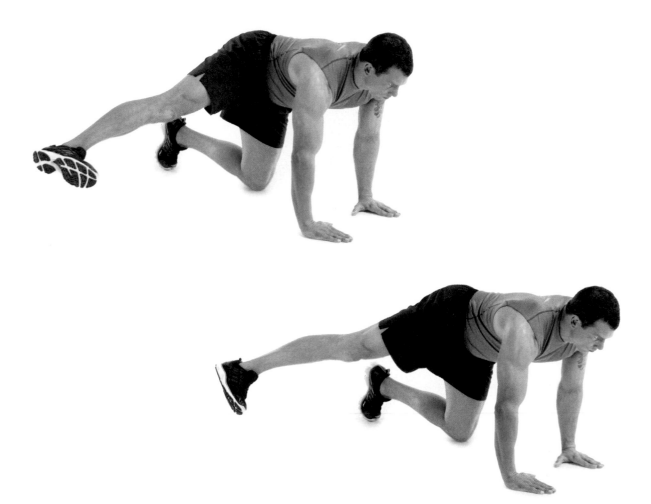

PROCEDURE: Same as with the last movement: Bring your right leg out to the side until it's almost perpendicular to your body. Depending on your degree of flexibility, you'll be able to go between 20 and 90 degrees. Rotate the leg clockwise and then counterclockwise.

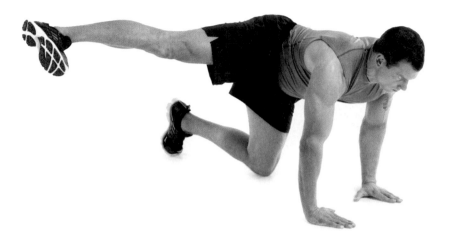

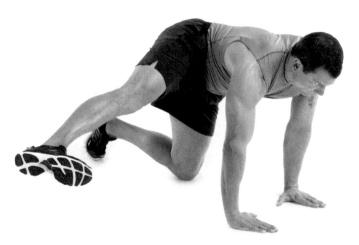

YOU SHOULD FEEL IT: In the side of your hip flexor.

12i. 4×4 MATRIX
Windshield Wipers

COACHING KEY: Move from the hip. This is not a kicking movement.

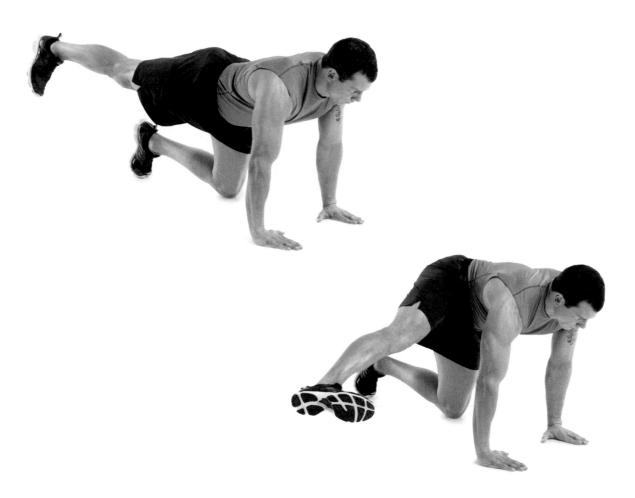

PROCEDURE: Extend your right leg all the way back, parallel to the ground. Rotate the leg to form a 90-degree angle with your torso (or as far as possible) and back, creating a windshield-wiper effect.

YOU SHOULD FEEL IT: In your hips and oblique muscles.

12j. 4×4 MATRIX
Karate Kids

COACHING KEY: Keep your weight evenly distributed in both arms.

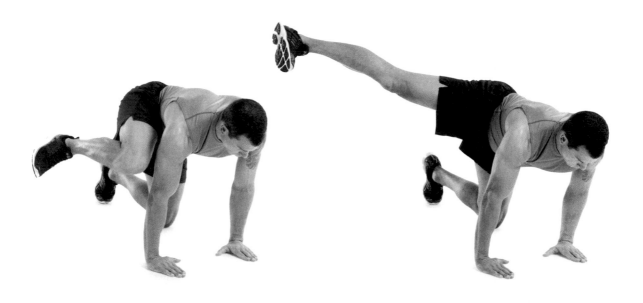

PROCEDURE: Bring your right knee to your right elbow and kick to the side. If you've had some martial arts training, you'll recognize this as a side kick. If you can't perform this movement with much power because of a lack of flexibility, do it as best you can within your range of motion, which will improve throughout the program.

YOU SHOULD FEEL IT: In your hips, obliques, and lats.

Now that you've done the 4×4 Matrix on the right side, go back and do exercises 12a through 12j on the left side.

REVERSE 4×4 MATRIX

At this point, we flip over into the "crab" position, which you might remember from grade school gym class if you ever played crab soccer. You'll be on all fours with your body facing up, with only your hands and feet making contact with the ground.

13a. REVERSE 4×4 MATRIX
Tabletops

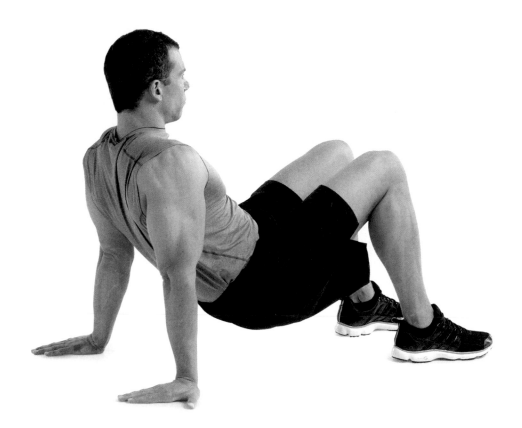

PROCEDURE: Bridge (lift) your hips toward the ceiling and then bring them down for the prescribed number of repetitions.

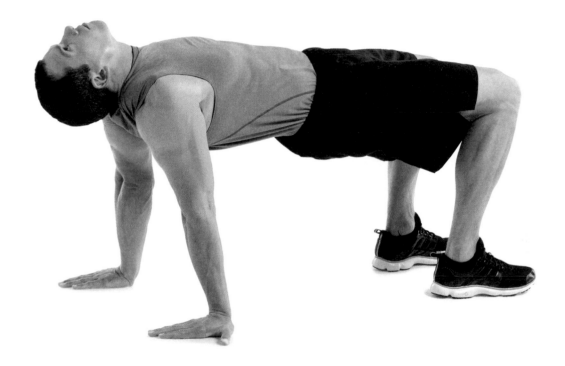

YOU SHOULD FEEL IT: In your hips.

13b. REVERSE 4×4 MATRIX
Crab Trees

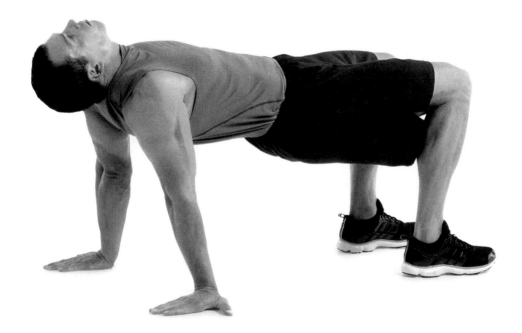

PROCEDURE: From the crab position, bridge your hips toward the ceiling. Keeping your hips raised, alternate reaching up with each hand as if delivering a high five.

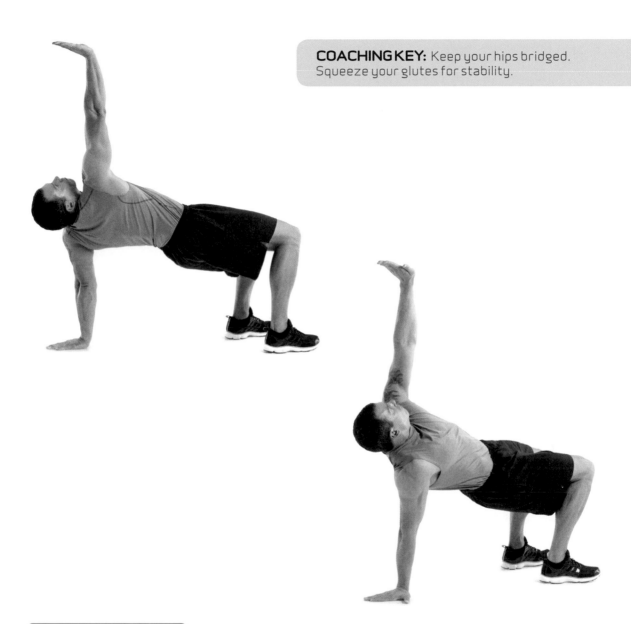

YOU SHOULD FEEL IT: In your hips and shoulders.

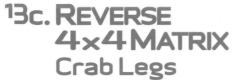

13c. REVERSE 4×4 MATRIX
Crab Legs

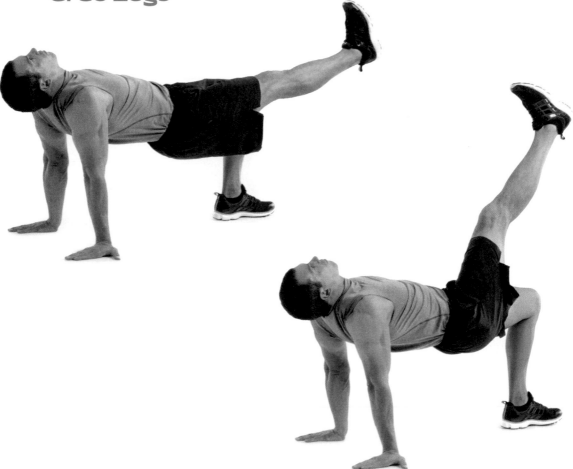

PROCEDURE: From the crab position, with your hips raised, straighten out your right leg and lift it up and down. Repeat with your left leg.

YOU SHOULD FEEL IT: In your hips.

13d. REVERSE 4×4 MATRIX
Crab Claws

COACHING KEY: Think in terms of delivering power from your hips, not your feet.

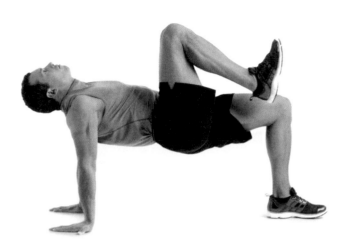

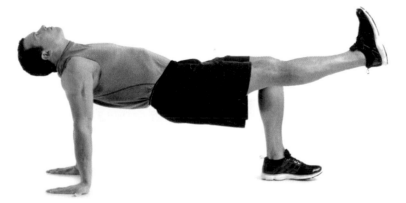

PROCEDURE: From the crab position, with your hips raised, bring your right knee to your waist, forming a 90-degree angle with your torso, and shoot the leg out piston-style for the prescribed number of reps. Repeat with your left leg.

YOU SHOULD FEEL IT: In your hips.

13e. REVERSE 4×4 MATRIX Running Man

COACHING KEY: Don't drop your hips. Keep them bridged by squeezing your glutes.

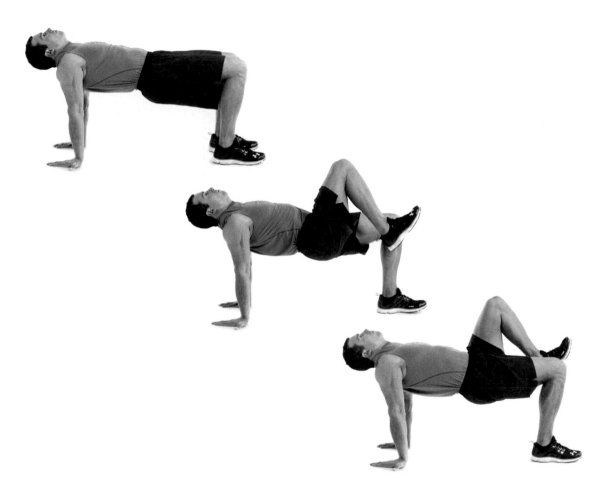

PROCEDURE: From the tabletop position (hips bridged toward the ceiling), run in place for 30 seconds.

YOU SHOULD FEEL IT: In your hips.

14. HIP LIFTS

COACHING KEY: Unless you're a gymnast, don't worry about getting your butt off the ground; it's probably not going to happen.

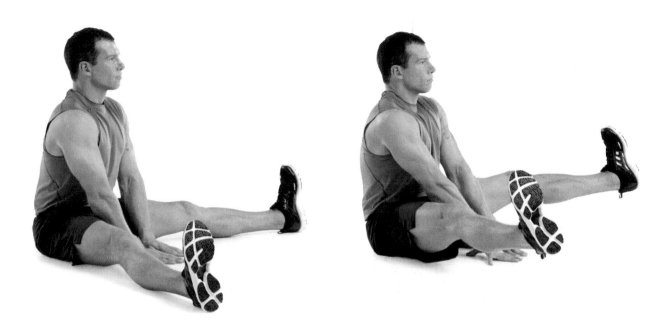

PROCEDURE: From a seated position, spread your legs as wide as you can. Place your hands on the floor in front of your groin and lift both legs at the same time as high and as fast as possible. Carefully lower to the ground.

YOU SHOULD FEEL IT: In your hips and groin.

15. ALTERNATING HIP LIFTS

COACHING KEY: It's okay if you can't touch your toe. Just reach out as far as you can.

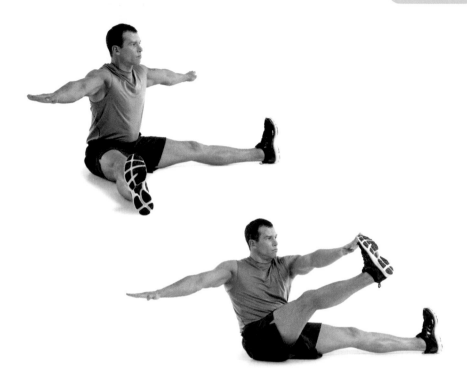

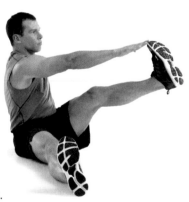

PROCEDURE: Same as Hip Lifts, only this time lift your legs one at a time.

YOU SHOULD FEEL IT: In your hips and groin.

On-Ground Matrix

This is a slight variation on the Reverse 4×4 Matrix. Instead of being in the crab position, we'll be lying flat on our backs. First we'll complete all of the exercises with the right leg, then we'll repeat on the left side.

16a. On-Ground Matrix Leg-Ups

COACHING KEY: Squeeze your right glute. This will make the movement easier and also is the natural way to move.

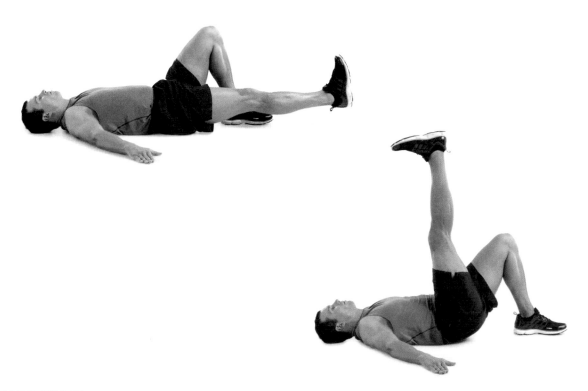

PROCEDURE: Lying on your back, raise your right leg as far as possible. Lower carefully and repeat.

YOU SHOULD FEEL IT: In your right hip and glute.

16b. ON-GROUND MATRIX
Reverse Pistons

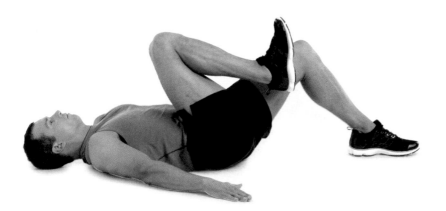

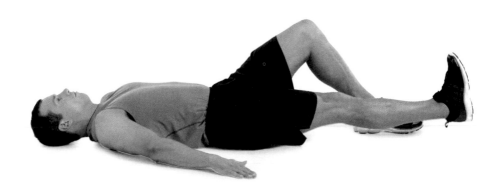

PROCEDURE: Lying on your back, bring your right leg to your body, bending the knee, and kick the leg out straight donkey-style, as if you're kicking in a barn door.

YOU SHOULD FEEL IT: In your hips and core.

16c. ON-GROUND MATRIX
Tick-Tocks

COACHING KEY: Think in terms of moving your leg from 12 o'clock to 3 o'clock. If you can only make it to 1 or 2 o'clock, that's fine. You'll improve as you progress in the system.

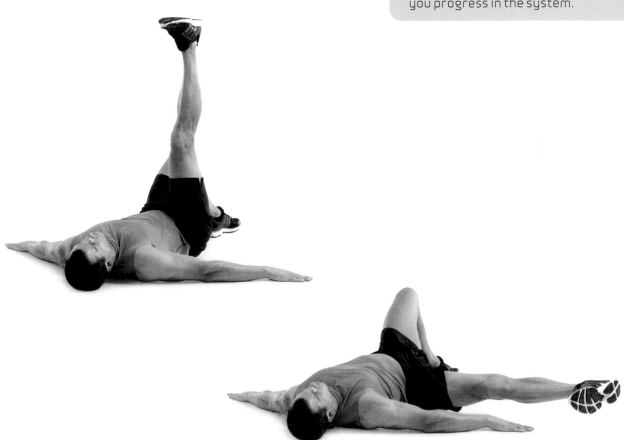

PROCEDURE: Lying on your back, take your right leg out to the side as far as possible and return to the starting position. Repeat with your left leg.

YOU SHOULD FEEL IT: In your hips and groin.

16d. ON-GROUND MATRIX
Pelvic Tilts

COACHING KEY: This is a subtle movement, but it's effective.

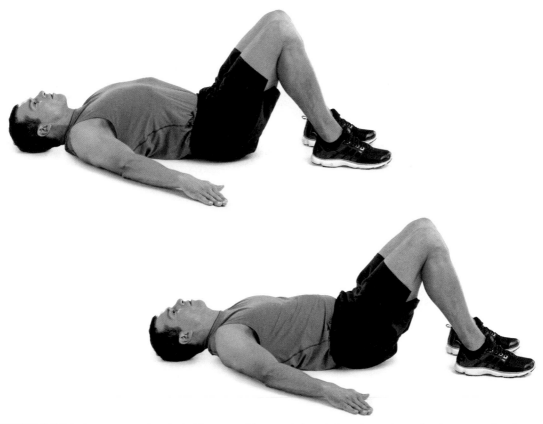

PROCEDURE: Lying on your back, bridge your hips and then bring them down for the prescribed number of repetitions.

YOU SHOULD FEEL IT: In your hips.

Do exercises 16a through 16c on the left side.

17. Cooldown

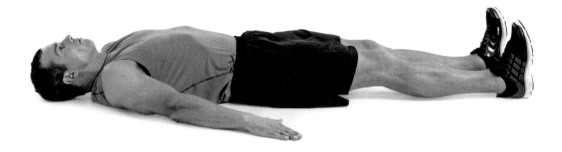

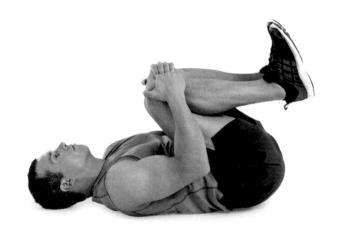

PROCEDURE: Lying on your back, hug your knees to your chest for 3 seconds. Return to the starting position. Stretch as far as you can from your toes and hands.

The following is a series of 10 movements designed to give you a phenomenal cardio workout in just 10 minutes. It's optional, and you might choose not to do it, especially in the early days of the program as you learn the 4×2 and 4×4, which will take 2 days apiece. As in the other workouts, do 10 to 20 reps of each exercise on each side unless otherwise indicated.

    You'll likely find, however, that you're looking for some active rest on Wednesdays or on the weekends. Active rest is the philosophy that your body recovers better when you put it through a light workout than when you do nothing.

THE CARDIO CORE WORKOUT

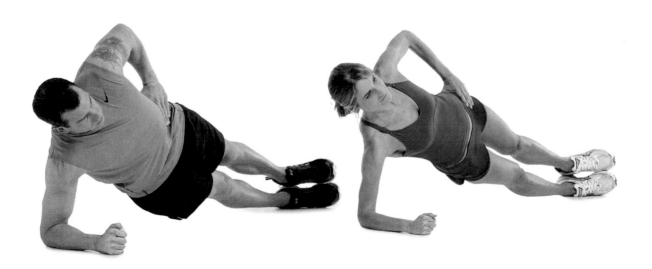

THE
CARDIO
CORE
WORKOUT
AT A GLANCE

2 times a week, 10–20 reps of each exercise
Wednesdays and weekends (or whatever 2 days you choose)

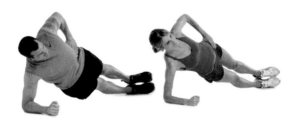

1a. SIDE MATRIX
Side Planks
(PAGE 192)

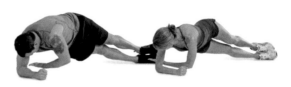

1b. SIDE MATRIX
Threading the Needle
(PAGE 193)

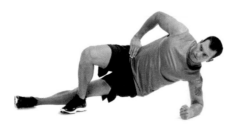

2. CROCODILES
(PAGE 194)

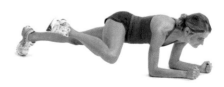

3. PLANK OUTS
(PAGE 195)

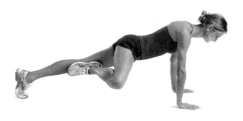

4. LOCK JAWS
(PAGE 196)

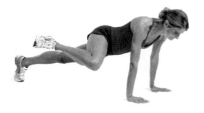

5. CIRCLE OUTS
(PAGE 197)

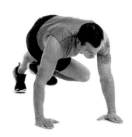

6. PENDULUMS
(PAGE 198)

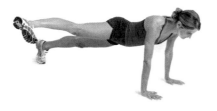

7. SWINGOUTS
(PAGE 200)

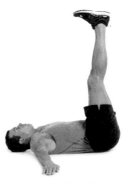

8. HOLD OUT HIGHS
(PAGE 202)

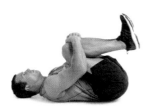

9. COOLDOWN
Knee Huggers
(PAGE 203)

SIDE MATRIX

This consists of two movements: Side Planks and Threading the Needle.

1a. SIDE MATRIX
Side Planks

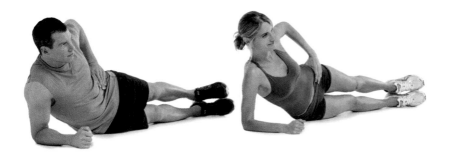

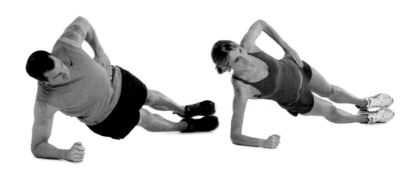

PROCEDURE: Lie on your right side with your right forearm on the ground, elbow under your shoulder. Your body should be in a straight line, with your toes pulled toward your shins. Push your hips off the ground so your body is in a straight line from ankle to shoulder. Repeat on the opposite side.

YOU SHOULD FEEL IT: Pretty much all over. This is a full-body exercise.

1b. SIDE MATRIX
Threading the Needle

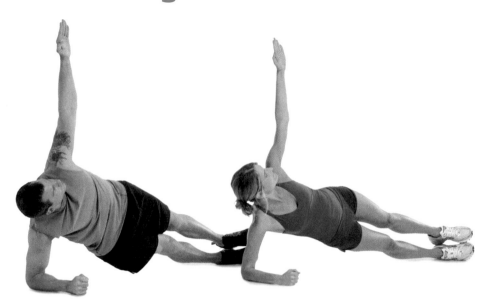

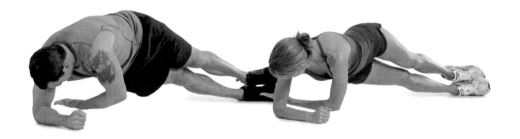

PROCEDURE: From the side plank position (hips raised) raise your top arm. Thread the needle by reaching between your torso and your stable arm. Repeat on the opposite side.

YOU SHOULD FEEL IT: Pretty much all over. This is a full-body exercise.

2. CROCODILES

COACHING KEY: Squeeze your glutes. Keep your body in an erect position. People tend to fall forward on this. The body must stay in an erect position. Everything from heel to head should be in a straight line.

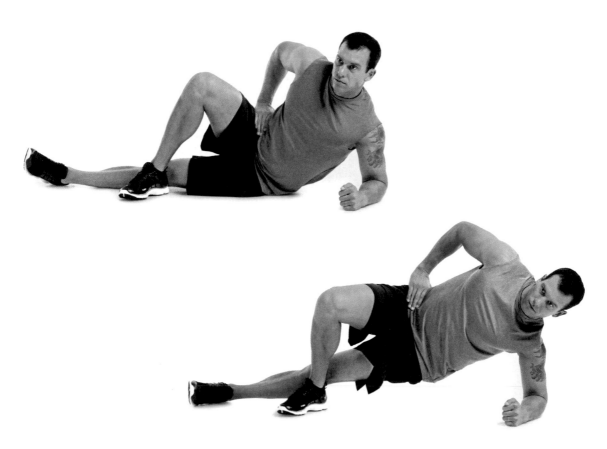

PROCEDURE: Lie on your left side with your left elbow on the floor for support. Place your right hand on your right hip with your right foot in front of your left extended knee. Your left leg is on the ground, along with your left hand. With weight on your elbow and heel, drive the hip as hard as you can off the floor. Slowly lower it. Repeat on the other side.

YOU SHOULD FEEL IT: In your hips and glutes.

3. PLANK OUTS

COACHING KEY: Move from your hips, not your knees.

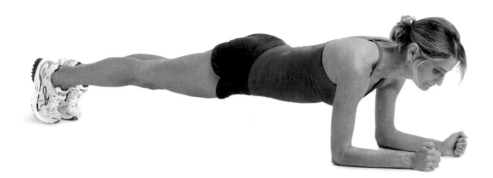

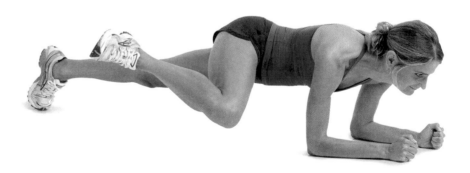

PROCEDURE: From the plank position (forearms on the ground), drive your right knee outside your right elbow. Alternate sides.

YOU SHOULD FEEL IT: In your hips.

4. LOCK JAWS

COACHING KEY: Keep your hips parallel to the ground. Your body should be in a straight line from head to heels.

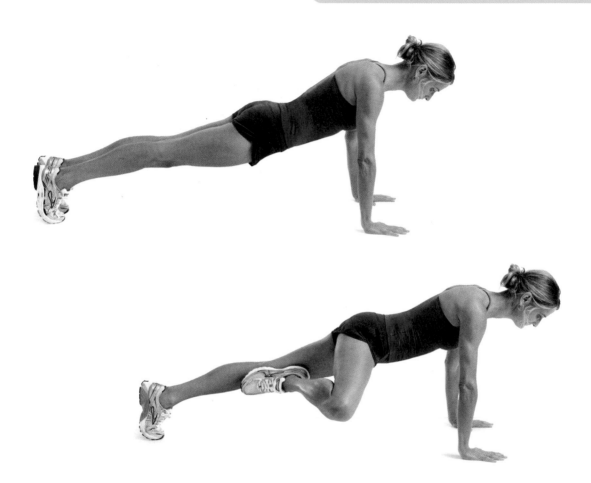

PROCEDURE: From a pushup position, slide your right heel up the inside of your left leg and hold. This is similar to the yoga tree pose, in which you do the same movement standing. Alternate sides.

YOU SHOULD FEEL IT: In your core, lower lumbar region, hip flexors, and shoulders.

5. CIRCLE OUTS

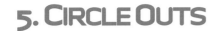

COACHING KEY: Synchronize your breathing with the movement. When the knee comes over, exhale. When it goes under, inhale. This will keep your body stable.

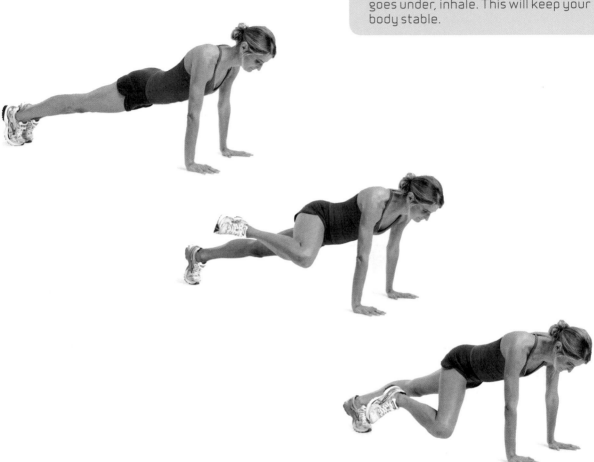

PROCEDURE: From the pushup position, lift your right leg as in the Fire Hydrant movement. Bend your knee and hinge from the hip. Perform circles with your leg. Repeat on the opposite side.

YOU SHOULD FEEL IT: In your hips, lower abs, and lower back.

6. PENDULUMS

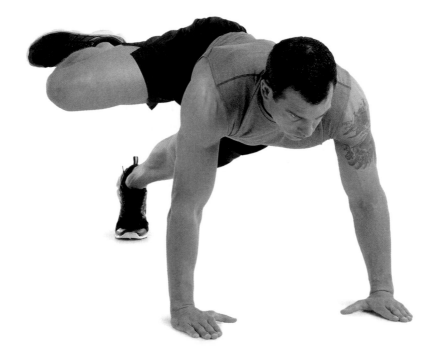

PROCEDURE: From a pushup position, bend your right knee and swing it out to the side, and then back across your body. Repeat on the left side.

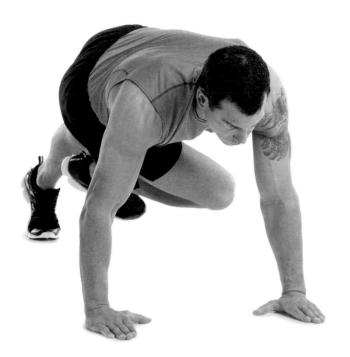

YOU SHOULD FEEL IT: In your hips and groin.

7. Swingouts

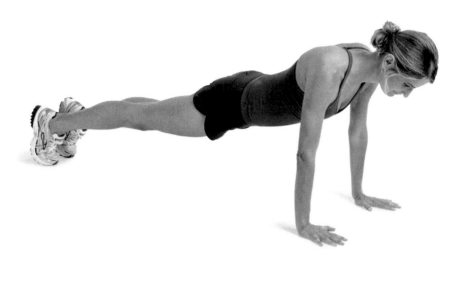

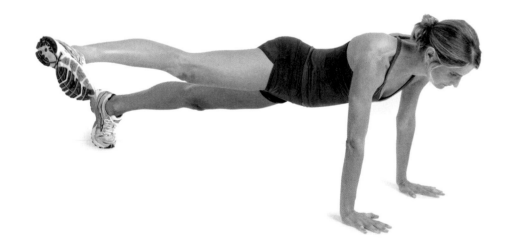

PROCEDURE: From a pushup position, swing your right knee from side to side. Switch and repeat.

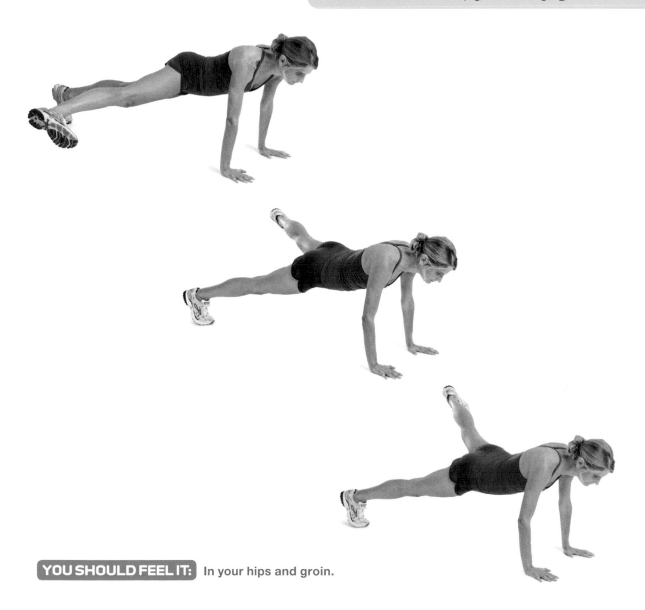

YOU SHOULD FEEL IT: In your hips and groin.

8. HOLD OUT HIGHS

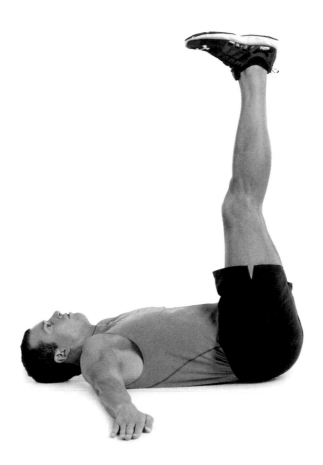

PROCEDURE: Roll onto your back, your arms out to your sides to stabilize your body. Raise your legs straight up in the air and dorsiflex your feet. Push your lower back into the ground. Squeeze your spinal erectors and ab region and "hold out high."

YOU SHOULD FEEL IT: Throughout your core.

9. COOLDOWN
Knee Huggers

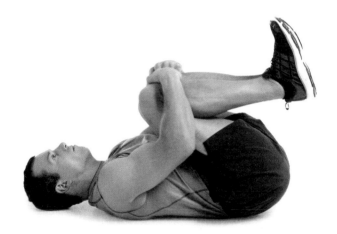

PROCEDURE: Lying flat, simply hug your knees to your chest for 3 seconds.

YOU SHOULD FEEL IT: Throughout your core.

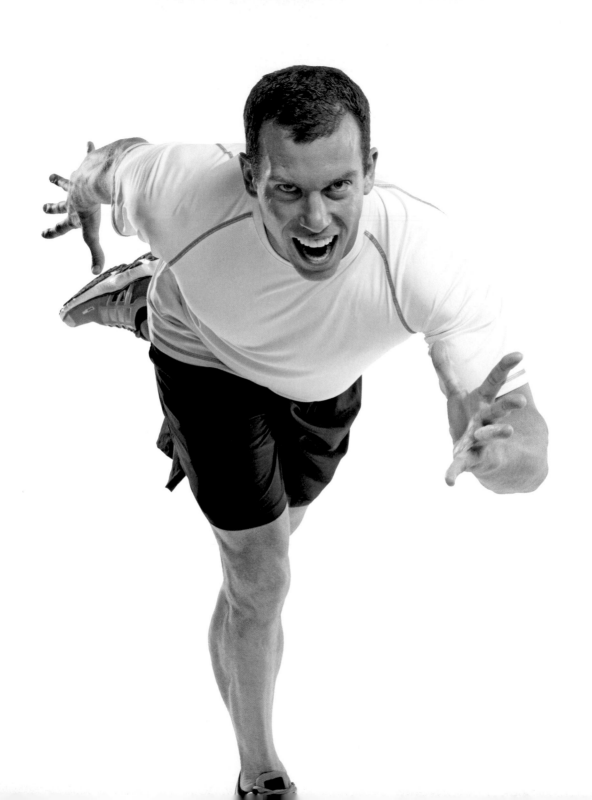

STAYING AT THE TOP OF YOUR GAME

By following Cardio Core 4×4, you'll get in the best shape of your life and have more energy. You'll create strength and stability in your shoulders, midsection, and hips, which will make you more resistant to injuries and long-term deterioration.

In short, you'll be healthier.

But what if I told you there are dozens of little things you can do every day to avoid colds, infections, and other ailments? I get accused of being a germophobe, and I plead guilty. There's nothing worse than coming down with some bug that knocks you out for a few days.

Fortunately, there are many home remedies and nutritional strategies to get you back on your feet. In this section of Fit Tips, we look at how you can avoid sickness and everyday ailments by taking some simple precautions.

We'll take a look first at some easy ways to cut down exposure to germs and bacteria, followed by some simple methods to improve your health using common items you probably already have around your home.

Let's start with lunch. Ladies, your worst lunch date might not be the person sitting across from you. It's your handbag. The bottoms of most handbags carry up to a staggering 10,000 bacteria per square inch, and one-third of bags carry fecal bacteria. Placing your bag on a table might add some icky bacteria to your lunch.

Even your menu can be a health hazard. A study in the *Journal of Medical Virology* reports that flu viruses can last for 18 hours on hard surfaces. Hundreds of people could be passing their germs on to you. Solution? Never let the menu touch the plate or silverware, and wash your hands after you order. To escape the bathroom without touching the door handle, simply palm a paper towel and use it to grab the handle.

You're no better off eating in at the office. Only 44 percent of office refrigerators are cleaned each month, and 22 percent of them

FIT TIP

Having a party? Stay healthy by following these tips: Opt for air kisses when greeting party guests, to avoid common infections such as cold sores; use disposable towels in the bathrooms, as sharing cloth towels with guests can spread germs; and place spoons by serving bowls to avoid guests double-dipping and spreading germs.

are cleaned just once a year. So the next time you're looking for a relatively clean place to store your lunch, consider your office bathroom, which is probably cleaner than the office fridge! (Just kidding.)

The gym also can be a danger zone. Avoid touching your face between sets. Most gym weight equipment is covered with rhinoviruses (instigators of the common cold), human feces, and sweat. That's because many gyms wipe down their equipment only once per day. Also, research has shown that higher bacteria levels are found on weight equipment than on aerobic equipment (73 percent versus 51 percent).

Ever wonder where the most germs reside at the gym? Look to dumbbells and stationary bikes. Sweat splatters on these pieces of equipment and spreads quickly. A particularly nasty one is MRSA, a staph bacteria resistant to some antibiotics. It can survive on surfaces for up to 3 days. So wash your hands and wipe down equipment before and after every workout.

It's amazing how quickly germs can spread. There are more than three million bacteria per square inch inside the average toilet bowl. When you flush, those bad boys get ejected into the air and land on everything—including your toothbrush. Always close the lid before flushing, and store your toothbrush in a drawer.

FIT TIP

Are your lunch cold cuts bad? Skip the sniff test and trash whatever meat you haven't eaten in a week. When you're ready to build your sandwich, slather on the mustard. Researchers at Washington State University killed off 90 percent of three potent pathogens—*Listeria, E. coli,* and salmonella—within 2 hours of exposing them to a mustard compound.

Remember the 5-second rule: Anything from food to the cap of your water bottle that you drop on the floor will be covered with bacteria within 5 seconds.

As for soap, studies have shown that there's absolutely no reason to buy the antibacterial formulation. There is no scientific proof that antibacterial versions are any better at preventing infection than regular soaps, and the antibacterial stuff might make bacteria stronger and more resistant to existing germ killers, which is doing more harm than good.

At least you don't have to worry about the

shower, right? Think again. The showerhead can spray such things as *Mycobacterium avium* and other germs known as nontuberculosis mycobacteria. To end this problem, tie a small plastic bag filled with white vinegar around the showerhead and soak for an hour. This will help kill much of the bacteria, making you feel a lot cleaner.

If you miss out on an annual flu shot, protect yourself the old-fashioned way by washing your hands. A recent study found that people who washed their hands at least five times a day had 45 percent fewer respiratory illnesses such as infection by the flu virus. Even though vaccination might be the best preventive measure, hand washing is a great alternative.

HOME REMEDIES

There's nothing more frustrating than a visit to the doctor. You feel lousy to begin with and then must sit in a waiting room to get a few minutes with a doc who is going to shuffle you out as quickly as possible with a prescription. All of which will be expensive and inconvenient regardless of your health insurance coverage.

Doctors go through medical school with only a few hours of instruction about nutrition. A study published in the *American Journal of Clinical Nutrition* found that only one in six doctors preaches to patients about nutrition's role in preventing disease, while other studies show that just 28 percent of doctors mention exercise. That's why their knee-jerk reaction is to medicate rather than to consider home remedies, many of which can be found in your pantry or refrigerator.

If you're one of the millions of allergy sufferers, try a spoonful of local honey, which comes from the same plants causing the allergic reaction. Taking in a small amount of the allergen works just like a vaccine and will help your immune system build antibodies against it.

Speaking of honey, pour a dab of honey on a cut before covering it with a bandage. Believe it or not, honey has powerful antibacterial properties. A recent study found that it was capable of destroying almost all strains of the most common wound-infecting bacteria.

Your condiments might be just as effective as anything in the medicine cabinet. The next time you nick yourself in the kitchen, reach for the black pepper. Run cold water over the wound to clean it, using soap if you were handling meat. Then sprinkle on the pepper and apply pressure. The bleeding will stop quickly, because black pepper has analgesic, antibacterial, and antiseptic properties. Just don't grab the salt shaker by mistake.

Salt *is* terrific for a sore throat. The mineral pulls excess fluid away from swollen tissues, which reduces inflammation and pain. Recommended dosage is half a teaspoon of salt in 8 ounces of warm water.

Got athlete's foot? Then get some garlic, which has properties that kill the fungus. Take several garlic cloves, crush or mince, and add olive oil. Let the mix sit for 3 days. (You also can buy crushed garlic in a bottle from the supermarket.) Soak your feet in warm water, dry them, and then apply your garlic mix.

Got a cold? Forget echinacea, which became a popular remedy a few years ago. There's no conclusive research proving echinacea to be effective against the common cold. What can you take? Vitamin D. Studies have found that D can stimulate the production of a virus-killing protein, and taking D supplements can lead to fewer viral infections.

If not vitamin D, then how about mushrooms? They contain proteins called cytokines that help the body defend itself against viruses, according to research from Tufts University. Which fungi have these benefits? Ordinary button mushrooms, available at your local supermarket.

Peppermint also can help with a cold. Thank the menthol in peppermint for the plant's ability to clear phlegm and mucus from the bronchial tract to facilitate easy breathing. It's also good for soothing indigestion, gas, menstrual cramps, and irritable bowel syndrome. Take peppermint to the gym as well. When you need a little energy boost before a workout, take a whiff of some peppermint. The scent alters the perception of how hard you're working, making workouts appear less strenuous and easier to complete. Simply chewing on a stick of peppermint gum should do the trick.

Speaking of sweet stuff, next time you get a

FIT TIP

The next time you're stuck with the hiccups, forget holding your breath or drinking tons of water. Instead, take an ice cube to your Adam's apple and rub for a minute. The cold temperature of the ice will interrupt the reflex arc from your brain to your diaphragm, which actually causes hiccups. Voilà! No more hiccups.

mouth ulcer, reach for sugar. Your mother might have told you ulcers are *caused* by sugar, but new research has found that granulated sugar can help cure them too. It does this by keeping wounds bacteria free. Microorganisms that thrive on raw flesh need water to multiply, but applying sugar draws fluid away, so they starve to death. Dab on the sugar twice daily.

To deal with cold sores, mix a crushed aspirin with a drop of water until you have a paste. Apply the aspirin paste to the cold sore and cover with a large bandage. Leave on overnight and repeat this process until the sore disappears. Placing a warm Earl Grey tea bag on the cold sore for 20 minutes also will do the trick. That's because the bergamot oil in Earl Grey tea aids in the healing of cold sores.

For headaches, try olives. Foods rich in healthy fats reduce inflammation, a catalyst for migraines. One study found that the anti-inflammatory compounds in olive oil suppress the same pathway as well as ibuprofen does.

Remember that old adage "Feed a cold and starve a fever"? This folklore dates back centuries and is untrue. Listen to your body instead. If you're hungry, eat a little but not too much. If you have a fever, stay hydrated. Hot and cold beverages can be soothing. Dairy products such as ice cream may thicken phlegm, but they don't increase bodily production of phlegm and may be one of the few things sick children will eat.

A temperature up to 102°F is considered a mild fever and can be treated by drinking plenty of fluids. But to quickly bring down a reading above that, put an ice pack under your arm or near your groin. Icing either spot will cool your body's core. It's uncomfortable, but it works fast. Then see a doctor.

For congestion, brew a steamy beverage or bowl of soup. Hot liquids lubricate the airways and loosen mucus in the chest and sinuses, making it easier to expel.

Have a cough? Consider over-the-counter meds that contain dextromethorphan. It helps raise the cough threshold in the brain so you'll be less sensitive to irritants like postnasal drip.

If you want to treat a cough naturally, keep in mind that theobromine, a chemical in

FIT TIP

Don't store prescription medicine in the bathroom. The constant exposure to light, heat, and humidity can cause it to degrade at a faster rate than it should. Opt instead for a cool linen closet.

chocolate, is as effective at soothing coughs as codeine, a key ingredient in many prescription meds. So choosing chocolate over NyQuil is not a bad idea. Just don't pretend to have a cough to indulge in this tip.

Does going outside with a wet head really cause a cold? Not so. Viruses cause colds, thus you need to be exposed to the cold virus in order to get sick. When someone sneezes or coughs, droplets containing the cold virus escape into the air. If you're close enough to some of these droplets, there's a good chance you'll soon be coming down with a cold.

As for the long-running debate over whether to use heat or ice for swelling: Use *ice* when swelling is present, after an injury occurs, and postworkout. Apply *heat* prior to physical therapy and preworkout to increase bloodflow. The recommendation not to ice beyond 48 hours following an injury is a myth.

SIMPLE LIFESTYLE CHANGES

It's funny how making a few simple lifestyle changes can have a profound effect on your health, productivity, and quality of life. I'm not talking about big-picture stuff such as smoking, alcohol consumption, and nutrition. Instead, making adjustments to routine, everyday aspects of your life can pay huge

dividends over time. It's the real-life benefit of compound interest.

If eyes are the windows to the soul, the mouth is the window to a person's overall health. Just ask a dentist, who with a quick glance down your yap can see not only gum disease but whether you're likely to have cardio-vascular disease and a host of other ailments.

Did you know that brushing with a dry toothbrush cuts tartar by up to 60 percent while reducing the risk of bleeding gums by up to half? Save your money and choose a soft-bristle, generic-brand toothbrush. Brushes with many bells and whistles will not make your teeth any whiter. It all comes down to regular brushing and keeping your gums healthy.

It's tough to get people to floss. Maybe if they knew flossing could improve their sex life, they'd be more motivated. Gum disease is seven times more common in men with erectile dysfunction than men who take care of their teeth and gums. The reason? Bacteria in gum tissue can travel throughout the body, causing inflammation that may damage the blood vessels that cause the penis to expand.

Teeth whitening can be expensive, whether it's done with tray kits for home use or laser treatments at the dentist's office. Why not try strawberries? Crush a strawberry to a pulp and then mix with baking soda until blended. Use a soft toothbrush to spread the mixture onto your teeth. Combined with baking soda, strawberries become a natural tooth cleanser. That's because strawberries contain malic acid, which acts as an astringent to remove surface discoloration.

Toothpaste isn't just for brushing and for patching holes in the wall to get your security deposit back. It's also a remedy for pimples. Apply a dab of it on your finger and spread over the pimple, keeping the paste on overnight. It's unknown which ingredients in toothpaste actually fight acne, but ingredients such as silica derivatives and zinc compounds may be helpful. Also, market brands work better than all-natural ones.

Moving on to the other end of the body, isn't it amazing how much grief our feet can give us? Knowing your foot type can help you choose

the right shoe. Simply wet the bottom of one foot and step on a brown paper bag. Trace over the wet image with a pencil and take it to your local running store. You'll be matched up with the correct fit and enjoy your runs a lot more.

If you're experiencing knee pain, perhaps it's time to check your shoes. To avoid injuries, write an "expiration date" on your shoes as soon as you buy them; 5 months is the ideal time to change shoes. Shoes last about 500 miles, so simply divide 500 by your average weekly mileage to determine how many weeks your shoes are likely to last.

Speaking of shoes, the best time to shop for a new pair of athletic shoes is late in the day. That's when your feet are the largest. Make sure there's a half inch of space in front of your longest toe and that you can easily wiggle your toes. Then slip off the shoes and compare them with your bare feet. If each shoe isn't obviously wider and longer than your foot, go half a size bigger.

As for high heels, they look good on the ladies but cause undue pressure throughout the body. In fact, a 100-pound woman walking in high heels produces 1,500 psi (pounds per square inch) of force. A barefoot 6,000-pound elephant generates just 75 psi.

By following Cardio Core 4×4 program, you'll increase your core strength, which—if you have back problems—should alleviate back pain. Another way to ease your pain, if you're a guy, is to lose the wallet. Sitting on a thick billfold can put pressure on your sciatic nerve, the major nerve running through the buttocks. Make it a point to squeeze your butt muscles when standing in place. You'll force your body into a position that automatically stabilizes your spine, which lowers the risk of back injuries.

Dealing with traffic can be stressful. When you reach your destination, place a cold towel or an ice pack wrapped in a towel on the back of your neck for 10 to 15 minutes. Cold temperatures increase the level of serotonin in the brain, making you feel calmer. Works great after a long day at the office.

Once it's time for bed, slip on some socks. The instant warmup widens blood vessels in your feet, allowing your body to transfer heat from its core to the extremities, cooling you slightly, which induces sleep. Remember: Getting 6 to 8 hours of sleep will help lessen your chances of becoming obese and developing weight-related conditions like type 2 diabetes and hypertension.

FIT TIP

Avoid air fresheners. Many household air fresheners contain phthalates, which have been linked to developmental or sex hormone abnormalities that include decreased testosterone and sperm levels, along with malformed sex organs in infants. Instead, try placing coffee beans, vinegar, or baking soda in a small bowl to help rid your household of everyday odors.

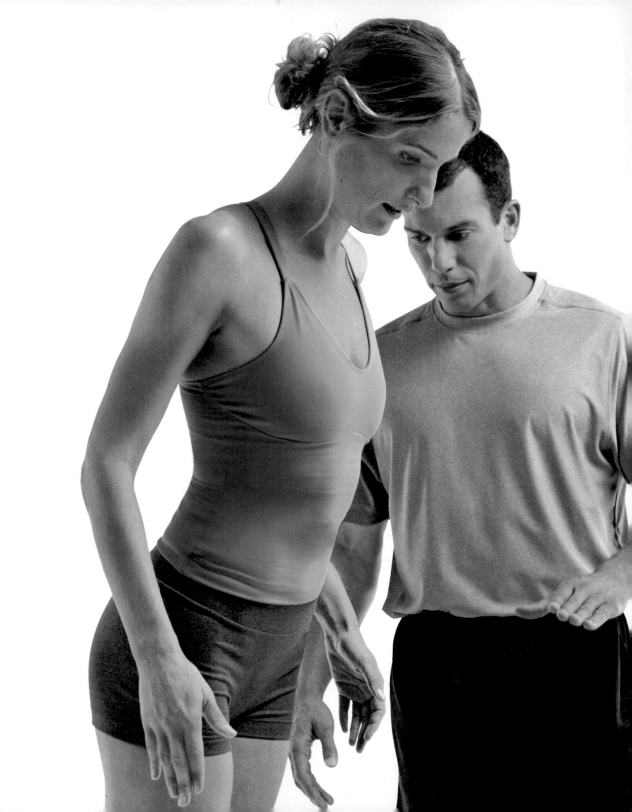

FAQs

Q: Will I gain or lose weight with this program?

A: It depends—and that's a good thing. By following Cardio Core 4×4 and the nutritional component of program, you'll burn fat and add lean muscle. Muscle is more dense than fat; it takes up less space. So even if your weight stays the same, you'll likely look smaller because you'll have more muscle and less fat.

With this program, you're going to ramp up your metabolism. You'll require more calories, and you'll keep your metabolism burning hot by eating five or six small meals a day. As a result, you'll lose fat and gain muscle. Some people might actually gain a few pounds, but most will lose some weight.

How much? That's not important, and you should not get hung up on the number. You can have two men, each 5 foot 10 and 185 pounds, who look dramatically different because of their body composition. One might have 8 percent body fat, the other 25 percent. The same is true of two women who are 5 foot 5, 130 pounds.

Did you know that a number of prominent female athletes make it a point not to divulge their weight? It's not because they're ashamed of it. Actually, they're proud of their rock-solid physiques. They just don't want women who don't exercise to think that they'll look the same carrying, say, 155 pounds on a 5-foot-9 frame.

A woman who trains can pull this off and look lean, even thin. That's not the case with a woman who does not exercise.

Bottom line: By following this program, you'll find that your clothes will fit better or you'll need to purchase smaller ones. When that happens, you won't care if your weight has gone up or down.

Q: Should I weigh myself?

A: If you're someone who checks the scale regularly, continue to do so. It's true that studies show that people who step on the scale on a daily basis avoid gaining weight. That's because they tend to make adjustments accordingly. But don't get hung up on a number. People who do not exercise but follow the losing battle of calories-in, calories-out tend to rely on the scale. You should be more concerned with how your clothes fit and how you look in the mirror.

Q: I've gone through Cardio Core 4×4 program several times. What's next?

A: Congrats! The great thing about Cardio Core 4×4 is that you can continue to add reps as you become more proficient with the program without going over 20 minutes. That way you'll constantly have more workout density and continually challenge yourself further. If that's not enough, try adding more time. I frequently give classes and go as long as 1 hour.

Q: Why does Cardio Core 4×4 not include weights?

A: I'm a big fan of resistance training, and you'll get plenty of it in this program, but that doesn't mean it has to include dumbbells. Cardio Core 4×4 was designed to be excuse-proof. That means it can be done with no equipment, in as little as 20 minutes, and in as little as a 4×4-foot space. You'll be amazed at how much resistance your body can offer.

Q: Won't women get "bulky" doing any kind of resistance training?

A: No. It's nearly physiologically impossible for women to bulk up lifting weights or with any other resistance training. That's because testosterone is responsible for a muscle's bulk, and women simply don't have enough of this predominantly male hormone to build Schwarzenegger-size bulges. Because muscle is denser than fat, strength training actually makes muscles shapelier. So resistance training, either with or without weights, actually produces a leaner, slimmer look.

Q: What's the best time to train?

A: The American Council on Exercise recommends working out between 4:00 and 6:00 p.m., when your body temperature is highest, thus making your workouts more productive. But it's more important to exercise consistently than to focus on a particular time of day. Some people can't get motivated in the morning, and others are too burned out after work. So pick a time of day that works for you. The most important thing is consistency.

Q: Can my kids do this program?

A: Absolutely! Most kids have yet to lose their natural flexibility due to inactivity. This program will build strength, stability, and flexibility.

Q: What should my heart rate be during Cardio Core 4×4?

A: Heart rate monitors are useful tools, and you'll find it telling to monitor your heart rate during this program. On the other hand, people have a tendency to obsess about the numbers. Working out

shouldn't be so complicated. You need to challenge yourself but have fun doing it. You'll burn calories all day long by dancing, getting dressed in the morning, going for a walk, or running with your dog.

Q: What fat-burning zone should I strive to reach?

A: Ignore the fat-burning zone. It's a myth that you must work out for 20 minutes before you begin burning fat. (We're finished in 20 minutes, after all.) The thinking once was that you needed to exercise in a range between 60 and 80 percent of your maximum heart rate. Your body uses more energy at high intensities—just look at the physique of a sprinter. Short, intense intervals will burn more calories and fat in as little as half the time. This program is all about short, intense intervals.

Q: Is it true that muscle will turn to fat when you stop working out?

A: Not so. Fat and muscle are two different substances, and one cannot turn into the other. Less of one simply means more room for the other. When you stop using your muscles, your body becomes significantly less efficient at burning calories, which allows the pounds, in the form of fat, to creep back on.

Q: How quickly will I see results?

A: The magic number in the industry is 20, as in 20 days into a program before you see noticeable gains. A 9 percent decrease in body fat after 12 weeks of any resistance training program can be expected. (No wonder many fitness videos promise fat loss within a 12-week period.) You'll begin to feel better from your first Cardio Core 4×4 workout, but by the end of 20 days, you should notice dramatic changes, assuming you've adapted a healthy nutrition program to match your dedication to the workout.

Q: What kind of music should I listen to during the 4×4?

A: Whatever music gets your blood pumping. But by the same token, being subjected to the wrong music could put a downer on your performance. Researchers found that the blood vessels of exercisers who were subjected to music they didn't like constricted 6 percent in just 30 minutes, reducing overall aerobic capacity by more than 10 percent. When exercisers listened to favorable music, their blood vessels expanded 26 percent, bringing in a 34 percent performance boost.

AFTERWORD

I hope you'll use Cardio Core 4x4 as the foundation of your success, not just for the next 40 days but for the rest of your life. Each day, be sure to revisit those goals you set for yourself in Chapter One. Place them on your mirror for daily inspiration.

The great thing about Cardio Core 4x4 workout is that you can continue to progress by adding additional reps as you become more proficient. Be on the lookout for JCORE DVD series, which will coincide with the release of this book.

I take great pride in helping prominent people succeed, but I'm just as proud of the folks I work with who are not household names. That's why I hope you'll share with me your success stories from using this program at www.cardiellofitness.com.

I look forward to hearing from you.

JAY CARDIELLO

ACKNOWLEDGMENTS

To offer the words *thank you* to the following individuals is so small compared to how honored I am to have each of them in my life.

First and foremost, to my wife, Paula, thank you for all your patience and understanding throughout this long process. Since the day we met, you have recognized my dream of helping people and have provided me with such confidence in making that dream a reality.

I cannot begin to express how thankful I am to all my friends and family, especially Stephan Hankin, Michael Baccaro, Mr. McBride, Gunner Peterson, and Peggy Lucas. You have shown the kind of love and support that one can only dream of having. Thank you for never giving up on me.

To my collaborator, Pete Williams, I hold myself forever in your debt. You are a man of passion, and I truly do not know how many Skype hours we spent working on this book, but we did it. We made it happen! And I say "we," for this would not have been possible without you.

David Larabell is a literary agent that any writer dreams of having. From our first meeting, you expressed to me that this book could forever impact fitness and create more than just a lifestyle change. Also, that this book would instill in people a greater sense of confidence in their capabilities. David, you were right!

Marc Guss and Richard Charnoff of Alpha Entertainment, you put together a great team. I am forever thankful for this opportunity.

To the entire team at Rodale, thank you for providing me with this opportunity and for your ability to see that this was not just an idea but a vehicle to change people's lives. Thanks to Shannon Welch for overseeing this project, while providing both Pete and me with a positive structure that ultimately made the difference in reaching our goals. Thanks also to Marie Crousillat, Chris Rhoads, and Nancy Bailey at Rodale! It was truly an honor to work with and be a part of such an amazing company. Thank you, Rodale.

Courtney O'Neill, you are more than just a publicist. You are a friend. I can truly state that neither my career nor this book would have happened without you. I am so thankful to have you a part of my life. I look forward to a long career together with you.

Lastly, to all of you whom I have had the honor of calling clients: You have made me who I am today and have taught me so many lessons of patience, forgiveness, and ability to see past aesthetics. I love each and every one of you. Thank you again for your trust.

ABOUT THE AUTHORS

JAY CARDIELLO, CSCS, is best known as the trainer for many prominent entertainers along with Fortune 500 executives and prominent Wall Street figures such as Meredith Whitney. Working with such time-crunched celebrities, often in movie trailers and other confined spaces with little or no gym equipment, Cardiello developed Cardio Core 4×4 routine, a full-body workout that provides the benefits of strength training, endurance work, yoga, and even martial arts training in one efficient 20-minute program.

Dubbed "Jay Cardio" by 50 Cent, with whom he lived and traveled for 4 years, Cardiello was a childhood martial arts champion growing up in northern New Jersey. He overcame a learning disability and 580 SAT scores to graduate with honors from the College of William & Mary. While previously enrolled at the University of Arkansas, he had suffered a devastating fall while competing in track and field. That ended his athletic pursuits but launched a coaching career while he was still an undergraduate at William & Mary, where he led the track and field team to

its first female national championship in the triple jump.

Always driven to overcome long odds and adversity, Cardiello in college wrote letters to every professional sports team, which led to a series of valuable (if low-paying) gigs in the NFL, XFL, Arena Football League, Major League Baseball, and UFC. At a career crossroads, he moved to Manhattan and took a position at the elite Clay Fitness. There he launched "NFL Training Camp," which led to coverage by CBS and the *New York Times*. While at Clay, he was hired to train several prominent boxers, eventually attracting the attention of 50 Cent.

While working with Cardiello, the hardworking rapper and actor developed a powerful, chiseled physique that caught the attention of other celebrities and the media. Cardiello has appeared in numerous television programs, including *The Real Housewives of New York* and 50 Cent's own *The Money and the Power.* He is regularly featured in media outlets such as the *New York Times, Elle, Details, InStyle,* Forbes.com, *Men's Fitness,*

EXTRA, BET, MTV, and Martha Stewart's Sirius satellite radio program. He is also the fitness editor-at-large for *Shape* magazine.

Cardiello and his wife live in New York's SoHo neighborhood, where he continues to train film and music stars, Wall Street financiers, and Fortune 500 executives.

PETE WILLIAMS is the author or coauthor of numerous books, including Mark Verstegen's *Core Performance* (Rodale, 2004), which popularized core training and led to four additional *Core Performance* titles, and Brody Welte's *Paddle Fit* (Vook, 2011), a fitness regimen centered on stand-up paddleboarding. Williams began his career as a *USA Today* sportswriter covering Major League Baseball, and his books include Mike Veeck's business motivational book *Fun Is Good* (Rodale, 2005) and his own *The Draft: A Year Inside the NFL's Search for Talent*. His work has appeared in the *New York Times*, *SportsBusiness Journal*, *Washington Post*, *Men's Health*, *Triathlon Life*, and *Competitor*. An avid triathlete, he's the creator of EnduranceSportsFlorida.com and the host of the Fitness Buff Show, an online radio program focusing on training and high-performance living. A graduate of the University of Virginia, Williams lives in Florida with his wife and their two sons. His Web site is www.petewilliams.net.

INDEX

Underscored page references indicate boxed text. **Boldface** references indicate photographs.

Crosscurrents / MODERN CRITIQUES

Harry T. Moore, *General Editor*

The Modern Italian Novel
FROM PEA TO MORAVIA

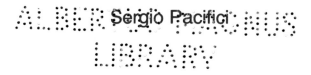

Sergio Pacifici

WITH A PREFACE BY

Harry T. Moore

SOUTHERN ILLINOIS UNIVERSITY PRESS
Carbondale and Edwardsville

FEFFER & SIMONS, INC.
London and Amsterdam

For Zee
"sweetiepie"
with much love
and thanks
for all the
new memories

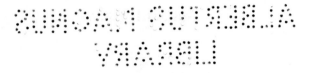

Library of Congress Cataloging in Publication Data (Revised)

Pacifici, Sergio.
  The modern Italian novel.

  (Crosscurrents: modern critiques)
  Includes bibliographies.
  CONTENTS: [1] From Manzoni to Svevo.—[2] From Capuana to
Tozzi.—[3] From Pea to Moravia.
  1. Italian fiction—19th century—History and criticism. 2. Italian
fiction—20th century—History and criticism.
PQ4173.P3   853'.03   67-13047
ISBN 0-8093-0873-8

Contents

Preface

Since its beginning in 1962, the Crosscurrents/Modern Critiques series has published more than one hundred volumes. Some of these have been written by already established critics, but we have been proud to present also the first books of younger writers. Some of our authors have even written three volumes for us (David Madden, Irving Malin, Siegfried Mandel), and now we present another of these authors to give us a third book, his conclusion of a triology on the modern Italian novel.

Its author is Sergio Pacifici who is Professor of Italian at Queens College of the City University of New York. His monumental work is unique in English presentations of twentieth-century Italian writers, above all for its admirable range; and within that it combines important information with expert evaluation. One of the book's achievements is its Selected Bibliography, which not only contains a full list of recent works on Italian literature, but presents useful critical commentary on these books.

The body of Dr. Pacifici's own book concerns such significant novelists as Cesare Pavese and Alberto Moravia, as well as others of great interest and importance. As already indicated, the material is helpfully factual, but it is never pedantically so. The necessary information is provided as essential background to the understanding of the authors in question.

Dr. Pacifici frequently uses synopsis, but not in such a way as to make his book a merely convenient "trot" or "pony." Rather, this author uses synopses to present a critical point of view, for he is highly selective in what he chooses to offer, and his selection of incidents in any story is based upon a need for critical exposition. This is seen most clearly in his discussion of a novel by Gadda, in which he demonstrates the necessity of a synoptic approach in a very necessary critical examination.

This is the kind of book which in its skillful treatment of all phases of its subject will be illuminating to those approaching the modern Italian novel for the first time; and this study, with its fresh insights and expert conclusions, will be helpful even to those already familiar with much of the material. At more than one level, then, Professor Pacifici's book is an exceedingly useful one.

HARRY T. MOORE

Southern Illinois University
October 9, 1978

Introduction

The present volume is the third and last and what was originally conceived as a one, then a two-volume study of the modern Italian novel. A realization that the abundance of the material would simply preclude the achievement of my objective led me to expand this project to three volumes. I am deeply indebted to Vernon Sternberg, Director of the Southern Illinois University Press, and Harry T. Moore, Editor of the Crosscurrents series, for supporting my decision.

The aims of this introductory study are simply to correct, modify and otherwise extend present knowledge of the Italian novel in English-speaking countries; to try to answer, insofar as possible, certain basic questions students inevitably ask in connection with the novel in Italy: Who are the enduring novelists that country has produced over the past century or so? In what ways did they improve the native tradition of the genre? In what specific manner can we read such works as reflections of the vast social, political, and economic changes undergone by the nation? What insights into the human predicament do they offer to the reader of today, and how significant and relevant are such insights?

This book hardly claims to offer any final answers to these and other questions. It does propose, however, to prepare the initiate to begin grappling with them, and, by providing him with a certain amount of factual information and interpretative comments, it hopes to enable him to begin formulating independent, if tentative, judgments.

The scheme of this volume, like the two that preceded it, is simple. I have chosen a number of writers whose work seemed to be particularly apt to illustrate the development of the novel in modern Italy. Rather than attempting to study their entire literary production, I have generally limited myself to considering only the book or books that are most persuasively indicative of their vision as well as of the thematic, stylistic, and structural innovations they brought to the genre. Within the limitations of space, I have also touched briefly on those important biographical and cultural events of my subjects when, by so doing, the meaning and significance of their work could be illuminated further. No detailed study of the selected number of writers included in this book has been attempted, and only three of them, for reasons which I trust my analyses will make clear, receive major treatment. The English translations of titles mentioned are given in brackets after the Italian titles. If the work has been published in an English translation the English title and publishing information appear in parentheses.

This book begins with Enrico Pea and ends with Alberto Moravia. With the exception of Moravia, the writers discussed here are no longer living.

I think it is only reasonable to point out that this history is in essence a sort of "Reader's Guide" to the Modern Italian Novel: being the first to appear in English in almost a half a century, it cannot claim to be an exhaustive nor, much less, a definitive account of its subject. There are omissions of names and facts; no doubt, some of my informed readers will want to challenge my selection, which has been at once critical and personal. Nevertheless, choices, difficult and troubling as they are, must be made. I offer no apologies for the writers left out other than to say that, even taking into account the nature of the present survey, I have rejected the alternative of presenting a *catalogue raisonné* of names and facts for a somewhat more detailed presentation of fewer novelists. Those readers wishing to extend their knowledge of the field will find the bibliographical references particularly helpful. They include the most lucid and penetrating studies that have appeared in Italy (many of them quite recently), as well as some of the best material in English—material, I regret to say, often overlooked by Italian scholars.

My analyses are based upon a reading of the works in the original. In order to make the text easier to read, I have generally quoted from the standard English translations listed in each chapter. In all other cases, the translations are mine.

It is my sincere hope that this volume will begin filling a regrettable lacuna in Italian studies and that it will contribute to a firmer understanding of, and discussion about the novel. If it achieves its aim, the effort that went in to writing it will prove to have been fully justified. I should feel doubly rewarded, however, if it will also stimulate others to restudy the relatively unexplored problems of the modern novel in Italy and offer fresh interpretations of its quality and achievement.

I should like to acknowledge with deep gratitude the help and assistance of the staffs of the Paul Klapper Library of Queens College, the Yale University Sterling Memorial Library, and of the Italian Cultural Institute of New York, and in particular Mrs. Mimi Penchasky, Mr. Harry P. Harrison, and Mrs. Maria Anita Gargotta. I am thankful to all those colleagues who, privately or in their reviews, offered suggestions for improving this study, and the many others who generously sent me offprints of their publications on my subjects. I owe a special debt to Mrs. Cecilia T. D'Agostino and the professional staff of the Word Processing Center of Queens College, for the skill with which they prepared the final manuscript copy of this book, and to Ms. Josiane Hayat for helping prepare the Index.

Parts of chapters 8 and 9, on Vittorini and Moravia, originally appeared in my previous volume, *A Guide to Contemporary Italian Literature: From Futurism to Neorealism* (Carbondale: Southern Illinois University Press, 1972), and are reprinted here with kind permission of the publisher.

SERGIO PACIFICI

Riverdale, New York
June 26, 1978

The Modern Italian Novel

FROM PEA TO MORAVIA

1

Background of the Modern Italian Novel

The twentieth century opened in Italy on several uncertain, if
not ominous notes. The enthusiasm for national unification had
spent itself, and a profound disillusionment vis-à-vis the possibility of creating a truly united Italy pervaded the work of Federico
De Roberto and Luigi Pirandello. Veristic fiction, whose best
practitioners had been Luigi Capuana, Giovanni Verga, and
Grazia Deledda, among others, was on the wane. The rhetoric
of Carducci, Pascoli, and d'Annunzio (the poets of "the third
Italy," as Benedetto Croce called them), with their nationalism
and narcissism, gave way first to the Futurists, headed by Filippo
T. Marinetti, with their faith in a machine society and a resolve
to make a *tabula rasa* of all traditional values, and then the "Crepuscolari" (the poets of "the Twilight") who focused on the dull,
gray, dispirited life in the provinces. On the political front, Italy
was undergoing her first, most difficult phase as a member of the
European community of nations governed by parliamentary rule.
The moderately progressive policies of men like Giuseppe Zanar-
delli and Giovanni Giolitti, who served as prime ministers before
1914, were instrumental in making possible certain basic social
reforms coupled with a promising democratization of the country's bureaucratic structure. The fragility of the fiber of social and
political institutions was to become apparent throughout the
chain of events that led to a world-wide war. In 1914, Europe,
and at a later stage Asia, found themselves entangled in a conflict
which involved the most powerful nations (England, France, the
Austro-Hungarian Empire, Germany, Russia, China, and Japan), and, some months later, the United States, as well as the
weaker countries, such as Belgium, Holland, and Italy.

Italy found herself in a puzzling, almost bizarre situation: having signed a pact (called the Triple Alliance) in 1882 with Germany and the Austro-Hungarian Empire, she was technically allied with her traditional archenemies. Thus, from August 1914 until May 23, 1915, Italy resisted the pressure from both the Right and the Left, which clamored for abstention or intervention for moral, practical, or political reasons. Finally, on May 24, 1915, Italy entered the conflict on the side of the Allies (which, we may note, had in the past shown little interest in Italy's struggle to achieve unification and freedom from Austrian, French, and Spanish rule), after receiving assurances that her claims to certain territories bordering on Austria and what is today Jugoslavia, as well as her demands of colonial land, would receive sympathetic consideration at the peace table.

When the war was finally over, three years later, the Great War, the Good War, or, more simply, World War I as it was eventually called, left its imprint everywhere: millions of lives had been lost, several million people wounded, billions of dollars of property, public and private, lost, destroyed, or severely damaged. The peace conference held at Versailles, and the treaty it produced after months of intense negotiations, turned out to be not much more than a document that redesigned the map of Europe, Africa, and Asia, and which all but guaranteed a bitterness and a discontent that would inevitably lead to another world war.

World War I left the whole world shattered and shocked: Italy, considerably economically weaker than most other European countries, found herself spiritually and psychologically devastated. Confusion, uncertainty, restlessness, and discontent intensified daily and, as a result, the already precarious political situation deteriorated visibly; faith in the democratic process came under a period of strain that would, but a few years later, lead to its rejection. Inflation, unemployment, workers' agitations, the increasing number of strikes, the strengthening of the Socialist party, posed grave threats to the world of industries, banks, and the middle class. The elections of November 1919 showed a clear movement of the electorate toward the Left, with the Socialists increasing their representation in the House of Deputies by 100 percent (from 78 to 156 seats), mostly at the expense of the right-of-center Liberal party. Even though the internal situation had stabilized by 1920, increasing concern with the dangers posed by the Socialists and the newly founded Communist party resulted in a fragmentation of political power, further weakening the government and making possible the meteoric rise of a party led by one Benito Mussolini, an ambitious politician whose positions tended to change regularly, according to the pressures and the shifting winds of public sentiment—a pattern that was to mark his career until his tragic demise in 1945. From a leftist, noninterventionist socialism, reluctant to see his country at war, he led his followers down the path leading to intervention, a switch that cost him expulsion from the Socialist party. This, of course, did in no way dismay the young leader, who seemed to have read and mastered rather well Machiavelli's political theories, accepting the conclusion that politics entails sleeping with strange bedfellows, and that the means, or any practical means, justifies the end.

Mussolini's rise to power might never have taken place had it not been for the shocking way in which Italy was treated at the peace conference at Versailles that proved to be the proverbial straw that broke the camel's back. Territorial claims (and, specifically, the annexation of the small city of Fiume, near Trieste) were rejected out of hand by the British and American delegations, on the pretext that they had not been discussed prior to Italy's entrance in the war, a stance that angered the Italians to the point of withdrawing from the conference in the spring of 1919. When they returned, after some stormy changes in political leadership, the more substantial question of the distribution of German colonies in Africa had already been decided, and Italy was left empty-handed.

The frustrations and irritations of the peace conference fueled the general dissatisfaction with the way in which Italy was governed, and particularly the widespread resentment toward the anti-imperialist policies of the Giolitti government, moving a large segment of the electorate toward such a nationalist party as Mussolini's Fascists. The strong tactics adopted by the Fascists —who resorted to the stick, castor oil, and murder to intimidate the opposition parties of the center and the left—created a situation of civil war, with violence escalating daily, and with no peace in sight. On October 28, 1922, after having systematically harassed leftist municipal administrations, and exploiting the indecisiveness of the cabinet headed by Giolitti, Mussolini decided to "seize" the government. Together with a squad of Fascists, several thousand men strong, he marched on Rome, offering King Victor Emanuel III, a weak and confused monarch, a "united Italy." Visibly impressed by the strength of the Fascists, the king asked Mussolini to form a new government.

Between 1925 and 1926, through series of "reforms" that were to continue until the outbreak of World War II, the structure of the state was radically changed, and the bureaucratic machinery dramatically overhauled to assure absolute, total control of power. All meaningful positions were assigned to faithful party loyalists who were responsible to the Duce himself, who in turn was accountable only to the king. Elections were abolished, replaced by plebiscites that were meaningless, since only the yes ballots were counted, the function of Parliament substantially downgraded (and eventually completely abolished by the Grand Council in 1938), local self-government abolished, freedom of the press greatly curtailed and finally eliminated, and the independence and integrity of the courts damaged beyond repair. A secret police, ostensibly created to protect the government, was turned into a repressive instrument with wide powers to strike down any "subversive" (read: "independent") element. The new corporate state, as it began to emerge in the late 1920s, was one where strikes were forbidden, disputes between employers and employees settled by special courts, and both sides were compelled to join government associations. Government "participation" in industries, both heavy and light, increased substantially. By 1931, through two holding companies, the government gained control of the banks.

The humiliation inflicted on Italy at Versailles was not easily forgotten, much less forgiven. "The Allies," as Massimo Salvatori remarked, "were accused of having deprived Italy of her legitimate fruits of the victory." As a consequence, much of Mussolini's foreign policy was fashioned in a way to lend support to all nationalistic movements (in Hungary, Austria, Bulgaria, Germany, and Spain), and was instrumental in helping Hitler and Franco achieve power in Germany and Spain respectively. The same policy led to the declaration of war against Ethiopia in 1935–36, the withdrawal from the League of Nations in 1937, and the signing of the so-called Pact of Steel with Germany and, later on, with Japan.

Fascism had come to power with violence, and violence, of

one kind or another, was what kept it in power. Harassing, beating, intimidating, jailing, and, whenever opportune, murdering political antagonists (Giacomo Matteotti, the Roselli brothers, Pietro Gobetti, and Antonio Gramsci, the founder of the Communist party in Italy, were the first of what would be a long list of victims) became regular practice. The voices of other distinguished political and academic personalities were silenced in other ways: Carlo Sforza, Gaetano Salvemini, Palmiro Togliatti, Giuseppe A. Borgese, and Ignazio Silone were forced to flee from their native country and seek political asylum in France, Switzerland, Russia, and the United States. Numerous other writers (Cesare Pavese, Carlo Levi, Corrado Alvaro) were sentenced to the "confino politico" ("political surveillance") in small, godforsaken villages of southern Italy. Other intellectuals (Alberto Moravia) were not permitted to sign their articles, or, as in the case of the future Nobel laureate Eugenio Montale, lost their jobs when they failed to request their membership card in the party. The losses to Italian culture did not stop here: Maestro Arturo Toscanini, who had been a sympathizer of fascism in its early stages, was beaten up by a gang of Fascist hoodlums angry at his refusal to play the Fascist hymn, "Giovinezza, giovinezza!" and left Italy in 1931; Enrico Fermi, an outstanding young physicist, married to a Jewess, left with his wife to travel to Stockholm to accept his Nobel Prize, and emigrated to the United States where he was to do important work on the atomic bomb.

What role did fascism play in the development of a culture consonant with its ideology and political aspirations? And how did it affect the quality of literature? The answer to both questions is negative: unlike other political ideologies, particularly socialism and communism, fascism counted on a very limited number of intellectuals to articulate its ideological and philosophical position. Indeed, aside from Giovanni Gentile (1875–1944), who introduced his special concepts of education, pedagogy, and philosophy through his reforms of the schools, no influential intellect dominated the scene. Similarly, and at least for several of its early years, fascism lacked a clear policy vis-à-vis the creative arts, although it favored certain styles in architecture and painting, and was partial to certain musical composers, such as Pietro Mascagni. Yet, with the passing of time, its edicts and position papers had an inhibiting effect upon writers: for example, the government did not look favorably on, and eventually banned, the treatment of suicide as well as other criminal acts that in any way cast an unfavorable light upon, or otherwise suggested that the spiritual, moral, and social health of the Italian people and their government was anything less than admirably perfect.

Despite his deep mistrust of intellectuals, Mussolini frequently succeeded in attracting if not their allegiance at least their passive acceptance through a variety of rewards and special benefits. Aside from the usual number of patronage positions in the Ministry of Education, and in the schools and universities over which it had jurisdiction, there was also the newly (1929) revamped Royal Academy of Italy, partially financed by private industries, and modelled on its French counterpart, founded by Cardinal Richelieu in the seventeenth century. Presided over by Giovanni Gentile, the official philosopher of the party, its members rated the title Your Excellency, a free, first-class travel pass, a prestigious-looking uniform, complete with decorative sash, sword, and impressive plumed hat, and a 3,000 lire monthly stipend. Luigi Pirandello, Alfredo Panzini, Gabriele d'Annunzio, Filippo Tommaso Marinetti, the scientist Gugliemo Marconi, the historian G. Volpe, and the musician Pietro Mascagni were among the first to be elected to the academy, conceived "for the purpose of preserving our intellectual life in its national character according to the genius and the tradition of the [Italian] race, and also to favor its expansion abroad." In addition, party members with proper credentials (and some without) could count on a positive examination and review of their applications for one of the posts in the many research and study groups that came under the umbrella of the National Institute of Culture, which included the Treccani Institute which produced an excellent encyclopedia, remarkably free of political ideology, and the film group L.U.C.E. Finally, there were also grants and subsidies for repertory companies (such as the one organized and directed by Luigi Pirandello), film projects, trips abroad, and special pleasant assignments. These and other advantages, however, did not come without a price tag: by 1931, the cost of pursuing one's vocation as a teacher, for example, required signing a loyalty oath to the king and the party, something which a few brave intellectuals refused to do since they perceived it as an intolerable abridgment of their right to speak their mind and dissent, when appropriate, from the gospel of

Mussolini and his bureaucracy. Fascism, as the historian Edward T. Tannenbaum confirms in his study of *The Fascist Experience*, "produced no original high culture of its own and had little influence on the main literary and artistic trends of the period." Whatever influence it did have was largely negative, preventing and restraining freedom of thought and expression.

It is fair to note here that naïveté, idealism, misinterpretation, or temporary inability to perceive the true nature of fascism led many a young writer to believe for a while that the movement born of a revolution sui generis was serious in its promises of social and economic reforms, and support its cause for nationalistic reasons and out of a growing impatience and dissatisfaction with the policies the Great Powers (especially England and France) followed vis-à-vis Italy. Vasco Pratolini, Elio Vittorini, Vitaliano Brancati, Alfonso Gatto, and numerous other writers who belonged to the left wing of the party, eventually understood the true nature of fascism, its shabby morality, its bombastic claims, its warmongering policies and its fraudulent schemes, and quit the party. Some of them became more and more active as critics of fascism and joined the Underground shortly after Italy's declaration of war against her former ally, Germany, in 1943. Yet, these defections proved to be the exception, not the rule. An analysis of what Enrico Falqui dubbed, without aspersion, "the black twenty years," leads us to agree with the stark conclusion reached by Fabrizio Onofri's question: "Must we condemn in toto art, literature, Italian culture of the Fascist twenty years?" The answer was: "From a broad historical point of view, the answer cannot be uncertain: Art, literature, Italian culture did nothing to oppose Fascism."

The quality, trends, and eventual achievements of Italian letters during fascism were profoundly influenced by the work done by some of the reviews, or "little magazines," which had flourished before and after World War I. Two of them, *La voce* (1908–16), edited first by Giuseppe Prezzolini and then by Giuseppe De Robertis, and *La Ronda* (1919–22), proved to be trend-setters. The first had worked hard to introduce European poetry, philosophy, and culture to what was still a parochial public. The second, with its "call to order," by which was meant a return to the classical limpidness of the masters of Italian poetry, Petrarch, Ariosto, Leopardi, and Manzoni, proposed a program of respect and respectability in literature and, by extension, in politics. In the words of the historian of literature, Natalino Sapegno, "*The Rondisti* [were] opposed to indiscriminate enthusiasm, the distinction and the sense of measure; [they were opposed] to impotent ambition, humility, and the exigencies of the craft; they concentrate their attention on the literary fact itself, in its formal meaning, as a restoration of technical values—grammatical and stylistic. They denied the myth of sincerity, of immediacy, insisting on the importance of the reflected and conscious elements of artistic elaboration; they looked with difference upon the contamination [of art] with morality and philosophy, pointing out precisely the concept of literature as a disinterested exercise and an absolute reflection of any content in terms of style."

The whole thrust of *La Ronda* was toward the *belle page*, the exquisitely written essay, the highly controlled "*elzeviro*," a sort of commissioned piece, fiction, criticism, or cultural report that appears in the "third page" of Italian newspapers. By contrast, 900 (or Twentieth century), directed by a gifted playwright and novelist, Massimo Bontempelli, for three brief years (1926–29) attempted to widen the points of contact between Italy and continental literature by, among other things, publishing its material in French, then the accepted language of diplomacy and culture. It is at least a proof of its daring and sensitivity that Alberto Moravia was first published, with an excellent short story, in the first issue of 900. Bontempelli's efforts proved to be short-lived, however, and with the demise of his review, the focus turned again not to the *città* (the city as symbol of urbane culture) but to the *paese* (or the rural town, as symbol of a national, and hence provincial, narrow culture), directions that took the form of two respective trends, "*Stracittà*" and "*Strapaese*" a kind of Italian "America, love it or leave it" point of view. *Il selvaggio* (literally Savage, or Primitive), published between 1924 and 1943, edited by a journalist-novelist, Curzio Malaparte (who, in the final months of the war, turned Communist and became a Maoist before his death in 1957), assisted by the poet-painter Ardengo Soffici, and the painters Mino Maccari and Ottone Rosai, served as a kind of bastion for all those who felt threatened by any corruptive influence on the healthy, admirable, genuine native tradition, even if such threats came from Fascist Rome.

Balancing the narrow cultural parameters of *Il selvaggio* was the Florentine review *Solaria* (1926–37), which, throughout its publishing history, dedicated itself to introducing in Italy some of the finest and most talented Continental and American writers. The roster of such artists is long and distinguished, and includes Marcel Proust, Paul Valéry, T. S. Eliot, James Joyce, Thomas Mann, Franz Kafka, as well as the Italians, among whom were Umberto Saba, Eugenio Montale, Giuseppe Ungaretti, and Elio Vittorini. As the founder of the review was to write, long after *Solaria* had ceased publication, "[*Solaria*] was anti-Fascist one might almost say because it was not fascist. . . . It was a review whose cultural tendencies found themselves in disagreement with official tendencies. . . . One might almost say that *Solaria* formed an island of cultural resistance, were it not for the precise historical meaning such a term has acquired today."

Financial pressure forced the closing down of *Solaria*. One year later (1938), another review, *Letteratura*, also located in Florence, brought out its first issue. For several years, until 1947, when numerous difficulties forced it to suspend publication, the magazine literally kept cultured readers in touch with some of the best, most innovative, and interesting writing being published in the free world, much as *Solaria* had done during its own publication history.

In the early twenties, just as the novel was experiencing a rebirth of interest, the debate about the genre was sparked anew by a confrontation between Ugo Ojetti, a journalist and literary critic, and Giovanni Papini, a self-taught man who was to leave his mark on literature for his fiery *"stroncature"* and his autobiographical *Un uomo finito* (1912; *The Failure*, N.Y., 1924). Papini took the position that, for reasons having to do with their cultural tradition, training and general dispositions, Italians were better suited to write poetry, essays, and biographies rather than novels. It is yet another irony in the history of the genre that such polemics should take place just as the novel, thanks to such writers as Tozzi, Borgese, Pirandello, and Svevo, among others, was beginning to experience its first success in Italy.

Meanwhile, general cultural conditions were transforming national life into something at last homogeneous and cohesive. Education was slowly making possible the teaching of a national language, thus breaking down the obstacles posed by the local dialects. Compulsory education, however slowly its provisions were enacted and enforced, began making dramatic progress in reducing the appallingly high percentage of illiteracy that had plagued the nation for centuries and which had slowed down considerably the mobility of young adults in their upward climb. New publishing houses, such as Mondadori, of Milan, were founded; new newspapers started, and new opportunities were offered to writers by the possibility of their contributing to the "third page" (or cultural section) of such dailies.

The advent of fascism, with its negative presence on the creative scene, discouraged the psychological type of narrative, while indirectly encouraging less taxing and controversial writing. As practiced by such artists as Pea and Palazzeschi, this type of novel relies heavily on purely autobiographical or fablelike material, to produce a work that is in general mildly critical of middle class values and standards. Stylistically and thematically conservative, its mission is still to amuse its readers, and for precisely this reason, coupled with a benign neglect of moral and social issues, it was found to be perfectly acceptable by the regime. Besides, as Moravia remarked in a recent interview granted to Federico Camon, "Fascism was so accustomed to such a depressed, stifling atmosphere that it attached no importance to literature, which it considered a bizarre, decorative, and innocuous activity, especially because of its century-old (at least in Italy) incapacity to have any influence whatever on society." Such a surprisingly detached attitude came to an end. Beginning in the early thirties, government supervision of anything printed grew relentlessly: anyone who published material thought to be even indirectly critical of life in Mussolini's Italy (including Moravia himself), found himself in great difficulties if not downright danger.

The undisputed masters of the novel in Italy in the first quarter of this century had been Italo Svevo, Luigi Pirandello, and Federigo Tozzi. The first dug into the subconscious and, through a subtle blend of irony and humor, poked fun at human foibles; the second conveyed, through an effective depiction of man searching for his true identity, the sense of the necessity of illusions (or masks) to shelter himself from the pain of living; the third revealed the tragedy of man's incommunicability through the torment of the father-son relationship. All three were restless artists, writers who were deeply aware of the changes in values, mood, and concepts of life emerging in their society, just as an-

other contemporary writer, Giuseppe A. Borgese, was able to cap-
ture and give form (in his novel *Rubè* [1921; *Rubè*, N.Y., 1923])
to the political confusions Italy experienced in the years following
the end of World War I.

All in all, the period that goes from the mid-twenties to the
mid-forties may be fairly characterized as one of preparation,
rather than one of achievement. The writers whose work attained
critical and popular recognition were by and large, men and
women who temperamentally, culturally, and politically were
anchored in the nineteenth century: Alfredo Panzini, Grazia
Deledda, Bruno Cicognani, Aldo Palazzeschi, Riccardo Bac-
chelli, Marino Moretti, Gabriele d'Annunzio. The new generation of writers, born shortly after the beginning of this century,
began publishing in the mid-to-late thirties, reaching a wide audience at the end of World War II. It was only then that it became
clear that three other novelists had emerged as the influential
maestri of their generation: Alberto Moravia, Elio Vittorini, and
Cesare Pavese. Like their predecessors, Svevo, Pirandello, and
Tozzi, they hailed from three radically different parts of the country: Moravia was born in Rome, Vittorini in Sicily, and Pavese
in Piedmont. Born within a few months from each other (in
1907 and 1908) the first two were self-taught, while Pavese was
in every sense, down to his college credentials, his critical essays,
and his teaching, a scholar and an intellectual. Their approach
to the art of the novel could hardly have been more different:
Moravia, from the very beginning of his career, was a "realist"
with moral and psychological pretensions, who found his major
theme in the schism between man and reality; Vittorini, after a
short-lived "realistic" period, sought to create what Donald Heiney
has felicitously called "the operatic novel"; Pavese, through his
use of myths and symbols, aimed at poeticizing reality, much as
Vittorini tried to poeticize ideology.

Moravia, Pavese, and Vittorini were by no means the only
novelists active in the period under consideration. In addition to
Brancati, Buzzati, Alvaro, Gadda (all discussed in the present
study), or Pirandello (discussed in the second volume of this survey), there were others, both talented and worthwhile: Guido
Piovene (1907–74), whose morbid, decadent tales were written
under the influence of d'Annunzio, as were the novels of Giovanni Comisso (1895–1969); Francesco Jovine (1902–50), whose

books showed almost from the very beginning a strong regionalistic interest, in the manner of Giovanni Verga; Tommaso Lan-
dolfi (b. 1908), a writer who steadfastly refuses to deal with reality
in the traditional sense, preferring to express his view of life in
Kafkaesque, at times surrealistic, terms, which yielded its best
results in books like *La bière du pecheur* (1953), *Le due zittelle*
(1945; *The Two Spinsters*, collected with *La moglie di Gogol*, in
the English edition *Gogol's Wife and Other Stories*, N.Y., New
Directions, 1963); Vasco Pratolini, a self-educated, prolific writer
(1913), whose production began in the early forties, with autobiographical, lyrical books such as *Il tappeto verde* [The green
rug] (1941) and *Via de' Magazzini* (1942), but who, only in the
post–World War II years produced his best novels, *Cronache di
poveri amanti* (1947; *A Tale of Poor Lovers*, N.Y., 1949), and the
ambitious, and extremely controversial three-part, five-volume
Una storia italiana ([An Italian story], composed of *Metello*,
1955, *Lo scialo* [The waste], 1960 and rev. 1976, and *Allegoria
e derisione* [Allegory and derision], 1966); Bonaventura Tecchi
(1896–1968), a profoundly humane, wise narrator, almost a kind
of Italian Thomas Mann, whose numerous novels, the best of
which are *Giovani amici*, 1940 [Young friends], and *Gli egoisti*
(1959; *The Egotists*, N.Y., 1964), reveal his unmistakable passion
for order, moral rectitude, and compassion, without ever giving
the impression of preaching or moralizing.

In general, honest, well-intentioned, and serious as most novelists of Fascist Italy were, even when necessity rather than true
conviction made them join the party, they shared a reluctance to
deal with the concrete reality of their time, to face the evil and
injustice they saw around them more clearly everyday. There
were exceptions, of course: Alvaro wrote of the poverty of the
shepherds of his native Calabria, Moravia looked at the decay of
the middle class with a clinical eye, unperturbed by the embarrassment of his readers and the regime, Carlo Bernari addressed
himself to the plight of the working class. The easiest way out of
this predicament was to retreat to autobiography, or escaping to
the imaginary, the fantastic. The possibility of "hermeticism,"
offered to poets such as Eugenio Montale, was not really viable
for the novelist. Few were courageous, gifted, or inventive enough
to compose allegories like Vittorini's *Conversazione in Sicilia*
(1940; *In Sicily*, N.Y., 1949) or Moravia's *La mascherata* (1941;

The Fancy Dress Party, N.Y., 1952). Others still, Borgese, Ferrero, Taddei, and Silone, chose exile over surrender, compromise, and silence.

The war, the humiliating defeats and destruction Italy experienced, destroyed all the illusions and myths of power Mussolini's rhetoric had sold to the nation. It also changed the position many an intellectual had occupied with respect to his duties and obligations toward society. Giaime Pintor, one of a small number of liberal critics, articulated his feelings in a letter written before his death shortly before the end of the war: "At a certain moment intellectuals must be able to transfer their experience onto the ground of usefulness, common usefulness; each must be able to take up his position in a fighting organization. . . . Musicians and writers, we must [all] renounce our privileges to contribute to the freedom of every person."

The time was ripe for a radical change. Beginning in 1945, and continuing with different vigor and intensity in the fifties, a unique renaissance began taking place in Italy. The movies of Roberto Rossellini, Luchino Visconti, Vittorio De Sica, together with the novels and fiction of Pavese, Vittorini, Moravia, Pratolini, Giorgio Bassani, Carlo Cassola, and the younger Italo Calvino, Leonardo Sciascia, Beppe Fenoglio—to mention just a few of an impressive group of writers—focused with unusual sensitivity on the tragedy of the social injustices, and of the war their country had endured for far too long because of the folly of Mussolini's policies. There was everywhere a sense of moral and social renewal, aimed at opposing corruption, tyranny, and at bridging the gap between every human being and his neighbor, thus lessening man's solitude.

The proposition that a literary artist should become involved, or engaged, in the life and politics of every day, became a matter receiving constant attention in the postwar years. It did not take too long, however, even for such a liberal and committed writer as Elio Vittorini, to perceive that artistic freedom could not, and should not be restrained by politics and that, as he saw it, politics and culture "constitute two, not one, activities." The intervention of the Soviet Union in Czechoslovakia and Hungary in the 1950s, proved that a nation's wish for change of political direction was ultimately determined by Russia's policies and strategy. As a result of such a repressive stance, which called for massive armed intervention, the political climate in Europe changed considerably, and the sympathy and support of the intellectual community began moving toward the center in the political spectrum.

The outburst of novels dealing with the war and with social conditions in Italy, significant as it was, did not take place without any preparation during the years of Fascist rule. After all, Moravia, Vittorini, Bilenchi, Pavese, and others, were known and their books admired for their polemical stance toward the ruling regime: they provided the example, the encouragement (which assumed more practical form when Vittorini himself was named editor of a new series of novels, "I Gettoni," written by young, promising writers) for the new generation of novelists to avoid flights into a never-never land, in order to avoid reality thus nurturing the concept of literature as evasion. And even the more mature writers began taking stock of the meaning the Fascist experience had had in their lives.

One of the elements that played a central, if subtle, role in fashioning a novel mirroring problems and issues of Italian society was the "discovery," in the middle thirties, of American literature, thanks primarily to the pioneering work done by Cesare Pavese and Elio Vittorini. To be sure, America had always maintained its presence in the hearts of the Italian people, many of whom had relatives and friends who had left their native soil in search of work and opportunities in the United States. A few intellectuals had actually visited and lived in this country for several months: Mario Soldati and Emilio Cecchi, the former a young, talented journalist, novelist and film director, the latter a sensitive, sophisticated essayist, translator, critic, produced two books, *America, primo amore* [America, first love] (1935) and *America amara* [Bitter America] (1940). The picture that emerges from their books is one that lends credence to the worst aspects of life in this country, an alienating, cold, money-dominated nation, a depiction that fueled Mussolini's hostile perceptions of America, and his ever-increasing contempt for its democratic government. The presentation of America was substantially distorted (in Cecchi's case) by a profound suspicion of every aspect of American life, and in particular, its lack of a firm literary tradition. Cecchi, in Leslie Fiedler's words found "in our quite alien culture the threat of anarchy, the nightmare of modernity," while, on the other side of the political spectrum, "younger anti-Fascist Italians like Pavese found in it a promise of cultural as well as political, clue to a new kind of literary tradition, 'a tradition of seeking tradition,' to set against their own official culture, the legendary Mediterranean past which, under Fascist auspices was being transformed from a museum to a prison."

Thanks to the labor of Vittorini and Pavese (neither of whom had ever set foot on these shores), a considerable part of modern American literature, including Melville, E. L. Masters, Sinclair Lewis, Sherwood Anderson, William Faulkner and Ernest Hemingway, became accessible to the reading public. The success American writers began enjoying was, no doubt, due to many factors: but, chief among them, was their lack of pretentiousness, the directness and honesty with which they dealt with universal human problems. In his ground-breaking book, *America in Modern Italian Literature*, Donald Heiney claims that "The vogue of American literature was assisted by a quite incidental fact: that the younger generation of Italian writers, their own creativity discouraged by the regime, turned to reviewing and translating for economic support." While the facts are correct, the conclusions are hardly justified if one bears in mind that the remuneration for such work was too modest to be of much consequence in the financial needs of a translator. Moreover, many of the substantial Italian writers whose works began reaching our shores and the international audience in the postwar years—from such poets as Eugenio Montale and Salvatore Quasimodo, both Nobel laureates, to Moravia, Vittorini and Pavese—had, by 1945, completed and/or published an important part of their literary production.

By the end of the forties, the intense love and admiration for American letters was unmistakably on the wane. In a book review of Richard Wright's *Black Boy*, broadcasted in May 1947, and in a subsequent article published in the Communist newspaper *L'unità* (August 3, 1947), entitled "Yesterday and Today," Cesare Pavese announced: "The days are gone when we discovered America!" Between 1930 and 1944, dozens of American books had been translated and avidly read by all those who, by their very act of reading them, had expressed their outrage toward fascism and their longing for new values. "Now it is all over." Once the presence of fascism as a ruling force had disappeared, America's role as a leader of the free world had been severely, if not irremediably weakened, by her capitalistic and atomic bomb policies. America and her culture could therefore no longer represent the oasis of freedom, vitality, and innovation it had been during the Fascist years. "Without Fascism to oppose," wrote Pavese, "without a progressive historical idea to personify, even America—for all her skyscrapers and automobiles and soldiers —will no longer be the vanguard of anybody's culture."

The decline of what for a good many years had been an intense love affair with American literature was balanced by a growing, and unusually productive, fascination with the life and problems of that large portion of the Italian peninsula south of Rome known as *il Mezzogiorno*. Social, economic, and political considerations helped make such a rediscovery inevitable. The appalling spectacle of the exploitation, manipulation, and neglect endured by the *Mezzogiorno* could hardly be tolerated at a time when Italy was proclaiming the beginning of an era of justice, freedom, and well-being for all its citizens regardless of geographical location. To be sure, the "Southern novel," with its insistence on social conditions and how they affect the individual, had already a respectable, if recent tradition, going back to the second half of the nineteenth century. Its recognized *maestro* is Giovanni Verga, its leading theorist Luigi Capuana, and its most effective practitioners count such names as Federico De Roberto, Grazia Deledda, Salvatore De Giacomo, among others. During the thirties with the possibilities of addressing oneself to the problems of poverty, injustice, and illiteracy all but foreclosed by the Fascist censors only a handful of writers managed to concentrate on depicting the miserable existence, without hope and freedom, to which the people of their native soil had been condemned.

In the early forties, and in the years following the end of World War II, a veritable legion of southern writers—from Francesco Jovine to Michele Prisco, from Domenico Rea to Leonardo Sciascia, from Luigi Incoronato to Giuseppe Dessí, Fortunato Seminara, Mario Pomilio, Saverio Strati, and many others, too many to be listed here—wrote novels that placed the urgent problems of the *Mezzogiorno* squarely on the conscience of the nation. And, at long last, a serious attempt to ameliorate the conditions of the South and improve the standard of living of its people was begun in 1950 with the establishment of a special fund, called *"Cassa del Mezzogiorno,"* to finance a massive plan of reconstruction and capital construction of roads, factories, housing, and offering special incentives to business firms to locate some of their plants in the South. One of the books that was extremely influential in reopening the whole question of *"il Mezzogiorno"* was, ironically enough, written between 1943 and 1944, by Carlo Levi, whose anti-Fascist activities had earned him a term in the desolate hamlet of Grassano, in the Lucania region. The book, a brilliant essay-diary entitled *Cristo si è fermato a Eboli* (1945; *Christ Stopped at Eboli*, N.Y., 1947) which became almost immediately a worldwide best seller, and stimulated American interest in Italy. By a remarkably strange and curious coincidence, it was Levi's first and only novel *L'orologio* (1950; *The Watch*, N.Y., 1951) that signaled the end of the all too brief period during which Italy had enjoyed the illusion that good fellowship, compassion, trust, and unselfishness would be the main forces that would uplift the nation and give it a sense of purpose in the difficult days ahead.

Toward the end of the 1950s Italy began enjoying a phase of economic expansion that brought about an unparalleled boom that greatly improved the standard of living for both the middle class and the working class. New factories opened, new business ventures were launched, millions of tourists flocked to the cities, the museums, the beaches, and the vacation places in Italy, improving still further the economic situation. The publishing industry also benefited from the "miracle" of the nation: it was not uncommon for works of fiction to sell upward of one hundred thousand copies, breaking most previous records. Yet, at that time books began being less precious, sacred messages between a writer and his public, than objects pure and simple manufactured according to the latest techniques that merchandised books as though they were soap and toothpaste, a deplorable situation that prompted Elio Vittorini to remark: "Books, in time of cultural industrialization, have become merchandise to be bartered like turnips, cotton or any diploma." The "industrial novel," dealing with life in the factories, the psychological impact of the new conditions upon an individual born and raised in a prevalently agricultural society, would make its entrance on the literary scene—and a new era would be at hand.

2

Three Writers in Search of the Novel

Enrico Pea

Even today, almost two decades after his death, Enrico Pea's friends recall him as a kind of legendary figure. A mere glance at one of the many photographs taken toward the end of his life would at once tell us why: his slender, ascetic body, his majestic, white, flowing beard, his round, thin black spectacles, his French cap, and his pipe, contributed to making him look less like a writer (who, in Italy, manages to look like a responsible, serious bourgeois) than like an ancient prophet, a pensive, distant yet curiously lively observer of life who could be seen seated at one end of his favorite local cafés at Forte dei Marmi, busy writing his plays or novels, or planning his creative activities.

At first reading, Pea may sound like one of the large group of writers hailing from the region of Tuscany, which has traditionally produced many of the finest raconteurs of Italian literature. But his *"Toscanità"* quickly vanishes just as soon as we read his work, or at least his earliest books. There is, to be sure, a genuine delight in the art of storytelling, a commanding ability to set the pace of the narrative. But the subject matter of Pea's books reveals his affinity with a special nucleus of writers (many of whom happened to have been born in Tuscany) who, whatever their differences of style, themes, approach to the art of writing, have an important experience in common. This special group includes such diverse personalities as Giuseppe Ungaretti (the master poet from Lucca), the fabulist Aldo Palazzeschi, from Florence, the poet-painter Ardengo Soffici, the poet-publicist Filippo T. Marinetti (founder and architect of Futurism), and others who were nurtured not in one but in two distinct cultural traditions, and came to appreciate their native heritage through, and thanks to, a prolonged residence in foreign soil. Thus, the fact that Pea, like Ungaretti, spent a considerable part of his formative years in Egypt, cannot be neglected in understanding the experience at the center of his writings, just as an awareness of the influence of the Bible and Oriental culture is essential to appreciate the tone of his work. Similarly, his living abroad developed in him a deep understanding of the condition of the uprooted individual lonely for his "home," yet often doomed to remain, even upon his return to his native land, a stranger, a pilgrim in his own country.

Living abroad, whether by choice or necessity, is an experience that sharpens one's sensitivity. In Pea's case, it also generated a deep yearning for companionship in a land where circumstances had forced him to live to earn his daily bread. As we shall see shortly, Pea endured more than his just share of pain and loneliness: indeed, so intense and dramatic were his personal experiences that they became central, if occasionally disguised, forces of the twenty or so books he wrote before his death at Forte dei Marmi in 1958.

Pea was born in the small town of Seravezza, located in what used to be, in pre-pollution times, one of the most lovely seashore resort areas on the western seaboard of the Italian peninsula. Pea stumbled on what was to be his true vocation only after a series of tragic personal experiences. Barely four, he lost his father who died as a result of an accident at work. His mother was forced to take a job as a maid in a nearby town, and Pea's grandfather, who had spent seventeen years in an insane asylum, took the responsibility for raising him, with consequences that were to shape and haunt Pea's imagination through much of his creative life. A mere youngster, Pea became a shepherd. He contracted smallpox and was hospitalized for several weeks. Once recovered, he chose to remain at the hospital as a cleaning boy. Under the guidance of a parish priest, he began, slowly and painfully, the long process of learning to read and write. When his grandfather died, he tried to enter the convent of St. Torpe, in Pisa, only to be rejected because of poor eyesight. He continued his life of jack-of-all-trades: he worked as an apprentice upholsterer, shiphand, carpenter, then in the Orlando shipyards at Leghorn. Unhappy with all these occupations, he decided—at the age of sixteen—to sail for

Alexandria, Egypt. There he worked first as a train conductor, then as a merchant trading in marble.

His contact with Near Eastern culture, which lasted until 1914, was to have a permanent effect on his creativity: the yellow sand dunes, the low, white houses with their terraces typical of many Mediterranean villages on the African coast, the color and scent of the sea, are persistent presences in his books. But what proved to be a turning point in his life was his experience in the hospital as a child: his long stay forced him to read and, at the same time, stimulated his desire to write. "I was seized by a passion to read, a kind of anger to learn, and so I filled my brains with whatever was accessible to my simple [power of] understanding. I was still a poor shepherd from [the] Versilia [region] who had emigrated to Egypt. After [learning to] read, I suddenly felt the urge to write, to put down on paper something of what rushed forth from my heart. But what a labor!"

Discharged from the hospital, he began trading first in wine (sold as genuine Tuscan "Chianti"), then in marble, and opened a small office in "La Baracca Rossa" ("The Red Shack"), a meeting place for many aspiring writers. There he met Giuseppe Ungaretti, who was to become one of the leading European poets of this century and a seminal figure in Italian letters. Pea's stay in Egypt gave him the opportunity of reading the Koran and the Bible, whose poetic character and the archetypal nature of its episodes became for him a most worthy model to imitate. As he confessed in his old age, "From that day on, I no longer laughed at God's fables: here is the book that lured me to [study] letters, revealed the universe and opened my mind."

In 1908, six years after marrying Aida Cacciagli, Pea decided to return "home." The next several years were spent working in a variety of occupations, many of which were connected with the theatre. He became a stage director, then an impresario. One of his noteworthy activities was the establishment of the so-called "Maggi," a type of popular theatre production whose tradition dates back to the Middle Ages and whose success lasted through the Renaissance.

His first literary efforts were prose poems, lyrics, and plays. The first work he published appeared in 1909, with the title *Le fole*, in an elegant edition illustrated with drawings by Lorenzo Viani. Highly recommended by Giuseppe Ungaretti, the slim volume was instrumental in giving its author a certain amount of recognition that persuaded him to continue his career as a writer. In 1912, Pea published *Montignoso*, in 1914 *Lo spaventacchio* [The frightened one], brought out under the imprint of the Florentine review *La Voce*, edited by Giuseppe Prezzolini with the assistance of Giovanni Papini and Ardengo Soffici. By this time, now a successful businessman and the father of three children, Pea, whose commercial activities required constant traveling between Egypt and Italy, was in Italy when World War I broke out. Called to military duty, he was excused because of poor eyesight, found himself without his business, but fairly well-known as a writer thanks primarily to the sponsorship of the group of *La Voce*. He turned to writing plays (publishing *Giuda* in 1918, and *Rosa di Sion* a year later), and devoting himself to the theatre. His *Judas* was not well received by the Church, and the polemics surrounding that work contributed to increasing his reputation.

One of the most intriguing aspects about Pea is that he began writing with an unusually limited cultural preparation. Still, this very factor, coupled with his unusual experience of living and working in two such diverse countries as Italy and Egypt, probably contributed substantially to making him a writer freer than most of his peers from literary conventions that frequently prevent an Italian artist from finding his personal style. From the moment he began his very first book, Pea turned his attention to the search for a genuinely new way that would enable him to paint his unique canvasses and weave the tapestries of his stories in an angelic way, allowing his own intuition, rather than study or calculated design, to be the guiding light to a more complete understanding of man's condition.

Moscardino (Engl. trans., Milan, 1955), the first "novel" by Pea, is in many ways illustrative of the works he produced during his early phase of creativity and of the qualities and flaws that have come to be typical of his writing. *Moscardino* is brief, somewhat disconnected, very much autobiographical: it is less a novel in the conventional sense, than a prose poem, whose unity is its unique cadence, at first lyrical and, toward the end of the book, biblical. If the range of the book is limited (a criticism that has been levelled at Pea throughout much of his life), its power of evocation, or what some of his critics called "the power of incantation," is admirable. The brief paragraphs that form the skeleton of the book gradually become the pillars without which the house of fiction Pea attempts to build could never become reality. And, as we approach the end of the work, we sense a definite movement toward something more sustained than a simple fictionalized autobiography, something to which many different readers can relate.

In brief, *Moscardino* tells the story of three brothers, children of Signora Pellegrina and her late husband, a physician: Moscardino's grandfather, and his two brothers—Don Lorenzo (whose sexual behavior was responsible for his not being accepted into a religious order), and someone whose name the narrator seems to be unable to remember, whose nickname is "il Taciturno" ("The Silent One") because he speaks very seldom. The tension between the three brothers is caused by the sensual passion they all nourish, to varying degrees, for a servant-girl, Cleofe. From the very moment Cleofe entered the house, a reserved, modest young girl from the nearby Mount Terrince, a place proverbially famous for the beauty of its women, life has not been the same for the three brothers. The grandfather falls passionately in love with the girl. His lust soon becomes imbued with violence, especially after he possesses her. Indeed, his love reaches such an intensity that he becomes literally unable to cope with his fear of losing her. It is his jealousy that turns on himself, as he tries to take his life by slashing his stomach—after which he is sent to a mental institution.

Love and violence become inextricably interwoven: and the grandfather's gesture seals his fate. Having Cleofe, has not been enough: and, in a sense, this becomes part of the symbolism of the story. We not only live in a society that has become increasingly more corrupt, turning to false or deceptive values, but has knowingly robbed itself of the possibility of peace with itself and its neighbors. Thus, the grandfather lives a life of fear, envy and anxieties (all clearly unjustified), but his brother Don Lorenzo (called *l'Abate* throughout the story) in what is an obvious irony (since he was deemed unacceptable for the priesthood by the Church) lives the agony of unfulfilled love, constantly masturbating, while the Silent One remains outside a life that, if it has a meaning, must be communication, compassion, and companionship. Not even the child born out of the union of the grandfather and the maidservant, resolves anything: on the contrary, rather than becoming a bond that might bring two people closer together, it is just another burden, one more factor that hastens her growing old, weakening her to the point of becoming ill.

The last part of the slim book focuses on Moscardino himself: the death of Signora Pellegrina and the illnesses in the family have increased the already precarious financial situation of the household. At one time Signora Pellegrina had been quite wealthy, but her husband had proved to be an ineffectual manager of the fortune she had inherited upon the death of two of her sisters, who were nuns. Moscardino's father is dead, his mother works as a maid in the city, and the grandfather has returned home from the mental institution, and now takes care of the youngster. Moscardino's younger brother, an epileptic, is being cared for by a charitable family in town.

Moscardino and his grandfather have established a certain rapport that allows them to savor life as much as possible, in full awareness of the briefness and frailty of human life. Thanks to their attitude they can face adversities and sorrow, and yet manage to preserve an astonishingly vibrant will to go on, and accept whatever life will bring them. And life is not particularly kind to them: unable to bear his emotional suffering, the Silent One hangs himself, while Cleofe, after years of illness and loneliness, passes on, some time after Moscardino's younger epileptic brother has also died.

These are the highlights of a tale that unfolds without being chained to a rigorous chronological sequence. The book moves toward its conclusion without ever destroying the illusion, carefully built up by the author, of fable and reality, the technique of developing a narrative "through explosions and lightnings."

Pea's semifictionalized autobiography is continued in *Il volto santo* [The holy face] (1924), considered by many critics one of his best books. In some significant ways, The Holy Face differs from *Moscardino*: the story is more unified, more objective and analytical at the expense of the lyrical tone of the previous book. Only seldom, however, is Pea able to reach a sustained level of narrative and, as a result, we are left with fragments that are often amazing for their power of synthesis.

Il servitore del Diavolo [The devil's servant] is, in my opinion, far more satisfying than *Il volto santo* and more successful as well. Written in 1928, brought out in 1931 after having been serialized in the review *Pègaso*, the book achieves what in the previous books had remained, willy nilly, an unrealized objective: the transformation of autobiographical matter into fiction while, at the same time, opening the experience to all readers by dramatizing universal feelings and values.

Once again, we follow the narrator-protagonist in his various jobs, first as a servant in the house of the Devil and Judas (both considered anarchists) then as a worker in the employ of Giovanni Sloder. Once again, the strength of the book lies not in its plot, which, however richer than in the previous books, is still relatively simple, but in its mood. The "Baracca Rossa" (the "Red Shack"), so persuasively depicted by Pea, is at once the primary physical and emotional locus of a story that glosses an important part of his Egyptian experience. But the Red Shack is more than a business address, so to speak: it becomes a sort of symbolic meeting place, international in character and universal in its function, where ever so many people—people who *become* characters—find a congenial atmosphere where that most painful of modern malaises, dislocation, may be assuaged temporarily. The people who converge on the Red Shack are as numerous as they are interesting: they are sailors, intellectuals, businessmen, adventurers of all sorts, and, most importantly, social rebels. But there are also the so-called enemies of the place: a man from Marseilles, one from Malta, and another from Greece. One or two figures among the habitués stand out: Pietro Vasai, a Florentine from a good bourgeois family, whose life has been ruined by his having been arrested, as a mere youngster, for disturbing the peace and resisting a police officer who had arrested him. From that day on, he had become a victim of police persecution no matter where he went: "He gave the impression of hating the world," notes Pea, "and he had a brotherly soul that was all romantic love as is generally true of all rebels. If a different teaching could have touched him in time, instead of a rebel who knows what could have become of this man, so eager to do voluntary social work, so willing to perform human assistance work without compensation." Then there is a twenty-year-old Greek, Percas, who falls in love with a charming Jewish girl named Rebecca, a recent arrival in Egypt from Russia with her family, fleeing from the impending Revolution. Despite their language difficulties (neither speak a common language), and a brief affair with a mature Jewess, their love manages to grow. The plight of those who have chosen to remain behind is realistically explained:

> The old folks do not budge: they will die there of deprivation. They are attached to [their] land, their things, even to danger. Those who are young leave, if they are not killed beforehand, jailed or deported. The old folks are chained by the Bible. Grown idiots by their prayers, they await the Messiah. The Government has no fear of them. But the young have broken the bridges between the New and the Old Testament: they laugh at the Patriarch and at the Rabbis alike. The fighting line is one: war against the middle class! Once compromised, it is better to flee, if one does not want to end up in Siberia.

As is true with many of his contemporaries, Pea writes primarily out of his personal, rather than intellectual and literary experience, thus driving to despair those critics who read more to satisfy their need for an exercise than for aesthetic enjoyment. Nevertheless, so prominent is the autobiographical element in Pea's work that we must speak of its achievement in different terms, perhaps as an exquisite ability to transform his subject matter into a *"fole,"* a word that is the contraction of the Latin *fabula*, or fable, a term he himself used as the title of his very first book, published in 1910. Pea never denied the autobiographical quality of everything he wrote. Indeed, in one of his last books, *Lisetta* (1946), he candidly warned the reader that "the story narrated here is a true one, stripped of many defects and details that would have made it prolyx." It may not be inappropriate to define Pea not so much as a novelist as a fabulist. Many of his books are permeated by a fablelike atmosphere and unfold in a manner that only tenuously links the various parts of the story they tell. Chronology is frequently discarded, chiefly, I suppose, because Pea is more concerned in giving us the feeling of the emotions than the impact of the facts. The past has a haunting attraction for him, even when it is not fitted in a structured picture: places and people, very real indeed, become symbols that evoke in us immediate recognition and sympathy. His books obviously reflect the approach and sensitivity of their author: what emerges are emotions bursting freely, cameo portraits, dramatic little scenes that at times explode, quietly, with a special intensity. "To narrate without feelings," Pea confessed, "is a difficult task for me. I am not a cold spectator, nor a cold collector of stories." "Most people," he added, "want to read the events of daily life in a way that makes it possible for them to find themselves in them."

His characters achieve their dimension both individually and collectively. They are an odd lot indeed: Egyptians, French, Italians, Greeks, Maltese, Christians, Jews, Atheists, Protestants, and Anarchists. They are the disinherited, the rejected, the lonely, the exploited, the peasants. They are held together by their love, and at times even by a bizarre hatred of one another, by their different passions and diverse beliefs. They are hippies *ante letteram*, damning the bourgeoisie and proclaiming the necessity of a revolution that will put an end to the false morality and cruelty to which the working class and the peasantry have been subjected since time immemorial. Their love of each other transcends national and religious barriers; they can relate to one another thanks to their basic qualities—decency, feelings of brotherhood, compassion—and their everlasting yearning for liberty.

Perhaps Pea is only peripherally a novelist in the traditional sense, and if one can speak of his special contribution to the novel as an art form one must be limited to speaking of his ability to transform "real" events into fiction.

Both in terms of the mood he creates and the uniqueness of his characters Pea deserves a niche of his own in the history of the genre. At his best, he writes a prose that has the music and rhythm of poetry; the settings of his novels have a personality that sets them apart from those of other writers. His novels are frequently "operatic." But if some of the events seem too melodramatic, or strained, they are always genuine. Overused, Pea's method can and does damage the effectiveness of his tales: when subtly used, however, it can and does produce magic, mesmerizing effects. In yet another way Enrico Pea should be remembered: in a period that demanded *la belle page*, he consciously worked to give the novel the cohesiveness it had lost. He also reaffirmed his faith in the genre without having to surrender or having to make concessions in either style or form, with the result that his novels have a substance, of feelings if not always of events, and a tone of exceptional quality.

Bruno Cicognani

As in the United States and many, if not all, countries in Western Europe, Italian writers have traditionally earned their living working in part of the sector of what we might call the cultural establishment: the schools, the publishing houses, the newspapers and periodicals, radio and television. There have been, and are, many exceptions, to be sure: Alessandro Manzoni and Antonio Fogazzaro came from relatively affluent families, and writing was a vocation for them, rather than a means to sustain themselves. In our century, Italo Svevo was a businessman, co-owner of a marine paint manufacturing concern; the poet Sergio Solmi a bank executive, Leonardo Sinisgalli an engineer, Paolo Volponi, the novelist, was until recently Olivetti's personnel director. The advantages of not working for the cultural establishment are evident, as are the disadvantages: all told, there may be something to be said for a position that does not inhibit a writer, and that places no pressures upon his creative process. In this sense, Bruno Cicognani was unusually fortunate: a lawyer with his own prosperous practice, he was able to lead a fairly independent life, devoting his free time to pursuing his creative interests. He shied away from personal involvement in literary groups, or schools, content to write only when he felt the need to do so, yet he managed to finish some fifteen books—plays, novels, autobiographies, and short stories—noteworthy for their seriousness and integrity. On two occasions did Cicognani surface in the Republic of Letters: in 1941, when he was named to the prestigious Academia d'Italia, and in 1955, when he was assigned the prestigious Marzotto Prize for Literature. While engaged in a very demanding profession, in the words of one of his critics, Piero Rebora, Cicognani "used the practice of law as a daily experience of humanity, a laboratory of psychology." He saw and depicted people with the logic and clarity of a well-trained lawyer, and the perception and compassion of an artist unafraid to delve into the baser instincts and actions of man.

Two of Cicognani's three novels, *La Velia* and *Villa Beatrice* are certain to rank among the better works of fiction published in Italy in the first half of this century. Both were composed in his middle years (born on September 10, 1879 in Florence, he passed away in 1971); both must be read with an awareness that its author's family was, in every conceivable way, very conservative. In one of his autobiographical books, he wrote about his father: "He believed, on the one hand, in the constituted civil authorities and in the infallibility of the Church; and, on the other hand, in the dignity of the individual vis-à-vis the masses; [he] also [believed] that the authorities had not only the right, but the sacrosanct duty to repress in any way, even with force (if force is the only thing they understand) the activities of those who rioted for the sake of achieving good [goals] only those in power are in the position to perceive and evaluate; [it is] the duty of the Church to eradicate [any attempt] of spiritual straying and to sacrifice even the body so long as the soul is saved." Although Cicognani has minimized the reactionary temperament of his father by underscoring the eminently antibourgeois nature of his upbringing, it is questionable, to say the least, whether his assertion can persuasively be supported by the world he wrote about and the manner in which he gave life to the world of his imagination. From his first work of fiction, *La Crittogama* [The cryptogram] (1909), written under the influence of d'Annunzio, Cicognani created a vast number of figures and figurines—petit bourgeois, artisans, workers, businessmen—and set them in the milieu he knew best, that of his native Florence. They are all solidly realistic and credible indeed, even if in Cicognani's early books their realism is based not on their psychological and social accuracy, but on the mimetic quality of their speech, with the result that we often hear Florence rather than understand it.

This is not the case of *La Velia* (1923), which has been characteristized as a novel of customs—the shabby, decadent, corrupt mores of the lower and middle middle class of Florence, with its greed and dishonesty. The novel is titled after its heroine, an Italian version of Madame Bovary, a sensual, ambitious, scheming woman, the natural daughter born out of a love affair between her mother, Nastasia, a seamstress, and Luigi Biagini, co-owner, with his brother Giuseppe, of a successful construction firm. Upon their death, Beppino (who is not, as generally believed, the son of Luigi, but of his brother Giuseppe) is left sole heir of a considerable fortune. A kind, naïve young man, totally unpre-

pared, temperamentally and professionally, to assume the direc-
torship of a demanding business concern, he becomes the easy
prey of Velia, whose appetite for money, status, and material
things is truly insatiable. Beppino is persuaded by the family lawyer to step down from his post and to ask the firm's chief engineer,
Soldani-Bò, to take over. Once Velia and Beppino are married,
Soldani-Bò moves into their home so as to be readily available
to satisfy Velia's sexual needs. Sexuality seems to run rampant
in the household, for it becomes a dominating force not only of
Velia's life, but of her mother's, her mother-in-law's, and of the
woman who compassionately took care of her in her final days, of
Beppino and, of course, of Soldani-Bò. As predictable, Velia
eventually becomes bored with her lover (who has been living in
Beppino's house in what tacitly at first, and defiantly later, has
been accepted as a *ménage à trois*). Soldani-Bò's strength deterio-
rates visibly under the various mounting pressures that control
his existence and for a moment he considers murdering Velia.
He has reached the end of the road: the only sane thing to do, as
he sees it, is to take his life. As the story closes, we find Beppino
resigned to his clerical duties, Velia turning to her new lover,
while her mother finds a position as the local priest's maidservant.

La Velia is a tortuous work, which moves in a dry, relentless,
uncompromising way toward its resolution. Everyone is doomed
in the novel, destined to be ultimately destroyed by the flaw of his
character that excludes lofty or idealistic values. Arrogance and
cruelty, of one sort or another, dominate the action. Love itself
is reduced to a mere affair of the senses, with no redeeming qualities; human relationships are determined not by feelings but by
selfish monetary equations. Yet, the schemings, cheating, and
violence that dominate the novel from beginning to end must be
understood against the background of Velia's upbringing, singu-
larly devoid of love and care and respect, coupled with the poverty
and other hardships she has had to endure. Throughout the unfolding of her story, we sense that the author is sensitive to her
problems, even though she is, as a character, not exactly pleasant.
The same can be said about the other characters who, however
weak or repulsive they might be, are depicted with unusual re-
straint and objectivity. There are two areas in which Cicognani

excels: the creation of many of the settings (particularly the home) in which the story unfolds, and feminine psychology, clearly understood and presented in the novel.

For a startling change in terms of characters and view of love, one must turn to Cicognani's second novel, *Villa Beatrice*. Where *La Velia* deals with obsessive annd eventually destructive sexual passion *Villa Beatrice* initially centers on a situation that may fairly be characterized by "absence of love," a puzzling condition that is endured, once again, by the novel's protagonist, Beatrice. The choice of her name has its own deliberate irony: its meaning is "bearer of beatitude," and is generally associated with the woman with whom Dante, still a mere youngster, fell in love and who was to inspire him to write his *Comedy*. Cicognani's Beatrice lacks the radiance of Dante's beloved, although she is capable, as we shall see momentarily, of an unusual act of love.

Originally subtitled "Story of a frigid virgin," *Villa Beatrice* offers a portrait of a sad, pathetic existence. As the book begins, we find Beatrice who has reached the age of thirty and is still unmarried, possibly condemned to spinsterhood. Her youthful days are rapidly sketched out. A combination of factors, mostly temperamental, have turned her into a capable person who rejects life and yet, surprisingly enough, demonstrates many of those qualities that reveal great inner strength and compassion. How did Beatrice become such an introspective, estranged person? What are the reasons for her fear of life? The evidence in the novel answers the question by showing that she is terrified by the prospect that life—by which we are meant to infer the sexual act—will soil what she is most proud of, her carnal purity. In this respect, we should note that the book opens with a surprising statement: "Who would want to love you? No one will love you: your mommy and daddy love you just the same, but as for the others. . . . Love breeds love. You will be loved as much as something made of stone. You are as arid as a pumice stone," comments one of her teachers. "What have you got in place of your heart?" No matter how much the reader is repelled by Beatrice's cold, withdrawn personality, it is difficult not to perceive that such comments will inevitably increase the young girl's insecurity and estrangement. Yet, her mother and father, two decent and honest people, realize that their daughter's persistence in continuing to lead an isolated existence will most surely not improve her chances for happiness and fulfillment. Thanks to the help of interested friends, they manage to find a good person interested in marrying their daughter. The man who, according to their middle-class mentality, they believe to be well suited as her mate is Romualdo, a moderately affluent businessman who owns a leather processing company. Now forty years old, a reasonable and open human being, he is a friendly, extroverted person, liked and respected by his peers and his workers alike, who yearns for a marriage with a woman who will be a loyal companion and a good mother to their children. He is not, to be sure, Prince Charming, but what he lacks in physical attractiveness is amply compensated for by his generosity, understanding, and goodness. Not surprisingly, Beatrice finds herself incapable of loving a man and cannot know what love is except in a childishly vague way. Such unpropitious circumstances make it unlikely that the two can enjoy a meaningful human partnership. As the story unfolds, knowing Beatrice's past, we realize that neither Romualdo's extraordinarily tolerant understanding nor his openness can change the situation. Beatrice is literally incapable of responding to her husband or to the overtures of friendship made by those who come in contact with her. As a matter of fact, she fails to relate to anyone: to her own parents, whom she would just as soon exclude from her life altogether, to her husband, who literally repulses her even though he is gentle and understanding, to the large household staff that had been looking forward to a strong and innovative mistress of the house, to her husband's friends, who try in vain to connect with her, and, finally, to the workers of her husband's factory. Through much of the book Beatrice feels and behaves like an animal raised only to be taken to the slaughter house, sacrificed to a marriage she does not really want with a man she cannot love. Her need for total privacy, physical and emotional, borders on a state of complete estrangement from the world about her, a world she feels has never taken notice of her as a human being with her own aspirations and problems. Beatrice's tragic condition, in short, consists not so much in her inability to feel but in her incapacity to articulate her feelings and be thus released of her emotions so as to lessen the pain of living. Time and again, she feels the need of talking about her feelings, but words are literally choked in her throat; other times, she chooses to react passively only because it happens to be the more honest way to express her alienation from life. Under such circumstances, she can hardly be expected to experience any joy; she can only look at herself with pity strong enough to cancel the world around her while that very world seems almost to be crying for her to become involved in life.

The turning event of the novel takes place when Beatrice conceives and gives birth to a child after a particularly difficult pregnancy. The little baby girl is promptly named Barberina, after Romualdo's deceased mother. In some cases the birth of an offspring can be instrumental in changing a woman's (or man's) outlook on life, triggering the beginning of a new relationship between a man and his wife. Not so in this novel; Barberina's presence succeeds only in driving her parents still further apart than they have been. Beatrice comes to look upon her daughter as a kind of rival, demanding the attention and love from her father that she has been unable to give to anyone. Furthermore, she begins to fear that Barberina might be eventually trapped in a similar psychic condition and experience the same agony and unhappiness she has had to endure since her childhood.

One day, Beatrice decides to take her problem to her parish priest, don Andrea. Thanks to his wisdom and sensitivity, she realizes the nature of her predicament; she understands at last that love breeds love. Nothing but frustration and unhappiness will touch her life unless she learns to open herself to those who are, or want to be, close to her. Life is giving, and giving is ultimately love, the major force of life itself and the element that makes life meaningful. There are no other choices before her; to continue living as in the past would only mean to follow a self-destructive course.

The opportunity to test her sense of commitment presents itself sooner than anyone would have anticipated, when Barberina falls ill with diphtheria and comes close to dying. She is miraculously saved by Beatrice's mouth-to-mouth breathing: unfortunately, the virus is passed on to Beatrice. Several months after her daughter's recovery, Beatrice pays the price for her courageous act with her own life, thus dramatically giving meaning to the verse of *The Gospel According to St. John*, "God is Love," the epitaph of the book.

Both *La Velia* and *Villa Beatrice* exemplify the qualities of Cicognani the novelist—a rare gift for depicting people and their basic emotions, even when, as in the case of Beatrice, they are essentially passive; an objective which, in a country as emotional as Italy, is nothing short of remarkable. The tragic ends of Soldani-Bò (in *La Velia*) and of Beatrice, are painstakingly described, with restrained compassion. Perhaps one of Cicognani's greatest strengths is his uncanny ability to see people as they really are, with no masks, no props that will permit them to hide from reality and truth. His strong points are accuracy of detail, a style that captures realistically the tone and substance of conversations, and, in his better books, a rare insight into the flaws of the human soul. He is especially convincing and effective when describing women (there are few, if indeed any men in his books worthy of the rank of protagonist), and particularly authentic when they are wicked. If his insistence upon portraying unpleasant, immoral women reminds us of Balzac, Flaubert, and Zola, his penchant for Florence as the setting of his fiction, and his focus on its inhabitants, places him in the tradition of the nineteenth century tradition of *"verismo"* and Naturalism. More precisely, Cicognani's work is particularly representative of the stage the Italian novel had to go through before reaching the broader scope and deeper significance of the European novel. It has often been said, with considerable justification I think, that the novel in Italy cannot help its being anything if not "regionalist," particularly in the period that goes from the Unification, in 1861, to World War II. Life in the provinces, the strong roots every Italian man of culture has in his native soil, its traditions, its history, its culture and its problems, has always been a source of inspiration too rich to neglect. In this sense, the work of Cicognani is traditional and conventional, with its insistence on Florence and its inhabitants. But he has also made a concerted effort to transcend the limitations of his predecessors and contemporaries by giving his main novels a psychological dimension that, without sacrificing the regionalist component, reaches out for a universality of meaning.

In a commemorative piece published shortly after Cicognani's death, one of his most loyal critics, Luigi M. Personé, speaks of him as "a great narrator," "one of the major, if not altogether the greatest Italian [novelists] of the thirties and forties." The assessment is too generous, particularly in the light of the limited number of novels he wrote, and the fairly narrow parameters of his vision. Cicognani's validity must be sought elsewhere: and it is not surprising that it should be found in his faithful, effective ability to re-create life in his beloved birthplace, in "his constant disposition," Luigi Baldacci notes, "to search for the good old times, witness of his honesty and document of his situation as man in society."

> Who am I? I am the clown of my soul.
> Aldo Palazzeschi, *Opere giovanili*
> Life is for the most part a merry-go-round
> of useless things.
> Aldo Palazzeschi, *I fratelli Cuccoli*

Aldo Palazzeschi

Writing about Aldo Palazzeschi, the brilliant critic Carlo Bo, while acknowledging that he had welcomed the opportunity of speaking about a writer who had been a close personal friend for several years, confessed nevertheless that he had not succeeded in "making a point" about someone he categorizes as a "major and least known" Italian writer. "Up to what point," writes Bo, "and to what degree is Palazzeschi part of the literary society of the twentieth century? . . . What substance is there in his relationship with those who matured in post–World War I [years] and, finally, is there a connecting link with the most recent creative writing as it has been shaped after 1945?" G. S. Singh in his lucid survey of Palazzeschi's work, places him in the group of "first-rate novelists and story tellers of the twentieth century," "even though in virtue of only two or three novels." Still another authoritative and demanding critic, Luigi Russo, after publishing a rather disparaging assessment of our novelist, not only toned down considerably his earlier reservations but indeed made a startling about face in the revised and updated edition of his valuable guide *I narratori (1850–1957)* originally published in the early twenties. Finally, Aldo Borlenghi, in a lengthy and comprehensive essay on Palazzeschi, writes that "*Le sorelle Materassi* [1934; *The Sisters Materassi*, N.Y., 1953] seemed at once a masterpiece, probably the summit of the Italian novel of our century"—an opinion which few serious readers would share without reservations. Similarly, many recent critics of contemporary Italian literature have willingly given lip service to an exaggerated evaluation of Palazzeschi's fiction, without adequately justifying critically their high esteem for him. Thus for example, Giuliano Manacorda, in his *Storia della letteratura italiana contemporanea, 1940–1965*, calls Palazzeschi "the most interesting writer" of the "generation of 1880–1890," yet devotes less than a paragraph to him, and mentions his name only four times in his history.

What is the reason that makes for a persistent lack of critical unanimity in assessing a novelist so widely loved, respected, and admired as Palazzeschi? Why does Carlo Bo call him an *"isolato"* (an "outsider") and why does a generation of writers, again in Bo's words, "find no possibility of being linked" with our novelist? Finally, what is it that makes Palazzeschi a maverick sui generis, who insisted in working within his tradition?

The answer to these questions is not simple, but it may be found, as is inevitably the case, in the record of the creative writing of our subject, placed in perspective now that his pen is still, after his death on August 17, 1974.

Aldo Palazzeschi, nom de plume of Aldo Giurlani, was born in Florence on February 2, 1885, into a moderately well-to-do bourgeois family. Being an only child, he received more than the usual share of parental attention and, surprisingly enough considering the rather inflexible social code in Italy at the turn of the century, enjoyed considerable personal independence. Supposedly that is the reason why Palazzeschi, like his good friend poet-turned-novelist Marino Moretti, began his artistic career not as a writer but as an actor, though he also completed his degree in accountancy. Soon enough, young Aldo abandoned the stage, always so uncertain as an occupation, and decided to devote himself to writing. His early poetry is not particularly profound, but it does shed light on the direction in which he was to move and on his originality as a novelist. Writing poetry in those days was the sign of a serious commitment to literature, and there was no lack of great poets to emulate—Carducci, Pascoli, and d'Annunzio among them. There were also the Futurists, a group led by Filippo T. Marinetti, with its exaltation of machines, speed, and violence—a violence that was directed chiefly at the past moral, artistic, and political values. Balancing the *Futuristi*, was the slim nucleus of the so-called *Crepuscolari* (or poets of the

Twilight), with their simplicity, their languid, resigned, and slightly morbid spirit that sang of the grayness of provincial life with words that reeked of the smell of hospital and disease. Alberto Frasson depicts this as a "poetry that seemed to lack any interests, devoid of vital impulses vis-à-vis the restlessness of the new generation: [hence] the need to break with the past, following a law that recurs inevitably every season; [the need] to break the exterior schemes of a rule by then exhaustively defined." Palazzeschi was able to graft these moods and needs into his poetry, whose dominating traits were a gentle irony, a playfulness, and a simplicity of language that were welcome antidotes to the baroqueness of d'Annunzio and the radical posture of the Futurists. He accepted the simplicity of the *Crepuscolari* together with the rebelliousness of the Futurists, and looked at life with considerable philosophical sophistication. There is no violence in Palazzeschi's lyrics, but there is a certain amount of sententiousness, softened by a pervasive touch of humor, "the nectar and the poison," as Enrico Falqui remarks, "of [Palazzeschi's] chalice." In this context, the famous, often quoted verse "Lasciatemi divertire!" ("Let me have fun!") provides the first, and perhaps most central clue to the magic of Palazzeschi's art, to his way of looking at the world in a manner that blends mockery and seriousness, fun and pathos, happiness and sadness.

While Palazzeschi has managed to retain the affection and respect of his readers, there is considerable disagreement about the quality of his work. Some decisively prefer the early production up to *La piramide* [The pyramid], others prefer his fiction of his "second period," particularly the novel *Le sorelle Materassi* (*The Sisters Materassi*) "destined," in the words of Enrico Falqui, "to remain unsurpassed." There is much to be said about the elusiveness, frothiness, and spontaneous fun in Palazzeschi's early work that commend themselves to the reader even though, as we shall see in the pages that will follow, a masterful handling and stylistic control do not succeed in making up for the absence of a serious, sustained vision of the world.

Most critics agree that 1914 marks the time that serves as the dividing line between the two periods of Palazzeschi's art, assuming that such a division is desirable and warranted by his creative writing. By 1914, in fact, Palazzeschi had behind him a respectable body of work: the collection of poems titled *I cavalli bianchi*

[White horses] (1905), *Lanterna* [The lantern] (1909), and *L'incendiario* [The incendiary] (1910, revised and expanded in 1913). Whatever one might think of Palazzeschi's verse (and it is not difficult to become unashamedly attached to its humor, to the detached manner in which human foibles and follies are depicted), it is clear that his poetry plays a conspicuous role in his later fiction. Indeed, some of its chief themes, such as the loneliness of existence and man's exploitation of other men, are clearly enunciated in many of his early lyrics.

During his first period, Palazzeschi also composed three novels: *Allegoria di novembre* [November allegory] (1907), *Il codice di Perelà* (1911; *Perelà, the Man of Smoke*, N.Y., 1936) and *La piramide* [The pyramid] (1914), all of which betray an obvious debt in theme and focus to Gabriele d'Annunzio. Thus, the first novel pivots around the love affair of Valentino Core, a Roman prince, with a British young man, with the symbolic name of John Mare. The opulence of its setting and the decadence of its subject and language recall d'Annunzio's *Il piacere* (1889; *The Child of Pleasure* N.Y., 1898). The protagonist, for example, is determined to keep his love free of any impurities so that it may remain always ideal and perfect. For this reason, the prince retires to his family villa, unoccupied for the previous fifteen years when his mother had taken her life, thus consigning to memory the burden of preserving intact, and therefore "perfect," a relationship life would have changed into something other than what it originally was. Every evening, the prince religiously goes out to mail his letter to John Mare and, with similar devotion, sets to explore one of the many rooms of the villa in a Proustian effort to recapture time past. Such efforts eventually fail to reach the desired goal. One day after the opening of the villa, the event is celebrated with a big party—a formal ball. But, much to the consternation of the two housekeepers, the Prince vanishes, presumably a suicide, never to be seen again. And with this, the first part of the novel comes to an end.

Part two is really a sort of a twenty-page appendix, consisting of newspaper reports, the gossips, the discussions, and opinions the mysterious disappearance of the prince has evoked.

If the title of the book *Allegoria di novembre* [November allegory] has justly puzzled many critics, I found no concrete evidence that they have come to grips with its significance. A working definition of allegory is: "a specific type of artistic expression, by means of fictional figures and actions, of truth or generalizations about human experience." When set against this definition, the artist's purpose becomes clear: his tale is an attempt to depict a love totally devoid of bodily contact. This intention makes the choice of the epistolary technique seemingly ideal as the most effective strategy to realize the author's intention, particularly since it affords him the greatest control over his material, while keeping the experienced suitably "distanced," as it were, from the hero-author of the story. Yet, while the form gives a semblance of reality to the theme of the experience, it also proves to be, with its one-sidedness and intellectualization of Valentino's passion for Johnny, the major flaw of the book. Determined to keep alive the memory of a love unstained by the temptations of the flesh, Valentino is ultimately content to feed his emotional needs with the memory of a love that was but will never be again. "In his attitude toward the English youth," notes G. S. Singh, "there is a characteristically curious admixture of refined sensuality and decadent sentimentality, an almost carnal version of Platonism or pseudo-Platonism. But this kind of a bond, and the psychological character it presupposes, is a serious limiting factor in a novel, because it does away with the need for any plot, dialogue, or dramatic incidents."

The homosexual character of Valentino's love for Johnny Mare (already adumbrated in their respective names) may be seen as a rather courageous effort to deal, implicitly and with great restrain, with a relationship hardly acceptable by the moral standards of the times. But what is even more interesting is that the novel seems to announce the score of weak, ineffectual, exploitable men and lonely, puritanical, sex-starved spinsters, and handsome, virile, aggressive adolescent males that people Palazzeschi's future novels.

Il codice di Perelà, Palazzeschi's second novel, has generally enjoyed the respect of the critics, many of whom consider it perhaps his best work. Certainly the novel has a complicated history: written between 1908 and 1910, brought out in 1911, it has since been issued in three different, "revised" editions (1920, 1943, and 1955), its title changed from *Perelà* to *Perelà uomo di fumo* to the present *Il codice di Perelà*. The author himself, in the short "Premessa" to the Mondadori de luxe *opera omnia* edition, calls it

"My light fable" ("la mia favola aerea"), "the highest point of my imagination"—an observation that is hard to dispute. Indeed, whatever its flaws, the book is unquestionably the best example of the inventiveness, the humor, and the pathos that are the hallmarks of its creator. The story itself is as odd as it is unusual: Perelà, whose name is made up of the first syllable of his three "mothers" (*Pena, Rete, Lama,* hence *Pe-re-là*) who for the past thirty-three years have fed the chimney from which Perela has come. The names of the three mothers are not idle choices: "pain," "net," and "blade," is their meaning, and it will become clear how Perela seems to fall in the net of his enemies, experiences pain, and will be cut off (with the blade of rejection) from this life. But, for the moment, he is ready to come out and step into the "real" world. At first he says nothing that is considered hostile or offensive to anyone. His lightness and gentle anarchy are seen as qualities unattainable by the average mortal. So great is the enthusiasm he stirs and the admiration showered upon him, that he is asked to work out a new "code of freedom" for the state. Alas, soon enough Perelà discovers, and is eventually victimized by, the incongruities, the paradoxes of society, and the insurmountable obstacles that lie in the way of anyone attempting to make a serious contribution to the public welfare. In this sense, one of his very first experiences is typical: the State finds itself in such precarious fiscal straits that it is on the verge of bankruptcy —a situation which contemporary history has taught us to be entirely possible, whether in the case of a large, and traditionally "rich" city such as New York, or a nation such as Chile.

A proclamation is issued to the effect that "The richest citizen, whoever he may be, who is willing to donate his *entire* private wealth to the coffers of the State" will be made king. Among the people who take part in this unusual contest is the town drunk, Iba. To the amazement of the townfolk, he brings to the royal palace sacks of gold, precious stones, and cash. By all standards, he has met the requirements of the edict and must therefore be crowned king. The populace is understandably stunned. Not only do the citizens refuse to participate in the festivities that are being arranged for the occasion, but they insult and vilify their new king. The following day, Iba's tenure is abruptly canceled when it is discovered that he failed to abide strictly to the requirements and terms of the edict. It now appears that several additional bundles of money have been found at Iba's house. The newly appointed king, on the basis of the evidence, must be dethroned and jailed. Perelà's fortune has run its course. But there are more surprises in store for the reader: Alloro, the supervisor of the royal staff of servants, has taken his life in a bizarre fashion. Alloro thought he might become, like Perelà, a "man of smoke." Perelà now becomes a threat to society since many people might wish to achieve his condition. Under the circumstances, Perelà must be removed from society. He is brought to trial, and, although forcefully defended by the Countess Oliva di Bellonda, who has fallen in love with him, he is found guilty and sentenced to life imprisonment. A special jail is built for him atop one of the highest hills near town, and, once inside, the door is sealed. Fortunately, thanks to the foresight of Oliva, there is a fireplace in the room and Perelà manages to escape, like a good man of smoke he is. His brief journey among mankind has failed in its objectives: he came to men to bring them humor and lightness, but all he has received in return has been insults and imprisonment for no good cause, thus forcing him to return to the realm of abstraction and myth from which he came.

As always, humor and irony are tools Palazzeschi effectively uses to make a statement about human nature. In the case of Perelà, they make us conscious of the unpredictable, erratic nature of our judgment, our morality. What was welcomed, praised, and admired yesterday can suddenly, mysteriously become a threatening element whose "abnormality," or uniqueness, must be condemned and eradicated from our midst. It is in this sense that some critics have been impelled to speak of Perelà as a Christ figure: His teaching of Love proved to be of no consequence when he was accused by his enemies and led to the cross. Perelà will also be confronted by the issues of war and love, and will be baffled by the contradictions of mankind that seems to yearn for peace, but furiously prepares for war, idealizes love, only to be frightened when its concepts are dashed against reality.

It is fair to say that Palazzeschi's third and fourth novels, *Due imperi . . . mancati* [Two empires . . . that came to nought] (1920) and *La piramide* (1926), served mainly to get rid of certain "ghosts" haunting him—the nationalism that looked to war and violence, as well as the glories of Italy going back to the Roman Empire, as hailed by Gabriele d'Annunzio and his followers, and the repressive posture of the Church. At the same time, his trust in the role of the man of letters in a world torn by war and social unrest was considerably strengthened.

Where *Due imperi . . . mancati* is somewhat abstract in its attempt to center on the specific malaise of contemporary society, the autobiographical volume *Stampe dell'800* [Prints of the nineteenth century] (1932), a collection of short stories, represents Palazzeschi's decision to deal with reality rather than with intellectual concepts or postures. The book was born out of a request made by the journalist Ugo Ojetti for a contribution to the review *Pègaso* about Florence toward the turn of the last century. Judging from the results, the idea seems to have appealed to Palazzeschi, who found the idea of writing a genre, the *bozzetto* (or sketch), that was new to him rather intriguing. As practiced by such modern writers as Serao, Di Giacomo, and Fucini, the *bozzetto* is a blend of the short short story and autobiographical recollections. It focuses on a single, simple event or person, and attempts to enable the reader to acquire a feeling for a particular historical era and place through the convergence of traits belonging to several people in a single personality.

If *Stampe dell'800* is unashamedly autobiographical in substance and almost Boccaccioesque in intention, *Le sorelle Materassi* is in ever so many ways Manzonian. It is unquestionably the best, most balanced and representative of Palazzeschi's novels, and the most satisfactory synthesis of his qualities and limitations as a writer of fiction.

Consider the story which unfolds in the book: Teresa and Carolina Materassi are two embroideresses of wide renown. Their marvelous artistic inventiveness, the high quality of their work, their feeling for beauty and superb craftsmanship, enable them to transfer on linen, cotton, and silk designs of unusual conception and originality. Their workshop in Santa Maria at Coverciano, near Florence, is regularly visited by a wide, affluent, and demanding clientele, drawn from the upper-middle class, the aristocracy, and the hierarchy of the Church. When the story begins, in 1918, the two sisters are fifty years old, soon to be joined by their sister Giselda, fifteen years their junior, whose husband of five years has abandoned her. Gifted with an indisputable managerial ability, Giselda assumes the function of contractor, supervisor, and general administrator of the not negligible family patrimony, which includes some land and rental properties. The task of running the house itself is in the capable hands of their maidservant Niobe, a good, generous, and compassionate woman whose life has been somewhat tarnished by two love affairs. A fourth sister, Augusta, is introduced briefly well after the story has begun. Six years younger than Teresa, she made her home in Ancona, on the eastern seaboard of the peninsula. Prior to his death, her husband had been a railroad worker; Augusta made their lot a little less precarious by working in a shoe factory and taking some sewing work home. Suddenly, she falls seriously ill; her two elder sisters rush to her bedside, barely in time to accept the responsibility of raising her surviving adolescent son, Remo. Little do they suspect what is in store for them! While barely fourteen, Remo has an almost insatiable lust for life and is hardly concerned with the problem of finding the money to pay for the good things of life he deems necessary for his lifestyle: Niobe will happily give him her life savings so that he may acquire a motorcycle and the sisters will be obliged to sign promissory notes to purchase an automobile and to pay other debts incurred to pay for his extravagances. Remo shows no less lust in his sex life: he has a strange friendship with a sixty-year old Russian countess (a friendship he uses to force his aunts to finance his new, thirty-five thousand lire automobile), then seduces a young girl who becomes pregnant, and finally marries Peggy, daughter of a wealthy American industrialist, leaves for the United States with his wife and his best friend, Palle, leaving his aunts bankrupt. At first, the sisters are all but devastated by their new condition of poverty. Slowly, with the help of Niobe, they begin their comeback, finding strength and unexpected inspiration from the memory of the many ways in which their nephew Remo brought them some of the happiness and fulfillment life had previously denied them.

In structure and strategy, *The Sisters Materassi* bears a strong Manzonian imprint. Like Manzoni, Palazzeschi (moderately but unctuously religious) is a methodical novelist, supremely concerned with the harmony and hence the beauty of artistic creation. The setting of the novel is described with admirable if somewhat excessive thoroughness. Similarly, his principal characters receive a detailed treatment: no intimate detail that might illuminate their temperament is spared. This is particularly true in the chapter devoted to the sisters, which contains observations at

times between the ironical and the sarcastic. When closely examined, the structure of the novel is shown to consist of a small
number of blocks of varying length (what Italian critics call *meda-
glioni*, or precise, complete portraits), chronologically arranged.
"There is in *The Sisters Materassi*," comments G. S. Singh, "as
in other novels by Palazzeschi, no straightforward narrative pro-
ceeding step by step; instead, what we have is a series of scenes
and situations which do not necessarily emerge one from the
other and are not always organically linked." Singh further believes that the "numerous descriptions, anecdotes and digres-
sions" constitute the links between the parts of the novel. The
point is well taken, even if I personally feel that *in fondo* it is
Palazzeschi's attitude toward his characters and his presence in
the unfolding of the story that gives continuity of tone and perspective to the book. Much like Manzoni, Palazzeschi accepts the
role of narrator, commentator, and, occasionally, wry moralist
in the book. The limitations of his story—ranging all the way
from the provincialism of its setting, the uncomplicated nature
of most of its characters, the narrow range of emotions portrayed
—and of his point of view, ultimately answer too many questions,
while refusing to deal forcefully with the problems at hand. Having excluded the reader from an overinvolvement in the story, we
find ourselves in a more or less detached position, without power,
mere silent observers and must accept the pace set by the narrator
—a pace that is particularly painfully slow in the opening section
of the book, where Palazzeschi assumes the role of the omniscient
narrator similar to Manzoni's: "Now that I have described the
[story's] surrounding landscape, I shall attempt to take notice with
you of the things that strike our curiosity at first sight." Or: "It is
necessary for us to observe carefully this room which is, one might
say, the [home] base of our very modest plot." With the author
always in firm control of his tale, there is always ample room and
opportunity for asides and ironical remarks à la Manzoni: "They
had not wished, and justly so, the boy [Remo] to wear mourning
clothes for his mother's death, [such being a] fragile institution of
bourgeois morality that bases everything on form and appearance." Or: "Simple people do not need a mouth to talk." When
Carolina takes to kissing Remo less like an aunt and more like a
lover, Palazzeschi remarks: "We must realize that for the first
time the fifty-year old spinster who was kissing a male, even

though just an adolescent, up to that time had kissed only boys much younger than [Remo], boys up to five or six years of age or a bit older, and that her kiss expressed the whole innocence and kindness of her condition of a virgin."

If *The Sisters Materassi* has long been considered Palazzeschi's best novel, there is ample evidence justifying the high marks received by the critics and the popularity it has enjoyed since its publication. It is not only a simple but effective tableau of Tuscany in the thirties, but a "convincing study of repressed femininity," in Ines Scaramucci's words. Unlike the early *Allegoria di novembre*, there is both diversity and interplay of the sexual motif: there is Teresa, whose femininity "reappeared only in the rare and brief moments of rest, and by now denied not by need, but by a habit of thoughts and of work changed into hard rule." There is Carolina, who, unlike her sister, "had preserved intact her external femininity," whose sensuality is revealed by and through such a common gesture as handling fruits; there is Giselda, with her hatred toward men because of her unhappy marriage; there is Niobe, who has experienced sex and is able to draw pleasure rather than pain, fear, or bewilderment, from Remo's presence. And, to complete the picture, there is Remo, with his aggressive, uninhibited sensuality that permits him to exploit anyone so as to satisfy his needs, and his pal Palle (whose name is revealing), a rough, ungraceful youth from a poor background, who is disliked by the two sisters mainly because he poses a threat to their possessiveness of their nephew.

Whatever action there is in the novel is either provoked or created by sex: even the two sisters' chosen profession, and the emphasis observed by the narrator on hand-made and embroidered lingerie, is symbolical of their need to compensate for an existence without sexual experience, while at the same time, it gives them a false sense of superiority and justifies their frequent acid comments about the women whose patronage has made their financial success! It is in the context of such a repressed life that it is understandable why Remo, with his energy, the sensuality he exudes, his magnetic personality should become their hope, their idol, their very *raison d'être*, and, eventually, their tragic downfall. But no matter: Remo has brought fire and vitality into the monotonous pace of the Materassi household, has upset its bourgeois values, and becomes at least a surrogate for a love the women were resigned never to experience. And that alone is worth the price they have to pay. After he has gone, Remo's presence continues, if only by means of a photograph (showing him in a daring bathing suit), suitably enlarged and prominently displayed.

Unlike his earlier works, *The Sisters Materassi* is a novel, not some sort of allegorical or frothy tale: it has a beginning, a middle, and an end, and a tenuous plot. The pace of the book and the direction it takes are suggested in the opening pages, with a reference to the fact that it was in the proximity of the place where the story takes place that Giovanni Boccaccio wrote his *Decameron*. The reference, complete with a quotation from the *Decameron*, is part of the strategy of our novelist, whose style, particularly in the book's first chapters, has an undeniable Boccaccioesque flavor to it, with its rich, leisurely rhythm, indicative of the fact that the author has nowhere to go. (We might think of Dante's *Comedy*, with its urgency, its purposefulness, its well-defined objectives as a suitable contrast.) But, while like Boccaccio, we feel Palazzeschi's *"gioia del raccontare,"* (the "pleasure of storytelling"), we must also be aware of the fact that the spirit animating the two writers could hardly be more different: Boccaccio preaches no lesson, favors no special way of life, except one of generosity and liberality of the spirit: his stories are in praise of the resourcefulness, cunning, and wit that permit men and women alike to enjoy life, touch and be touched by human emotions as fully as possible. In Palazzeschi, on the other hand, behind the appearance of fun and nonchalance, there is an implicit criticism of middle-class values and of the ways with which people deliberately allow themselves to be used by other human beings—all in the name of "love." Perhaps here is the most critical point of Palazzeschi's novels, for love is invariably presented in its most bizarre ways: the almost incestuous love of the Materassi sisters for their nephew, the love of Remo for Palle, with a hint of homosexuality suggested by the fact that the two sleep in the same bed (elsewhere we learn that Remo sleeps nude), the sensual love of Niobe for Remo, usually satisfied by voyeurism, the unhappy love of Augusta for her husband. There is no instance in the novel—as there is none in the others by Palazzeschi —of a happy, tender, satisfying love: even when Remo becomes engaged to Peggy, there is no acknowledgment as to the meaning of a significant relationship. When asked by his aunts whether he loves Peggy, Remo exclaims: "'In love! . . . Ah! Ah! Ah! . . . indeed, of course, of course I love her, no question.' . . . That word 'love,' had such a different meaning for him and for them, that provoked laughter when speaking about it, and he could not resist from laughting about it with all sincerity: 'Yes, of course . . . Ah! Ah!'"

What about Palazzeschi's own attitude toward his themes and characters? He can be sympathetic without being too involved, compassionate without being uncritical. He manages to look at human follies and cruelties and see the pathos of life through the unnecessary pain man inflicts on his fellowmen. He is at times guilty of making caricatures of his personages, and accept the inevitability of suffering so long as there is some beauty in the world—the godlike beauty of a Remo's splendid, angelic physique, the sensitivity of a Valentino Core, the innate goodness of Perelà. Through his detached stance, and a humor that culminates in *The Sisters Materassi* in the joyful "Ah! Ah!" with which the book comes to an end, Palazzeschi has succeeded at least in giving us a glimpse of the rationality and irrationality of human beings. And the expression of laughter represents, in essence, the only real judgment he wishes to make on the decade that brought love, tears, and havoc to the unforgettable Materassi sisters. "His outlook on life," writes Thomas G. Bergin, "seems to combine that of a small boy at a circus (and probably one who has sneaked under the canvas) with that of a sage who knows that wisdom begins but does not necessarily stop at melancholy."

3

The "Southern" Novel

"The depth and intensity of the problem of the Italian South must be seen to be believed." Roughly a third of the country, the lower end of the peninsula, which is usually called the *"Mezzogiorno,"* has suffered for centuries "a condition of severe economic depression and social distress," so wrote an eminent historian recently. Yet, despite an incredible social and economic backwardness that has long plagued the South, the region has produced, in what is surely one of the most puzzling anomalies of Italian history, a wealth of artists—painters, poets, philosophers, playwrights, sculptors, musicians, and, in recent decades, novelists.

The tradition of the Southern novel goes back to the second half of the nineteenth century. Indeed, a large share of Italian fiction of that period is "regional," which is to say, set in specific locales that play a prominent part in the plot, often to the point of making it inconceivable that the story could have taken place anywhere else. In the case of the better novelists, Giovanni Verga and Luigi Pirandello among them, their themes have an unmistakable universal ring: the hunger and nobility of character of Verga's Malavoglias, the pettiness and humanity of the inhabitants of Aci Trezza, the pessimism and introspection of Pirandello's characters—victims of social prejudice and persecution know no boundaries—are at once local and universal. It is to the credit of the many Southern writers who have followed Verga and Pirandello, that they have succeeded not only in creating stories full of insights into the conditions of poverty, exploitation, hunger, but also works that have placed on the table some of the burning issues of our time for everyone to study and understand.

In this sense, at least, literature has proven to be a most convincing instrument of "knowledge."

It should be made clear that interest in the *Mezzogiorno* has not been limited to novelists. Since the end of World War II, a score of poets and essayists (Carlo Levi, Danilo, Dolci and Rocco Scotellaro among them), have explored many of the problems of the South. By the same token, many writers born in the North (Pavese, Ottieri) have composed novels with Southern settings, while still others, born in the South (Vittorini, for example) have preserved a deep attachment to their native towns in the South without writing Southern fiction exclusively.

The three novelists chosen for inclusion in this chapter, may be said to represent three different tendencies of the Italian "Southern novel." Corrado Alvaro, journalist, poet, essayist and novelist, was born in Calabria and, by and large, wrote in the tradition of the nineteenth-century master Giovanni Verga; Vitaliano Brancati, born in Sicily, distinguished himself for the humor and biting satire with which he gave concrete form in his books to certain aspects of life in the *Mezzogiorno*; Giuseppe Tomasi di Lampedusa, a member of an aristocratic Sicilian family, wrote only one book in his lifetime, leaving it "unfinished" in the sense that he had no opportunity to revise his novel, as he died of cancer in a Roman clinic, still awaiting the response of the publishing houses that were considering and debating the merits of *The Leopard*.

Given the diverse background of these three writers, it is not surprising that their different interests and concerns should be lucidly reflected in their writing. Alvaro's strong moral sense, his sensitivity toward the backward, unjust conditions stoically endured by the peasants, shepherds, and working people of the South, and the prospect of violence as a way to correct the grave injustices perpetuated by the ruling class, constitute the flesh and blood of his writing. Vitaliano Brancati, a bourgeois in fact but not in persuasion, dedicated himself to depicting the boredom, laziness, and *"gallismo"* of a bankrupt middle class. Lampedusa, for his part, centered on the fateful decades that followed the political unification of the nation, and concentrated his attention on the traumas of having to adjust to a new social and political reality.

Corrado Alvaro: The Tradition of "Verismo"

I must say that I have never aspired to the reputation of being a Southern writer, and I hope that this is proven by the work I have produced up to now. In other words, I have never, save in the proper place, in a few articles and essays, set out to cast light on the conditions of my region, Calabria, or to illustrate its more or less current problems. I have never intended to engage myself socially, but rather to depict reality and to find a poetic, that is literary, dimension.

These words, excerpted from an essay entitled "Fitting into the Present," are eloquent and clear in their definition of how Alvaro sees his own place in the history of his native culture.

Alvaro was born on April 15, 1895, in a small village of San Luca, in the southernmost region of Calabria. He received his early education in Jesuit boarding schools in Rome and Umbria, completed his secondary studies at Catanzaro, and received his university degree in Milan, in 1919. After serving as an officer in World War I, he began his career as a journalist. His first books, *Poesie grigioverdi* [Graygreen poems] (1917), the color reference is to the army uniform, *La siepe e l'orto* [The edge and the truckgarden] (1920), *L'uomo nel labirinto* [Man in the labyrinth] (1926)—all failed to attract much attention, a situation that changed with the publication of *L'annata alla finestra* [A year at the window] (1929) and *Gente in Aspromonte* (1930; *Revolt in Aspromonte*, N.Y., 1962) which, together with *La signora dell' isola* [The lady of the island] (1930) and *Vent'anni* [Twenty years] (1930) were awarded the coveted Stampa Prize by a jury that included the future Nobel laureate Luigi Pirandello. Newspaper assignments took Alvaro to countries both near and far from his own: Germany, Greece, Turkey, France, and the Soviet Union, the last of which inspired his volume *I maestri del diluvio* [The masters of the deluge] (1935). In 1940, he won the Italian Academy Prize for his entire work; in 1951 further recognition came to him with the award of the Strega Prize for his autobiographical *Quasi una vita* [Almost a lifetime] (1950). He continued being a prolific writer until his death, on June 11, 1956. Among his fiction, *L'età breve* [The brief age] (1946) and *L'uomo è forte* (1938; *Man Is Strong*, N.Y., 1948) are regarded as outstanding.

The bulk of Alvaro's literary production, which ranges all the way from autobiography and poetry to essays and fiction, is often rooted in his native Calabria, particularly his own *paese*, the village where he grew up and which left such an impression on his sensibility. His more mature work, on the other hand, reveals a shift of emphasis to the meaning of the encounter of a Southern intellectual with the bureaucratic civilization of the North, more specifically, that of Baroque and decadent Rome—thus following a trajectory that moves in the opposite direction to that of Giovanni Verga's final and greatest phase of his literary creativity. Verga's masterworks, *I Malavoglia*, *Mastro-don Gesualdo*, and the unforgettable stories of *Vita dei campi* pervasively influenced the character and scope of Alvaro's Southern novels, with a major exception: the role the city plays in the development of the stories of the two writers, and the meanings and implications it acquires could hardly be more different. In Verga, the city is portrayed as a temptress that lures and finally corrupts the young generation, uprooting it from its home nest and ultimately contributing to its tragic downfall. In Alvaro's work, the city, with all its Babelian aspects, comes to represent the ultimate conquest for his characters, engaged in their special search for the pot of gold at the end of the rainbow. The difference in the vision of the two artists is larger than it may appear at first: in Verga's stories the choice between *paese* and *città* is made on sentimental and ethical grounds and becomes a matter of allegiance to the time-honored tradition of the "home." In Alvaro's stories, the choice is a telling sign that the world does not begin and end with our native town. The question is no longer a matter of belief in, and respect for, certain traditions, but a conscious realization of changing economic conditions and of the opportunities offered by the mushrooming industries in the northern regions of a politically united nation.

By general critical consensus, *Gente in Aspromonte* remains, despite the passing of time, Alvaro's masterpiece, the most persuasive, moving book he wrote in his four and one-half decades of literary creativity. Much like Verga's *I Malavoglia*, the story centers on the difficult life led by a small family in Calabria and on their constant struggle to survive the adversities that threaten, and ultimately destroy, their modest dreams. The opening of the book has a markedly muted almost tragic tone about it:

It is no easy life, that of the shepherds of Aspromonte, in the dead of winter when swollen streams rush down to the sea and the earth seems to float on the water. The shepherds stay in huts built of mud and sticks and sleep beside the animals. They go about in long capes with triangular hoods over their shoulders such as might have been worn by an ancient Greek God setting out upon a winter pilgrimage. The torrential streams make a deafening noise and in the clearings, amid the white snow, big black tubs, set over wood fires, steam with boiling milk curdled by a greenish ferment and a handful of wild herbs. The men standing around in their black capes and black wool suits are the only living beings among the dark surrounding mountains and the stiffly frozen trees. But even in this icy cold the nuts are ripening under the oak bark for the future delight of rooting pigs.

To a considerable extent, the shepherds are at the mercy of nature; water is possibly one of the most important factors in their harsh existence, followed by the danger posed by the terrain to which the animals are exposed when grazing on the rocky mountains. It is not infrequently that some of the animals fall into a gully, and their meat must be sold at once by the shepherds so as to recover at least part of the loss sustained.

Protagonists of the story are Argirò and his son Antonello. One day, the two set out to try to get a bank loan that will permit them to purchase and till a small plot of land, while their other parcel is allowed to rest for a year. As fate would have it, on that very day four of the animals (whose co-owner is Filippo Mezzatesta) are lost when they fall into a gully. Filippo will have none of Argirò's explanations of the accident and serves notice that he expects to receive all the money realized from the sale of the meat, including what normally would be Argirò's share. This last indignity persuades Argirò that he will never work for someone else again. With the help of Camillo Mezzatesta (Filippo's brother), a well-known usurer, he purchases some land, but bad weather destroys its harvest. The one remaining hope for his family's future is to send his youngest son, Benedetto, away to school at a seminary, and prepare himself for the priesthood. Education is quite expensive and the oldest son, Antonello, is sent away to work with a construction gang: his earnings are sent to the family so that his father's dream may come true. After the tragedy of his farm, Argirò buys a mule and becomes a private carter. Just as he is getting back on his feet, thanks to his hard work, three children, youngsters of Pirria (Camillo Mezzatesta's mistress) set the stall, where the mule is kept, on fire and the animal is burned alive. The motivation of this dastardly act is pure envy, as Argirò sees it: "Fortune is blind and envy has eyes to see. That is the way people are made—they can't bear to see someone else get on." To add insult to injury, Camillo's children, with Andreuccio as their leader, parade "about the square holding a mock mule's funeral, one of them pretending to be the tearful Argirò." "Argirò watched them without understanding, saying over and over to himself: 'Oh, the pain they've given me! Is there no end to man's cruelty!'"

The new misfortune adds more pressure to the already precarious economic situation of the family: Antonello now sends his whole salary to his father, but, physically weak and sickly, loses his job and returns home. Much matured by his experiences away from his village, he is no longer willing to accept the gross inequalities of the social system into which he was born. The stage is now set for the final act of the tragedy: only violence is seen as the instrument that can change the order of things:

The evening was dark and gloomy, with signs of a coming storm. There were flashing red lights in the sky like those that usually came in September, and it looked as if the downpour would flood the newly sprouted wheat. In this part of the country the rain can be an enemy of man. The rain that began that night continued to fall for several days, as if to tell Argirò that even if his mule were still alive, the roads would be impassable. It seemed as if the rain would never stop, and its endlessness dulled the edge of Argirò's sorrow as he stared at it listlessly like a prisoner staring at the bars of his prison.

Antonello's days as an honest, hard-working person are over. He turns into a brigand who slaughters Filippo Mezzatesta's herds, gives away the animal's meat, pillages his harvests, burns his precious land—all this while most of the villagers, held at Filippo's mercy for so long, refuse to come to his aid and indeed enjoy the spectacle of the fire voraciously destroying what had been valuable property. Filippo Mezzatesta himself comes down from the mountains where he has waged a courageous but hopeless fight to save his property from total destruction, his eyes lost and two streams of blood rushing down his cheeks. Justice, or the kind of justice the villagers welcome because it appears in the guise of fair retribution for past wrongs, has been done. Now at last Antonello can meekly surrender to the authorities—his violence has satisfied the villagers' anger. "When he saw the gleam of the carabinieri's caps and their guns pointing at him from behind the trees, he threw down his only weapon and stepped forward to greet them. 'At last,' he said, 'I have met Justice face to face. It's taken me long enough to meet Her.'"

The English translation of the book makes an ideological point the title in the original did not make. Indeed, it is questionable whether Alvaro himself would have wanted the word "Revolt" to appear on the book's cover during a period when the Fascist regime was making so much of its ability to restore "law and order" in a nation beleaguered by internal unrest and discontent. Yet, the novel's message is clear in proposing violence as the one effective instrument capable of changing an odious social order, and submit the values of the establishment to stringent tests challenging their fairness and justice. This notwithstanding, another central question is left begging: if we admit that changing the structure and values of an unjust society is a highly desirable goal, can such a goal be achieved by the terrorist acts of a lone individual, without arousing the consciousness of the peasantry (and the working class) to the point of making inevitable their becoming actively involved, rather than remaining silent spectators, in the struggle against the middle class and the landowners? What is the meaning of the villagers' willingness to accept as a gift the meat of the animals slaughtered by Antonello or killed in the fire that has devastated Mezzatesta's property?

By a remarkable coincidence, in another country, Switzerland, another writer, who was to achieve world prominence, was writing a book with a theme similar to that of *Revolt in Aspromonte*. His name was Secondo Tranquilli, his nom de plume Ignazio Silone: his novel, *Fontamara*, (1930; N.Y., 1960) was to appear in a German and English translation long before it could be published in the original Italian. *Fontamara* has been called a political novel: it tells of the exploitation and hardships endured for centuries by the inhabitants of a small town after which the book is titled, "Bitter Fountain." The novel, remarkable for the simplicity of its theme and form is framed in terms of the old struggle of the city (or landed gentry, the governments, and the bureaucratic apparatus through which the villagers' lives are controlled) and the *cafoni* (the peasants who till the soil, and who must submit to the injustices of the rich and the powerful). What happens in the course of the story produces an awareness that nothing will ever change unless the *cafoni* join forces with all dispossessed and working people to fight the miserable conditions they have endured for far too long. The goal, then, is the formation of a militant force capable of bringing about change—by violence, if necessary. Since politics is a way of life, life itself must be politicized: the masses must be educated politically, led (and this is a most important aspect) by leaders developed by the masses themselves, and not, as in the past, by the bourgeoisie. After all, is it not the bourgeoisie that has set up the standards, the values and the structure socio-political-economic the peasants are struggling to change?

None of these implications are part of the narrative or thematic fabric of Alvaro's novel, in which the central theme receives a conventional structural treatment. Once again, the landowners exploit the peasants and no amount of suffering seems to have any effect: things do not change at all, and when they do it is only as the result of the actions of a man gone berserk, actions that are ultimately unproductive, since the destruction of property brings only temporary relief to an anger that will be passed on from one generation to the next.

The novel is, in every respect, in the best tradition of *"verismo."* Its language is simple, direct, and yet poetic. Southern society is painted in somber colors: the rich are presented as unmovable bastions of power, devoid of understanding of and compassion toward poverty; the others—the shepherds and the peasants—are hopelessly weak, silently accepting the traditional relationship with the landowners; the country is hard, the city a beautiful, enviable heaven filled with every comfort, even if it does not enjoy the pleasure of savouring the fruits of the land with quite the same joy as the peasants. But this is a small consolation indeed; injustice is evident everywhere: in the way the peasants are treated, in the hardships imposed on Antonello so that Benedetto can be educated and move up the social ladder, in the way he must struggle in school he has entered without adequate preparation, in the exploitation of Pirria (Camillo Mezzatesta's mistress), in the many setbacks and sorrow (which include two deaf-mute sons) Argirò must endure, including the derogative nickname "Pumpkinhead." With all this, Argirò retains his dignity and pride, as does his family, even in the moments of disappointment and sadness. There are tears and cries to be sure, and there is pain that at times cannot be contained. But, as in Verga's *I Malavoglia*, there is strength and a stubborn resolve to persevere in the human search for a good, honest life—a dream that just will not be. As in Verga's *I Malavoglia*, once the first accident takes place, there is no way the tragedy can be stopped from unraveling: one remedy follows another, to no avail, for the end is predictable almost to its last detail. The fabric of the family unravels almost mercilessly: the departure of his son to school makes Argirò proud, but also avoided by his envious peers, and in the end rejected by his very son; Antonello, whose help makes possible the financing of his younger brother's schooling, comes home only to take revenge on a cruel society by way of his violence. But, while the novel follows the pattern of events of Verga's masterpiece, it also offers a new insight into the ideological form and structure of Southern society. Antonello's brother is sent away to school, because, as Gramsci remarked apropos of Pirandello's theatre, "there is no 'mechanism' that can raise life from a provincial level to a collectively national and European one." The awareness is in sharp contrast with traditional thinking on this issue: in Alvaro's book, the school diploma is turned into the very weapon by which someday Benedetto (and, by extension, the educated peasant) "will be able to humiliate the powerful," as Giuliano Manacorda persuasively suggests in his essay on our novelist.

A passage early in the book reveals the depth of his understanding of the way in which historical developments have and will continue to change the South:

Just as mummies fall into dust when they come into contact with the air, so this ancient way of life is breaking up as it comes into touch with something new. We have here a disappearing civilization. Let us not weep over its eclipse, but, if we were born into it, let us store up in our memory as much of it as we can. The liberation of the Kingdom of the Two Sicilies superseded an order of things that had been established for centuries, and the redistribution of feudal property not only increased some already swollen private fortunes. This village remained what it had been from time immemorial, a cluster of one-story rustic houses on earth foundations with fireplaces hewed out of natural rock—all built around one nobleman's palace, with its gates, stables, gardens, kitchen and servants. The common people's interests and struggles centered about this palace, near the church, for it was the focal point of all the wealth, all the good and evil of the village.

In the context of the tradition of the "regionalistic" novel, the novelty of the passage just quoted is undeniable: unlike Verga, Alvaro is capable of giving his work a more clearly explicit historical dimension, without making it a historical novel, as De Roberto had done in *The Viceroys*. Alvaro's conceives the artist as "a man who has the power to write harmoniously about life," and adds: "Pain is for the artist the key that opens all doors." Thanks to his creativity and power of synthesis, the artist, having witnessed an important event, gives it life and meaning, preserving it on the printed page for posterity. The society depicted by Alvaro in *Revolt in Aspromonte* is a closed one, permits no failures, respects only success. The equation is unacceptable to our writer: he looks for understanding and compassion, even though he knows how rarely society exhibits them. "A primitive and at the same time an intellectual," wrote Emilio Cecchi many years ago, by which he meant, if I read him correctly, a man deeply rooted in the primitive character of civilization of his native Calabria and yet capable of understanding intellectually, as well as poetically, his "world."

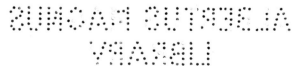

Vitaliano Brancati: Regional Fabulist?

"Would-be moralist and master of the 'baroque' and 'grotesque' prose style . . . far more than a merely regional writer," claims Claire Licari Huffman; "not an intellectual animal . . . Brancati had the breadth of a great writer without [his] intellectual power of articulation," notes Angelo Guglielmi; "a 'witness' of the spiritual and moral failings of Italy under Fascism and in the immediate post-war years," remarks Louis Tenenbaum. Over two decades after his death on September 25, 1954, Brancati's place in the history of the contemporary Italian novel is still the subject of considerable debate among the critics. Such failure is rooted in the complexity of his work as well as in its unevenness, both which are, in turn, traceable to the personal and political schisms that characterized his existence as well as the intellectual uneasiness that victimized him.

Vitaliano Brancati was born in the small town of Pachino, near Syracuse, on July 24, 1907. His father was a civil service employee clearly ill at ease with Fascist authorities, a difficulty that was to prove financially and morally costly, particularly when he was displaced from his position in Catania and reassigned to a minor post in the prefecture of Caltanisetta. Growing up in Sicily has never been easy: the island's social structure and its severe and archaic traditions are hard to bear; its sexual mores are antiquated and repressive; culturally (and here is a rub, considering the impressive number of first-rate men of letters Sicily has produced, from Verga to Pirandello, from Lampedusa to Vittorini) the island has always felt to be outside the mainstream of artistic creativity of the "mainland." Brancati belongs to the generation brought up under fascism, a generation that includes Alberto Moravia, Elio Vittorini, Cesare Pavese, and Vasco Pratolini, among others. Much like many of his contemporary fellow-artists, Brancati grew up as an admirer of d'Annunzio and a believer in the bold commitment of a social revolution made by the Fascists. Eventually, he, too, understood that the alliance of the party with the middle class, the industrialists, and the Church would never allow a radical change in the economic structure of the country to take place, and broke with fascism in the early thirties. Attracted to literature (his father had written poetry and was a talented lecturer), Brancati began his career by writing several plays, and published his first novel in 1932, *L'amico del vincitore* [The friend of the winner]. He finished his university studies at Catania, with a thesis on the Southern novelist Federico De Roberto—a choice not without its ironic cultural-political implications—and followed the route of other Sicilian intellectuals to the "continent" (mainland Italy) and its opportunities. He was fortunate in having good connections who, like himself, were Sicilians and favorably disposed toward their *paesani*; their friendship opened new doors in the labyrinthian maze of the publishing world. The journey to the North was to have other, and central, consequences. Not only was Brancati exposed to another world, the world of Fascist corruption, but to the ideas and ideals of two men who were instrumental in changing his political and literary orientation: Giuseppe Antonio Borgese, critic, writer, and professor of aesthetics who was to leave Italy in 1933 after he had refused to sign a loyalty oath to the Fascist party, and Benedetto Croce, whose career and work Brancati idolized until his death.

By 1935, Brancati's break with fascism and its culture was complete. The change of political posture was to carry a heavy price. Again and again, Brancati's books were ordered withdrawn from circulation by the Fascist censor, obviously sensitive to, and annoyed by, Brancati's implicit criticism of many social institutions held sacred by the government.

The mature phase of Brancati's literary career begins in the mid-thirties, and coincides with the change of his political posture noted above. With several books behind him, he set himself to compose *Gli anni perduti* [The wasted years], completing it in 1936, after two years' work. Serialized in the magazine *Omnibus* in 1938, the novel, by and large, has been unjustly treated by his critics. Claire Huffman, in her sensitive assessment of our author, calls it "the true turning point in Brancati's artistic, and not merely political, development," a view with which I agree completely. The setting of the novel is the imaginary city of Nataca, a persuasive geographic and social recreation of Catania (spelled backward). The first nine chapters serve to introduce us to a group of young men who have been away to the "mainland," and, having returned home, are so disillusioned by the slow, provincial, unbearably boring life there that they begin making plans to go back North as soon as circumstances will permit. The hero of the story, Leonardo Barini, returns to Sicily because he is nostalgic about his birthplace, but regrets his decision almost as soon as he has carried it out. This is something of a recurrent theme in the work of Brancati, built upon the contrast, and thus contrasting forces, between the North (sophisticated, efficient, open) and the South (repressive, apathetic, closed). Today, such a comparison would be considered justifiably stereotyped. Sicilians can be astute, aggressive, and resourceful; they are also (as depicted by Giovanni Verga and so many of his "followers") hardworking, generous, honest, and very much conscious of their roots. But Brancati's world turns on a different axis, specifically that of the comfortable middle class that spends much of its time fantasizing about afternoon siestas and sex.

In the case of the group of *Gli anni perduti*, an unusual dream is introduced: the building of a tower from which the tourists and the natives will be able to enjoy the magnificent view of the surroundings, a proposal that comes from a certain professor Buscaino, and thus, by virtue of its intellectual sponsor, deemed most worthwhile pursuing. The suggestion is accepted, and some thirteen years later, after overcoming all sorts of difficulties and delays, the project is completed. The end of the story is quite unusual: the tower cannot be opened to the public, and indeed must be demolished, because it violates city ordinances no one bothered to take into account; all that will remain, as a memory of the undertaking, will be a heap of rubble and dust! Ridiculous? Perhaps. But, when seen from a more Olympian perspective, aren't many actions of men absurd and laughable? It may well be that the failure of the project is presented too covertly as one doomed to fail because of the ineptness of its sponsors (all Sicilians), and as such limited in its commentary about human nature in general. However one might choose to see it, it does manage to open the curtain on the motifs that are central in the narrative of Brancati: apathy, indolence, laziness, and a certain sense of futility—conditions presented as being deeply ingrained in the temperament of Sicilians, seldom willing or ready to change their existence.

If the novel is read against the background of Brancati's personal and political evolution, however, the tower can well be seen as a phallic symbol typical of fascism (which the novelist was repudiating in those years); large and no doubt impressive, it is incapable of performing its most basic function! Seen from yet another angle, the long undertaking of building the tower serves as a metaphor of the stuff of which human dreams are made: it is an expression of the understandable human wish to create something that will survive its builders and become a legacy to future generations. An illusion it may well be, but how appropriate that the story should end with the demolition of the tower, and the symbolic consignment of the project to a heap of rubble and dust, an ironic disposal of a dream manufactured by Fascist mentality!

The central "problems" of *Gli anni perduti* reveal the extent of Brancati's debt to the poet Giacomo Leopardi and to the novelist-playwright Luigi Pirandello. Man can escape boredom and forget time by his becoming involved in projects whose difficulties absorb his mind and sap his energy, and thus be spared the metaphysical awareness of the pain of existence. Deep down, man also knows that such compromises are nothing if not illusions, which help us create a special niche in which we may feel relatively safe and protected from the cruelty of human actions. Yet another major theme, sex and eroticism, emerges and blossoms in Brancati's successive novels, constituting a sort of "Trittico Siciliano": *Don Giovanni in Sicilia* [Don Juan in Sicily] (1941); *Il bell'Antonio* (1949; *Antonio the Great Lover*, N.Y., 1952); and *Paolo il caldo* [Paolo the hot one] (1954), left unfinished when Brancati died in 1954, and published a year later, accompanied by a long Preface by Alberto Moravia, Brancati's long-time friend. The theme that links the three novels is *"gallismo."*

Just exactly what is *gallismo*? Taken in its most obvious manifestations, *gallismo*, or "roosterism," is a combination of male exhibitionism and exuberance, conveying the idea of sexual aggressiveness that may be real or imagined. Practiced by men young and mature alike, roosterism is frequently an attitude toward, or even a way of, life, with its rituals and strategies to be employed in amorous adventures, its obsession with women, its constant discussions about past, present, or future sexual exploits —to the point of being turned into a kind of symbol of a way of life. Last, but not least, roosterism accompanies men from their adolescence to old age, becoming a needed crutch for sexual insecurity or a much needed booster for battered or sagging egos, particularly convenient to cover up sexual impotence. Brancati himself, in a survey of the South commissioned by an important newspaper in the immediate post–World War II years, wrote: "[Gallismo] is considered the most noble and heroic act of life. One can be a thief, or flee before the enemy, lie, flatter, bend to tyranny . . . but the act for which one will never be forgiven is that of one's not having sufficiently respected . . . one's own dignity as a rooster."

It would be wrong to think that roosterism is simply an invention of writers or observers of the social scene. On the contrary, it is firmly rooted in the history of Sicily, dating back to the Arab domination and the strict separation of the sexes. The woman was relegated to a position of inferiority, forbidden to have any contact with members of the opposite sex without the most rigid supervision, with little or no voice in choosing her husband, usually if not always selected for her by her parents for economic, social, or political reasons. For centuries the woman in Sicily has been regarded as a mixture of the divine and the diabolical: the bearer of our children, regarded since the Middle Ages as a kind of angel who leads Man to salvation and Heaven, she can also distract us, tempt us, and cause our perdition. Man hardly enjoys a more comforting condition: torn by his respect for the sanctity of sex for the purpose of procreation, and by the temptation of the flesh, he frequently turns to houses of prostitution or to married women to satisfy his sexual needs. These, and other factors, tend to make of the sexual experience something forbidden outside the marriage, and as such, particularly tempting and desirable. If Brancati had limited himself to writing about roosterism, he would have been just another humorous writer. His originality rests not so much on his uncanny ability to depict *gallismo* with a firm hand and a considerable amount of feeling, but on his connecting it, as Claire Huffman observed, with "the questions that this phenomenon raises: . . . the great human questions concerning the nature of honor, love, happiness, fantasy and reality." With *Don Giovanni in Sicilia*, a mordant satire of the social and sexual mores in Sicily, Brancati felicitously blends the erotic motif of his earlier work with that of contemporary politics: roosterism and fascism are now presented as two sides of the same coin.

The hero of the story is Giovanni Percolla who, for the previous ten years, has lived with his three unmarried sisters, Rosa, Barbara, and Lucia. The opening situation reminds us immediately of Aldo Palazzeschi's *Le sorelle Materassi* (*The Sisters Materassi*): here, too, we have three good, honest spinsters pampering a man who is the substitute figure for the husband they never had. The pleasant, easygoing relationship they have enjoyed for many years is due, to a large extent, to the love and care they have given their brother, ever since the day when, upon the death of their parents, they were recalled home from their grandfather's with whom the three had been living. Giovanni finds himself spending long periods of time in the mainland, ostensibly on business or on vacation, but really trying, together with his best friends Scannapieco and Muscara, to educate himself sexually. Many of the first chapters of the book—the best of the work—depict in gentle, mocking way Giovanni's bashfulness toward women, his excitement at the sight of feminine undergarments, his frequent sessions with his friends talking about sex and women, and last, his adventures with prostitutes. "On the other hand," comments Brancati at one point, "if their experience of pleasure was enormous, that of women was extremely poor. Undressed of the lies, of what they told as having taken place and that had instead been only a wish, or had happened to someone else, their and Don Giovanni's past could be told in ten minutes. Shall we say it clearly? At the age of thirty-six, Giovanni Percolla had never kissed an honest girl . . . had neither written nor received a love letter, and the telephone receiver had never caressed his ear with the word 'my love.'"

After an extended sojourn in the North, where he has gone for business reasons, Giovanni returns home and one day the inevitable takes place: he falls in love (or so he thinks, at least) with an attractive girl from a fine family, Maria Antonietta dei Marconella. The event marks an important change in his lifestyle: for one thing, he breaks from his friends, whom he now deems vulgar and insensitive, and, for another, he decides to take his own apartment (a handsome villa in the outskirts of Catania). His sisters, who worship him, are baffled by the changes in his behavior: why should he want to bathe more than once a week, or why should he object to their cleaning drinking glasses with the ashes of the stove (where the cat urinates!), or become so fastidious in other ways? Unlike Palazzeschi's Remo, who mercilessly exploits his aunts and drives them to bankruptcy, Giovanni reassures them that he intends to continue his financial support—a commitment he honors as promised.

The depiction of Giovanni's love for Ninetta allows Brancati to touch other aspects of *gallismo*. While Giovanni fantasizes about his falling in love with Ninetta in a romantic way, it is really she who leads him to the altar and, as though this were not enough, stipulates in advance the numerous concessions she will enjoy after the marriage ceremony. They consist of what at first she calls the "five freedoms," one for each finger of the hand: the freedom to go out unescorted; to go skiing every year; to go on a trip every year; to go horseback riding; the freedom to take full charge of furnishing and decorating their home according to her taste, "because the woman is the queen of the house." Further concessions are easily won by Ninetta: the right to subscribe to a Swiss magazine; the right to use Elizabeth Arden beauty products. . . .

Shortly after their marriage, the newlyweds decide to move to Milan, where Giovanni gradually becomes "de-Sicilianized," welcomes men of letters to his apartment, enjoys the company of artists and professional people. The couple's stay in Milan is brief, even though Giovanni is at least partially successful in making do in terms of his earning a living and coping socially. And a short-lived love "affair" with a lovely, young woman (Eleonora Lascasas) almost threatens his marriage. Shortly after Ninetta announces that she will give him a child, the two agree to return to Catania, on a brief visit which turns out to be longer than either had anticipated. As the novel comes to a close, we find Giovanni back in his sisters' home enjoying the overlong afternoon nap that reminds him of bygone days, while his wife is visiting with her family. The story has come full circle: nothing has really changed, and perhaps it cannot be any other way. Anticlimactic the end surely is: but if Brancati means what he says, then it befits a book that shows that, for all the exposure to a different social milieu, Giovanni remains very much the "Sicilian" he was before his marriage. Since it is impossible to refashion his personality, he concludes that the two will be better off staying with their respective families as long as they remain in Catania!

The simplicity of the novel is somewhat deceptive, for at least two important points are advanced by the book: the first is that it is exceedingly difficult to break certain social and philosophical patterns embedded in the consciousness and life-style of a people since time immemorial. Almost twenty years later, the same point is made with greater intellectual lucidity and ideological depth by yet another Sicilian novelist, Giuseppe Tomasi di Lampedusa, in his masterwork, *The Leopard*. The second point is only obliquely made: the protagonist of the story is presented as an antihero, thus defying the wishes of the Fascist regime, weak, indolent, and apathetic, totally lacking the aggressiveness that was one of the party's chief characteristics. The main character is skillfully used by Brancati to paint an effective canvas of Sicilian manners. The chief element of the author's strategy is what may be called Pirandellian humor, whose objective is not to ridicule or to make us laugh, but to evoke understanding and compassion. The technique is based on the conflict between reality and appearances. Thus, Giovanni, portrayed as "good, serious, cosmopolitan," soon is seen by the reader for what he really is: weak, lazy, devoid of ambitions and ideas, capable only of fantasizing about love affairs that never get off the ground. Comic he may be to a point: for we realize that the culture into which he was born and educated is largely responsible for molding his character.

Il bell'Antonio (*Antonio the Great Lover*, N.Y., 1952) belongs to Brancati's second, mature period. Written in 1948, in a climate of hope after the end of World War II and of fascism, published in several installments in the weekly political-cultural periodical *Il mondo*, winner of the prestigious Bagutta Prize, *Il bell'Antonio* is the last novel completed by Brancati. The novel takes up, once more, the theme of *gallismo*, fortified by a political motif, this time explicitly presented. The novel is told by a "*cronista*," or a newspaperman covering city stories, whose professional scruples impel him to be as accurate and objective as possible.

The action is set in 1932, when its hero, Antonio Magnano, is twenty-six. The choice of the time is significant for it coincides with the moment when fascism completed its takeover of power at all levels. Antonio's main asset is his extraordinary physical beauty: ironically enough, it is his handsomeness that proves to be the element that eventually brings out his tragic flaw. Antonio's problems begin early in life: at the age of sixteen, he is accused by a young servant girl of having made love to her—an accusation she quickly withdraws. As Antonio grows up, his sexual magnetism proves to be irresistible. At age twenty-six, his photographs are exhibited in the fashionable Piazza di Spagna, in Rome. After having obtained his university degree, Antonio takes a job, working for the government (his family has moved back to Catania), with a brilliant career ahead. But one day he is almost seduced by a young girl, Luisa Dehler, daughter of an ambassador. At the suggestion of his uncle, Ermenegildo, he decides to go back to Sicily, so as to avoid possible future unpleasant incidents.

Shortly after his return home, his father suggests that he marry Barbara Puglisi, a girl from an affluent local family. Actually, Antonio's father Alfio points out, Barbara "is rich, she loves you, and she is honest." After a suitable period of engagement, the marriage, duly arranged by the respective families, takes place. Three years later, the couple is yet to be blessed by the birth of any offspring, and no one, especially Signor Alfio, is especially happy, let alone proud, of it. But an even more shocking revelation is yet to follow: Barbara's father informs Alfio that his daughter is still a virgin! Since the marriage, in the eyes of the Church, has not been consummated, it must be dissolved. Barbara soon afterwards is wedded to the duke of Bronte, while Antonio, still in love with her, returns to live with his family, and finds in his uncle Ermenegildo an understanding and compassionate consoler. But Signor Alfio finds it difficult to live under the terrible cloud of his son's sexual failure. One evening, in 1943, he ends up in a brothel which is hit during an air raid, and is killed. His death is viewed as a way to erase, however partially, the black mark that Antonio's sexual impotence had made on the family's honor and pride.

The story ends in an anticlimatic if not sordid note: Antonio returns to Catania, expecting to find his home destroyed by the aerial bombardments to which the city has been subjected. Instead, not only does he find his home intact, but in the process of being cleaned up and straightened out by a maidservant, to whom Antonio, in a dream, makes love.

What is the "point" of the novel? The message of *Antonio the*

Great Lover is, with some modest changes, the same Brancati makes in his previous work: eroticism considered per se, is clear evidence of the spiritual and emotional emptiness of a human being, a façade shielding a repressive political system. Under such circumstances, proving oneself a man becomes a meaningless exercise in futility. Robert Dombroski's comments are pertinent here: "Here rather than existing side by side the erotic becomes fused with the latter giving rise to the obvious analogy between sexual and political impotency. Antonio Magnano, a young Sicilian Adonis, has the frame of being an irresistible conqueror of women, whereas in reality he is actually impotent. . . . But after three years of marriage, the bond has yet to be consummated. . . . Then the regime falls and the war ends. The novel ends with Antonio desperately obsessed to at least prove himself a man. Applied to the [Fascist] regime, the analogy would go something like this: one who is impotent (fascism) but believed to be potent because it enjoys the favours of the various individually potent (those who benefited by it). Thus the link between appearance and reality, and the corollaries of the liability of potency and the impotency of those who oppose the potent and so on."

While it is tempting to read Brancati's novels for the political views they espouse, I prefer to read them as diverting stories which have the force of broad indictments of antiquated and irrelevant traditions of the South that are fundamentally inhuman: the widespread attitude toward sex, the tenacious at times arrogant resolve not to allow any change in the social structure to take place, the unbearable provincialism pervading much of the life and thinking in the *Mezzogiorno*, and, finally, a system of values that puts appearances before truth. My reading of Brancati persuades me that he is more successful when the moral implications are allowed to emerge naturally, not as programmed elements of the plot. My preference goes for a long short story, written in 1944, "Il vecchio con gli stivali," [The old man with his boots], considered by many critics to be one of the best pieces by our novelist. The story deals with a modest city employee, a clerk by the name of Aldo Piscitello, who, despite his seniority in the system, has been unable to achieve tenure. When the tale begins, the Fascists have been in power for several years. In their drive to consolidate their hold over the central and municipal bureaucracy, they make membership in the party a condition for employment. Piscitello, warned by the town mayor to enroll, at first balks—for he considers himself a nonpolitical person—but eventually reluctantly accepts the condition imposed by his superiors. Married to a cantankerous wife, who constantly complains about his job and voices her disappointment over his insignificant status and lack of progress in his career, Piscitello is sympathetically treated by the author: admittedly weak and in some ways inept, he is slowly built up into a symbol of the oppressive treatment the poor and powerless must endure to survive. Piscitello, in addition to all the other indignities, has to don his Fascist uniform (down to the required black boots and wide leather belt), and is expected to attend meetings and the various "spontaneous" demonstrations of approval and support for every idiotic blunder Mussolini and his entourage of misfits is about to make. A terrible anger begins building up inside him, and his sensibility is deeply offended. His anger, however, cannot take any form other than the one abuse to which he subjects his Fascist lapel pin in a moment of rage. The war comes, the Italian and German armies suffer humiliating defeats in Africa, and the American and Allied troops land in Africa and eventually in Sicily. With each day, the horrors of war come closer and closer to Piscitello's town. After a long bout with the plague, he returns home only to find that his job has been taken away from him because of his long and well-known association with the Fascists! The ending of the story is supremely ironic, but not without pathos: the reader, but not the world at large, knows about Piscitello's deep-seated contempt toward fascism and its values, since he has never articulated his opposition to the regime. It is precisely in this stance of non-commitment (or a commitment that remains locked in the mind) that we may well find Brancati's flaw as a novelist. Just like the "old man with his boots," Brancati had neither the passion nor the courage to "see" reality and be resolute enough to take a hand in shaping it. He remained content to trace his own political evolution in his books —from an enthusiastic Fascist in his youth, to a leftist conservative in his mature years. His books reveal him as an acute observer of the social scene of his native island, a writer whose irony and ability to satirize a world he knew intimately commend him to today's reader. What he lacked, as Vanna Gazzola Stacchini pointedly remarks, was the capacity to offer solutions to the problems he posed in his fiction: for this, his own values were ultimately to blame.

Giuseppe Tomasi di Lampedusa: The View from Within

By all standards, *Il Gattopardo* (1958; *The Leopard*, N.Y., 1960) surely ranks as one of the most extraordinary and written-about novels to have appeared in post–World War II Italy. Together with such works of the creative imagination as Gabriele d'Annunzio's *Il piacere* (1889; *The Child of Pleasure*, N.Y., 1896), Luigi Pirandello's *Sei personaggi in cerca d'autore* (1921; *Six Characters in Search of an Author*, N.Y., 1952), and Alberto Moravia's *Gli indifferenti* (1929; *The Time of Indifference*, N.Y., 1954), it is also one of the most controversial books of fiction to have been published in Italy during the last one hundred years. The polemics sparked by *The Leopard* split the literary establishment in diametrically opposed factions, exalting the work as one of the most important, meaningful, and beautifully written in recent times, or condemning it for a variety of sins, usually as reactionary, fraudulent, structurally and stylistically archtraditional in an era of experimentation and openness.

Most readers will not disagree that the historical, ideological, and moral stance characterizing the novel is conservative and narrow at best, reactionary at worst. All would agree that the issues raised by the novelist's political, social, moral, or religious positions have always and will continue to haunt us as readers. David Daiches, the well known British critic, put the problem in perspective in his excellent handbook A *Study of Literature* (N.Y., 1964) in these words: "What is to be our attitude toward a poet whose beliefs differ radically from ours . . . ? At what point . . . does our disagreement with a writer's ideas interfere with our appreciation of his work as imaginative literature? . . . One does not need to share a writer's beliefs," Daiches continues, "before appreciating the meaning of the words he employs," and goes on to suggest that, if we wish to be serious about what we read, we must suspend our beliefs and look at the book before us for what it is and what it attempts to say. Ultimately, we must make of the perfection with which the vision is expressed (which is to say, the completeness, the depth, the range, the beauty) the test on which the book will stand or fail. This is no easy task: meeting a writer on his own terms, particularly when religion and politics are involved, frequently becomes an obstacle few readers can easily overcome, with regrettable consequences, for in such conditions the reading of practically any serious novel is hopelessly compromised.

The publication of *The Leopard* was followed by so many objections (to some extent balanced by vigorous praise) that future historians of literature may well have ample evidence of what can happen when the "ideas" contained in a work of fiction clash with the ideologies of the critics and the readers. The reactions that followed the publication of the novel constitute a veritable dossier, covering every one of its aspects: some critics complained that the work displayed an appalling lack of interest in social problems of the *Mezzogiorno* in general, and Sicily in particular; others, such as Enrico Falqui, a prolific and articulate book reviewer, traced the book's structural and thematic flaws to the author's "squalid ideology"; others still, such as Vittorini, remarked that the posthumously published novel, along with its sixty-one-year-old author, were doomed to remain anomalies of creative writing in a period marked by experimentations that infused new vigor and vitality in Italian fiction of the 1950s. Many of the questions raised then are still very much debated, but hardly resolved today. There is some comfort in this, for it attests to the vitality of *Il Gattopardo* and its strangely magnetic interest.

The author of such an unusual novel was a member of the Sicilian aristocracy, Giuseppe Tomasi, duke of Parma and prince of Lampedusa, born on December 23, 1896. His family's roots go back well over a millennium, and its presence in Sicily dates back to the Renaissance. Don Giuseppe's great grandfather, Don Giulio Maria Fabrizio, was a distinguished mathematician and astronomer, whose scientific work earned him a prize at the Sorbonne; he was also an influential political leader, member of the Sicilian Chamber of Peers. Relatively little is known about Don Giuseppe's father, Don Giulio Fabrizio, from whom he seems to have been estranged. Lampedusa (for such is the name Tomasi wanted his readers and friends to use) served as an officer in

World War I, was taken prisoner, but managed to escape and make his way home on foot from the Balkans. He met his wife-to-be, Alessandra von Wolff-Stomersee in London, shortly after leaving the service in 1925. The step-daughter of the Italian ambassador, a gifted, highly cultivated woman, she was to become one of the leading Freudian analysts in Italy.

Don Giuseppe's interests in literature were both wide and deep: he was particularly well versed in French literature—his favorite authors were Montaigne, Rabelais, Stendhal, and Proust—and English letters, particularly Shakespeare, Dickens, Virginia Woolf, and T. S. Eliot. He was also a great admirer of such European masters as Tolstoy, James Joyce, and Thomas Mann. Lampedusa was seldom heard discussing Italian writers, but his rare comments indicate that he was unusually well informed and highly selective in his taste. In this connection, he is reported to have remarked that Federico De Roberto's prolix novel of Sicily in the last half of the nineteenth century, *I vicerè* (1889; *The Viceroys*, N.Y., 1962) was a "picture of Sicilian aristocracy seen from the servants' hall," hardly a complimentary assessment prompted in all likelihood by his dissatisfaction with De Roberto's treatment of the theme of his own book.

After his marriage, Lampedusa settled in Sicily. Unlike many members of the upper class, he declined to participate in any way with the Fascist government of Mussolini, and spent most of his time reading and managing his estate. In the summer of 1954, Don Giuseppe decided to accompany his cousin, the poet Baron Luigi Piccolo, to a literary congress at San Pellegrino Terme where he had been invited to receive a prize. The event would probably have remained inconsequential were it not for the fact that, some time after his return home, Lampedusa decided to sit down and write a novel he had carried within him for over twenty years. Regrettably, the work was to remain unfinished: the author never had the opportunity to give to the final chapters of the novel the same loving care he had given to the first part. As a result, there is some imbalance in the concluding section of *The Leopard*.

The Leopard was begun in the second half of 1955; by the end of the following year the first draft, as yet untitled, was completed. There followed a period during which the author set himself to revise and complete his work. According to the reports of a number of people who have a direct, accurate, first-hand knowledge of the evolution of the book, the original version consisted only of what are chapters 1, 2, 3, and 4 of the definitive edition. That version lacked several episodes that were to cause much controversy—namely, the love episode of Tancredi and Angelica and, most importantly, the long section describing the visit of a special emissary of the national government, the Cavaliere Aimone Chevalley of Monterzuolo, secretary to the prefecture of Girgenti. Finally, a longish section dedicated to Father Perrone (a chapter that has been called a story within a story, not really justified by the structure and theme of the book, according to some) and the final two chapters.

The story of how *The Leopard* came to be published is also intricate and, in some ways, troublesome in that it touches on the question of the integrity of the original manuscript. The printed edition was based on the copy of the novel owned by Elena Croce, daughter of the eminent philosopher Benedetto Croce, augmented by chapter 5, taken from a handwritten copy prepared by the author, and chapter 6, furnished by the writer's widow, after Don Giuseppe's death. In 1957, after the author had done a good deal of work on the novel, the manuscript was submitted to two of Italy's most prestigious publishing houses, Mondadori of Milan, and Einaudi of Turin. Both publishers, guided by an excellent editorial staff, headed respectively by Vittorio Sereni and Elio Vittorini, firmly turned down the book. By that time, however, the author was taken ill with cancer, and died in a Roman clinic on July 23. Shortly thereafter Signora Croce brought the work to the attention of Giorgio Bassani, himself a sophisticated poet, novelist, and essayist, and senior consulting editor at Feltrinelli, a Milan-based, aggressive publishing house. Bassani went over, and slightly retouched the novel's punctuation, thus adding unconsciously another element of confusion to an already bizarre story. Brought out in 1958, *The Leopard* became quickly a best seller as well as one of the most discussed books in this century, a development that would no doubt have surprised its aloof, ironical author. Some ten years later, Feltrinelli published the complete text of the work, based on the 1957 manuscript, without any alterations so as to put to rest past innuendos regarding the extent of the editorial revisions.

What is *The Leopard* about? Is it history, autobiography, or fiction? Like many novels, it is a little of all three: but the three elements have been masterfully blended so as to give some rare insights into the nature of change and death. Life is a constant exposure to change—human, political, intellectual, historical— and in this respect the changes, which are the very elements of the fabric of existence, and as such part of life as well as of our preparation for death. Lampedusa is exceptional in feeling, and giving form to the preoccupation with death. To create a believable world in which his synthesis can be dramatically shown, rather than intellectually discussed, he takes us back a full century, to a delicate and central moment of the history of modern Italy and of the Salinas, a respected and powerful Sicilian family.

As the book opens, in that unforgettable May of 1860, about one thousand legionnaires, led by Giuseppe Garibaldi, the most celebrated and colorful hero of the Risorgimento, are about to land at Marsala and free the island from the rule of King Ferdinand II of the Bourbon family. The chapters that follow, 2, 3, and 4, are set respectively in August, October, and November of the same year; chapters 5, 6, 7, and 8 take place in February 1861, November 1862, July 1888, and May 1910—spanning over fifty years. About two thirds of the novel are made up of the first four chapters, widely acknowledged to constitute the more solid and impressive part of the book, which falters a little as it reaches the end.

The cast of characters is relatively small, but unusually well portrayed. There is, first of all, Count Don Fabrizio Corbera, prince of Salina, on stage during much of the story: "very large and very strong. . . . In his blood . . . fermented other German strains . . . an authoritarian temperament, a certain rigidity of morals, and a propensity for abstract ideas; these, in the relaxing atmosphere of Palermo society, had changed respectively into capricious arrogance, recurring moral scruples, and contempt for his own relatives and friends," fastidious in his habits, an excellent mathematician, and astronomer; his two sons, Francesco Paolo, duke of Querceta, the heir, interested in his horses and in his lady-friend, weak and shallow; and Giovanni, "the second son, the most loved, the most difficult," who vanishes, preferring a "modest life as clerk in a coal depot [in London!] to a pampered (read: 'fettered') existence in the ease of Palermo"; his three daughters, Concetta, Carolina, and Caterina, inexorably doomed to spinsterhood; Don Fabrizio's ambitious nephew Tancredi

Falconeri, whom he loves more than his own children; Angelica (the beautiful daughter of Don Calogero Sedara, an astute speculator, and businessman, now mayor and future senator)—"Under the first shock of her beauty the men were incapable of noticing or analyzing her defects, which were numerous; . . . She was tall and well made on an ample scale; her skin looked as if it had the flavor of fresh cream, which it resembled; her childlike mouth, that of strawberries. Under a mass of raven hair, curling in gentle waves, her green eyes gleamed motionless as those of statues, and like them a little cruel"; finally, Father Perrone, the prince's private confessor.

The plot of *The Leopard* is unusually simple, a fact that has led more than one critic to complain that the book is very static. On the surface at least, the work would appear to be a historical novel: it is, after all, set in the 1860s, at the end of the *Risorgimento*, chronologically developed, and told from the vantage point of the actual date of the publication of the work, a point that permits the author to enjoy considerable detachment and insight. But the impression soon proves to be wrong, as we perceive that what we are going to get is not the reconstruction of a pivotal period in modern Italian history, but an interpretation of how those historical events have affected the characters in the story and, by implication, the entire nation. The changes about to take place are numerous and far-reaching; the very title of the book suggests, in an oblique manner, the irony of the situation: a *"gattopardo"* is a cheetah, or a crossbreed of lion and panther. But the prince is no longer the fast, sly, powerful and much-feared killer of the jungle: in point of fact, he is about to be dislodged by the jackals and the hyenas, two animals that came to symbolize the new rich that are making their entrance on the political scene, and take complete charge of the leadership.

The *"gattopardo,"* in short, is an "old" man watching history run its course without his being able to determine in any significant way the direction it will take. Hardly a "positive" hero, he is a skeptic who holds few illusions about life, and actually prepares himself for death which alone can free man from the suffering life compels him to endure. The only way open to him, if he is to preserve at least a measure of the power and influence he and his family have always enjoyed is by the alliance, through marriage, of his nephew Tancredi with Angelica—a union which is not without its share of irony. It is Don Fabrizio, born of a mixed marriage (a Sicilian father and a German mother) who lays the groundwork for the union of Tancredi (also the offspring of a mixed marriage) with Angelica. No one can predict, of course, how successful any human scheme will be. An intimation of this stance is found early in the novel, when the prince, in his daily visit to his garden, is attracted by a "somewhat crude," strong offense to his nose: "The Paul Neyron roses, whose cuttings he had himself bought in Paris, had degenerated; first stimulated and the enfeebled by the strong if languid pull of Sicilian earth, burned by apocalyptic Julies, they had changed into things like flesh-colored cabbages, obscene and distilling a dense, almost indecent, scent which no French horticulturist would have dared hope for." The comment might seem innocent: but when we complete our reading of the book, we realize how pointedly ironic (like so much of the novel) it is: the Sicilian soil (or Sicily itself) is not often receptive to flowers (or customs and ways of life) imported from the mainland. This notwithstanding, the marriage represents a chance worth taking, if for no other reason than that there are few other alternatives.

Alas, just as the marriage of the two lovely young people means a further thinning down of aristocratic blood, the "purity" of the Salinas is further weakened by Tancredi's unavoidable alliance with the forces of the national government. And, in a way, this is what the book is about—at least, in part. In the face of sweeping changes, just how does the ruling class adjust to the new facts? "If we want things to stay as they are," proclaims Tancredi at one point, "things must change," an observation that reflects accurately the scheming and turmoil of the 1860s and the decades that followed the realization of political unification. Indeed, it is precisely Tancredi's inventiveness, his determination not to allow himself to be drowned by the tempest of the *Risorgimento*, and his pragmatism, that attract the affection and faith of the prince in his nephew:

> Conquered for ever by the youth's affectionate banter, he [the prince] began during the last few months to admire his intelligence too: that quick adaptability, that world penetration, that innate artistic subtlety with which he could use the demagogic terms then in fashion while hinting to initiates that for him, the

Prince of Falconesi, this was only a momentary pastime; all this amused Don Fabrizio, and in people of his character and standing the faculty for being amused makes up four fifths of affection. Tancredi, he considered, had a great future; he would be the standard-bearer of a counterattack which the nobility, under new trappings, could launch against the new social State. To do this he lacked only one thing: money; this Tancredi did not have; none at all. And to get into politics, now that a name counted less, would require a lot of money: money to buy votes, money to do the electors favors, money for a dazzling style of living.

The impelling necessity to find ways to preserve the status quo, springs not only from an understandable desire to retain the family's influence, but also from a deep-seated conviction that Sicilians (or, for that matter, Southerners in general) do not really want any change, a thesis many Italian critics rejected outright. The prince's own skepticism toward the whole issue of change is symbolically depicted through his love of the stars and his impatience with the realities of everyday existence. A dedicated astronomer of an aristocratic sensitivity, he would like nothing less than to believe in the absolute permanence of the cosmos. As a serious scientist and mathematician, he knows that changes do occur in the "fixed stars," but such changes cannot be detected by the naked human eye as they occur over a time span measurable in terms of thousands or millions of years, thus justifying what is aptly called "permanence in transience." The prince's only hope is that all the changes in the sociopolitical order of the South will proceed at the same rate of speed as the stars'. His views on this question are carefully and candidly articulated in the long interview he has with Chevalley, the special emissary sent by the government to seek his commitment to the idea of political unification soon to be presented to the people by way of a referendum:

"I am a member of the old ruling class," he observes, "inevitably compromised with the Bourbon regime, and tied to it by chains of decency if not of affection.

"I belong to an unfortunate generation, swung between the old and the new, and I find myself ill at ease in both." And in what surely ranks as an absorbing historical analysis of the temperament of the Sicilians, he adds: "In Sicily, it doesn't matter whether

things are done well or done badly: the sin we Sicilians never forgive is simply that of 'doing' at all. . . . Sleep, my dear Chevalley,
sleep is what Sicilians want, and they will always hate anyone
who tries to wake them, even in order to bring them the most
wonderful of gifts; . . . All Sicilian expression, even the most
violent, is really wish-fulfillment." The analysis does by no means
stop here: cultural and geographical factors are summoned up,
history and psychology provide additional points to the desperate
equation of change. But I think it is vital to point out that it is
not change per se that the prince fears, but the futility of change
that generally comes too slowly to be truly effective in molding
the temperament of a large segment of the population. The
prince's actions reveal his philosophical consistency: cognizant of
the necessity of change, he goes no further than arranging the
marriage of Tancredi and Angelica, which ultimately means little
or nothing in the standing and fortune of the family. As a matter
of fact, despite the prince's willingness to change the economic
and personal relationships that have long prevailed between himself and his tenant farmers, we are given to see the apathy and
incompetence the ruling class shows in its efforts to come to grips
with the conditions of the new times.

The novel's interest in reality, in the world of objects, tangible
things, and people, balances what is the other pervasive theme of
the story, Fabrizio's love with death, carefully interwoven with his
healthy sensuality. The insistence on death is evident from the
words that open the book: "*Nunc et in hora mortis nostrae.
Amen,*" and the final scene, in which the prince's faithful dog
Bendicò, properly stuffed and preserved with other relics of the
family, is thrown out of the window, "flung into a corner of the
courtyard visited every day by the dustman."

The slow, agonizing death of a political order that for centuries
shaped the quality of life in the *Mezzogiorno* is revealed through
numerous, striking images of the death of people, animals, and
nature. Indeed, in one way or another, the author manages to
keep death prominently before us, particularly in the first part of
the book: "Enclosed between three walls and a side of the house,
[the garden's] seclusion gave it the air of a cemetery." "The real
problem," so reasons the prince when thinking about the uncertain political situation, "is how to go on living this life of the spirit
in its most sublime moments, those moments that are most like

death." Death constantly haunts the prince, particularly when violence is its cause. What repels him in particular, however, is not the philosophical question of death, which his religious faith has enabled him to accept with a certain amount of serenity, but its visible horror, as when the body of a dead Royalist soldier is found in his garden, "his face covered in blood and vomit, his nails dug into the soil, crawling with ants," or the gruesome sight of a rabbit, killed during a hunting event with his accountant Ciccio Ferrata, or the open wagon, "stacked with bulls killed shortly before at the slaughterhouse, already quartered and exhibiting their intimate mechanism with the shamelessness of death," the prince sees as he returns from the ball in honor of Tancredi and his fiancée, Angelica.

While a great era is slowly dying around him, the prince is himself preparing for his own death. That he esteemed and loved few people is implicit in his attitudes and behavior. He is, however, consoled by the understanding that it is the fact of human mortality that serves to redress the mistakes we commit while we live, and teaches us to be more forgiving toward the failings of society as well as of the individual. With death, comes the end of all those illusions that give us mortals a reason for enduring the suffering life so generously bestowed upon us. "Growing old," notes Richard Kuhns in a brilliant essay on "Modernity and Death" in *The Leopard*, "approaching death, he [the prince] realizes that the earthly realm is no more his to rule in accordance with his will than the heavenly; both obey laws beyond human desire. The Prince ends his life more keenly, self-consciously aware of the necessities in both earth and heaven."

Ultimately, the novel, through its various characters, addresses itself to the question of fulfillment, a problem that must take into account the sufferings man must endure in his quest on earth. And here the picture becomes very clear indeed: no one has really attained the best he or she could and should have attained by reasons of his preparation, character, circumstances: Tancredi accepts the role granted him by the new government; Angelica turns out to be too absorbed in herself to be capable of giving of herself; Concetta, sacrificed by her father when her genuine love for Tancredi is brushed aside, is condemned to live a spinster; Stella, the prince's wife, is constantly excluded from any meaningful feeling, while her two other daughters live out their existence without ever being touched by love, marriage and a family; even the prince, for all his sensitivity, intelligence, power and so-called wisdom, takes one last glance at all the years he has lived, at all the things—good, bad or indifferent—he has done, and attempts to draw "a general balance sheet of his whole life, trying to sort out of the immense ash-heap of liabilities the golden flecks of happy moments. These were: two weeks before his marriage, six weeks after; half an hour when Paolo was born, when he felt proud of having prolonged by a twig the Salina tree (the pride had been misplaced, he knew that now, but there had been some genuine self-respect in it); a few talks with Giovanni before the latter vanished (a few monologues, if the truth were told, during which he had thought to find in the boy a kindred mind); and in many hours in the observatory, absorbed in abstract calculations and the pursuit of the unreachable. Could those latter hours be really put down to the credit of life? Were they not some sort of anticipatory gift of the beatitudes of death? It didn't matter, they had existed."

With these words, the prince sums up his entire existence, leaving us with the distinct awareness that little, if indeed anything, is changed by man's actions. They are far from encouraging words, just as the vision of life they express is anything but positive. His notions are not the ones we are likely to entertain and agree with. Taking issue with the prince's view of history, Andor Gomme comments: "There is corruption at the heart of the new regime because the heart is always corrupted. This is not only a message of despair, because of the breeding which allows one to look on it with good natured but supercilious cynicism." Unquestionably, the novel by Giuseppe Tomasi di Lampedusa is pessimistic in the extreme. Perhaps, as Furio Felcini suggests, we ought to see the novel as a kind of metaphysical correlative of Lampedusa's own existence, lived in full knowledge that there would be no heir to carry on the illustrious family name. I prefer seeing it as a book whose very conception and creation was an affirmation of life, and as a brave and rare acceptance of the nobility of death.

4

Dino Buzzati: The Gothic Novel

Aloof, mysterious, haunting: these are probably the first adjectives that come immediately to mind to someone trying to characterize the literary production of Dino Buzzati—six novels (of uneven quality), several collections of short stories and poetry, and eleven plays. But generalizations or labels, convenient as they may be, are dangerous simply because they leave too many doors open, too many questions unanswered. If called to refine the characterization just offered, one might say that much of Buzzati's fiction presents us with situations that exploit, with varying degrees of success, the natural sense of fear people feel when they find themselves in situations within or outside the common range of their existence. The element of fear—of impending disasters, of death, or simply of the unknown—dominates Buzzati's work and view of life. Indeed, fear is the chief ingredient of the strategy of our writer, intent in keeping us waiting for something catastrophic to happen, thus forcing us to remain in a state of perennial alert, ready to jump off the boat that may be going down at any moment, or, even worse, suddenly aware of being locked in a situation from which the only exit leads to death. To achieve the condition of anguish that is produced by uncertainty, terror, or the inevitable that strikes without warning, Buzzati moves toward a denouement by way of a carefully calculated route, conscious that, to succeed, fear must be effectively translated into a statement about life that transcends the natural demands of the plot.

We may know fear through many kinds of personally lived experiences. What the artist must do is to show its significance in terms of the human condition, relate it, that is, to our fate: thus, to apprehend it, at least in literature, it must be shown in all its dimensions. A clever writer does not find it inordinately difficult to create suspense: what is difficult is stretching it into incontestable illuminations of the mystery all around us, and part of our soul as well, and give it order and place in the re-creation of life in the written page. When Buzzati is successful (and that is not too frequently) the anxiety generated by his tales takes the form of a symbolic waiting for something that will change the meaning of our existence, only to become suddenly aware, often when the goal may well be within our reach, that time has passed, little has changed, much suffering has been endured, and we are confronting the end. Buzzati assumes that all human beings crave love, peace, security, and companionship. He also knows that we deeply wish to fulfill ourselves, generally by doing things that will bring recognition, admiration, success, all in direct proportion to the capabilities and ambitions of each individual.

Yet nothing in life is guaranteed: on the contrary, everything is constantly in jeopardy, always at the mercy of uncontrollable events. At times, the slightest error, innocently made, may cause great havoc, as in the short story "Il crollo della Baliverna" [The crash of the Baliverna], which tells of how the accidental removal of a support of a famous building, much to the consternation of the protagonist, causes the sudden, total collapse of the edifice! In another story, "Sette piani" [Seven floors], Giovanni Corte enters a clinic where the patients are sent to one of its seven floors according to the seriousness of their illness. Ostensibly hospitalized for precautionary reasons, Corte never understands the nature of his malady, which is never diagnosed and therefore defies medical treatment, and dies after he has progressively been moved to lower and lower floors, in what turns out to be a symbolic treatment of man's descent to his grave.

If we are doomed to live an existence riddled with anxiety and trepidation, always expecting "something" that will harm or even destroy us, we must search for a reason that justifies our earthly pilgrimage, particularly if we become aware that the idea of life as a journey is central in Buzzati—as in *Il deserto dei Tartari* (1940; *The Tartar Steppe*, N.Y., 1952), or *Il grande ritratto* [The large portrait] (1960). Our compass must be readjusted: what really matters must not be the end, but how we wait, or how we prepare for the end. At times, hope, love, and companionship help lessen the anguish of waiting and the forlorn settings of Buzzati's fiction

—the rocky, angular mountains, the junglelike forests, the lonely, frightening deserts, the silent, alienating, labyrinthine cities.

What elements in the life of our novelist contributed to shaping a sensibility that created so many unorthodox stories and landscapes? Searching for clues to these question may prove somewhat disappointing, since Buzzati led as conventional and as uncomplicated an existence as one could imagine.

Born near Belluno, a small northern city, on October 6, 1906, Buzzati lived most of his life in Milan. The proximity to the Dolomiti mountains fired his enthusiasm for skiing and mountain climbing, and his awe of Nature's beauties. Living in the somewhat gloomy, efficient, culturally sophisticated Milan, drew him closer to the introspective, somber, philosophical literature of central Europe rather than the lyrical, romantic vein of his native tradition. The son of a well-known jurist, Buzzati received his advanced education at the University of Pavia, where he took a law degree so as not to disappoint his father, who had hoped his son would follow in his footsteps. His family's affluence permitted young Dino to pursue, early in his adult life, his real interest— writing. He embarked on a career that began in 1928 and was to continue until his death, on January 28, 1972, as a journalist, literary and art critic, special correspondent and, of course, writer of fiction. His assignments took him to distant, often unusual spots for long periods of time. His travels rounded out his experience of life, broadened his interests, and provided him with rich and unusual material for his fiction: with the passing of time, Buzzati has filled his tales with historical personages (ranging all the way from Churchill to Khrushchev, from Pope John XXIII to Brezhnev) and such timely problems as the cold war and the prospect of atomic warfare. This may give the impression that Buzzati is a writer engagé. Nothing could be further from the truth: he uses world renowned figures and issues not so much to add an extra measure of realism, but simply to heighten the irony of his vision of a world teetering on the brink of madness. "The optimum of journalism coincides with the optimum of Literature," he once stated; and it is a view of dubious validity that frequently tends to make his work too connected with the present, too facile, too historical and too little visionary, of limited scope and depth.

Buzzati's best and most enduring novels were written in the first few years of his extended literary career. It was in two of his early novels that he found the themes that were to haunt his imagination: *Bàrnabo delle montagne* [Bàrnabo of the mountains] (1933) and *Il deserto dei Tartari*.

Bàrnabo delle montagne took him several months to write, between assignments at the newspaper *Il corriere della sera*, where he was working as a reporter. The story the book tells, in a language unusually plain and lucid, is simple enough. But simplicity —as in much of Buzzati's fiction—turns out to be deceptive, for the emotions and issues depicted in the novel range all the way from duty, virility, and courage, to cowardice, remorse, violence, and compassion.

Bàrnabo is a young forest ranger, a member of a team of twelve men, and a leader, whose duties include guarding a small cave where a sizable amount of explosives has been stored. At one time, the explosives were supposed to be used in connection with a construction project, scuttled by its high cost and limited strategic importance as well as by the protests of environmentalists. Eventually, it is decided that the explosives and the ammunition that has been added will be kept at the disposal of troops patroling the border areas nearby, and all such material is to be placed in a hut near the new residence of the forest rangers, so as to make it easier to guard. One day, quite unexpectedly, two brigands storm the hut, and leave the head of the rangers, Antonio Del Collo, mortally wounded. A search for the killers proves to be fruitless: months go by, and no progress is made. One day, Bàrnabo and Berton, returning home after their patrol, find themselves under fire by a group of brigands attacking the storage house. While Berton makes his way to rescue another ranger, Franze, Bàrnabo stops briefly to take care of a small crow, hurt by a gunshot, and then finds himself at gunpoint distance, threatened by a brigand. Berton's generous efforts to persuade his superiors that in no way did Bàrnabo behave cowardly prove futile. Bàrnabo is asked to resign.

He goes back to nearby San Nicola, and takes a job at his cousin's farm. After many years, during which he has suffered much, unable to forget his fear on that fateful occasion, he is able to go back with his friend Berton (who has spent several months abroad) to visit his former buddies. Things have changed much during the years that have passed, and now the rangers live in the barracks of the county force. A new residence for the rangers is in the process of being completed, and Bàrnabo accepts the task of guarding the old house, up on the mountains, mindful that the brigands, who have attacked the depot again with no success, have promised to strike again in a year's time. After waiting, in vain, for the rangers to join him on that fateful day, Bàrnabo takes up his position in a strategic place from which he can keep the depot under surveillance. When the brigands come, and are within perfect distance from him, he is unable to pull the trigger of his rifle, even though his action could redeem him in the eyes of his peers, wiping out once and for all the shame of the cowardice he has had to bear for so many years. Killing would no longer make much sense: it would be another act of violence against people toward whom he feels neither anger nor hate. And, at last, Bàrnabo's soul is filled with peace.

Much of the best of Buzzati is in his first novel: his deep love of the mountains, the woods, Nature; the theme of waiting ("always protracted and deluded," as Enrico Falqui once remarked); the mysterious sounds that add to the suspense of his tales; the careful arrangement of events in a manner calculated to produce the maximum of tension. There is also the tendency to make of his characters and plots allegories of the human condition. Bàrnabo, for example, is one of a thirteen-member team of forest rangers. His act of cowardice has clearly violated the code by which they (and, by extension, society) live. He must pay the heavy penalty for his guilt, and spends several years in the jail without bars to which outcasts are condemned. Ultimately, he redeems himself through what is surely nothing less than an act of Caritas, of Christian Love for our fellowman. Time has not brought Bàrnabo much happiness: but, in the end, it does at least give him the much needed perspective that enables him to understand the absurdity of the price society often extracts of those who, without meaning to, might break its laws. Love of Nature, particularly the mountains and the forests, together with the presence of the explosives, are part and parcel of a symbolic dimension carefully built into the story. The tranquillity of natural surroundings is what permits man, at last undistracted by the frenetic rhythm of city life, to come to terms with himself, with those elements that have a special relevance in his conception of what life should be like: the explosives are frightening reminders of potential destruction, the end of life itself, with which we must all live, a reminder all the more dramatic for its being situated in the center of so much peace and quiet.

In *Il deserto dei Tartari*, most of the ingredients that give *Bàrnabo delle montagne* its unique character are perfectly blended and enriched, so as to yield not only pathos and anxiousness, fear and resignation, but also metaphysical implications (what Emilio Cecchi felicitously called "metaphysical *angst*") that deepen considerably the dimension of Buzzati's vision.

Giovanni Drogo, the hero of *The Tartar Steppe*, is a young army career officer who has just received his new assignment: a tour of duty at the Bastiani fortress, situated in a strategic spot between two mountain chains, a godforsaken place, as we soon find out, that seems to be located on another planet. Geographically, the fortress is about twenty miles from the nearest town: psychologically, it seems like a place where time has completely lost its importance, and where no real, normal human relationship is possible.

While many aspects of the story are purposely left vague, the reader can, on the basis of certain details of the plot, make some assumptions at least about the historical time of the action. To begin, we know that Drogo's country is a monarchy and, based on the reference to a King Piero III and other information, we assume that the time of the action is the nineteenth century. In fact, Drogo reaches his destination on horseback, and the weapons in the fortress do not appear to be modern. Much of the anxiety caused by the presumed incursions of enemy troops, or the suspicion (which only in the last pages of the book proves to be perfectly justified) that an underground trail leading to the fortress has been completed, could easily have been detected by some of the more sophisticated technological instruments of our century. Even communications between the fort and the headquarters seem to be handled exclusively by messengers, and kerosene, not electricity, provides the light. But such minutiae are out of order once we perceive that the historical dimension is unimportant in the novel: what happens, and the people involved in the story of *The Tartar Steppe*, demand to be seen and understood literally, of course, as well as symbolically, as we shall see.

Presumably, the principal mission of the fortress and its garrison is to defend the country against possible enemy raids, and from being attacked by unfriendly troops coming from beyond the desert that stretches at the feet of the mountains. The garrison, and the officers in particular, are so conscious of the importance of their mission that they refuse to leave even when their health justifies relief from hazardous duty. One day, their expectations appear about to be fulfilled: the general alarm is sounded. The alert proves to be unjustified, as the enemy troops presumably sighted in the vicinity of the fortress turn out to be patrols surveying and checking border territories. The events depress the members of the garrison, deeply disappointed by the opportunity just missed. Even Drogo entertains the possibility of requesting a transfer to a more active fort. His furlough to his hometown makes him conscious of the wide gap that exists between himself and his old friends, whose lives and activities have little or nothing in common with his. Tempted by the possibility of a deep relationship with a woman, he finally requests a new assignment. But his application is turned down by the authorities and he is ordered back to the fortress. Time passes quickly: fifteen more years have now elapsed in addition to the other fifteen already spent at the fortress. Drogo is now an old man, whose failing health needs medical attention of the kind only a well equipped city clinic can provide.

Ironically, as he leaves, news comes that the enemy has been sighted on a road built secretly during a period of several years. The big moment has finally come, but Drogo's health does not permit him to participate in the military operations against the enemy. On his way home, Drogo stops at an inn to spend a night of rest: and there death will pay its visit. Having been denied the satisfaction of fighting the enemy on the battlefield, he welcomes death with a smile. Unable to savor the one challenge for which he had sacrificed gladly the best years of his life, Drogo perceives that there is no rhyme or reason why he should want to go on living. The acceptance of this fact—an act which in itself requires as much strength, courage and determination as he needed during all the years during which he waited for the big moment of his existence—is in effect what sustains him in the last hours of his life, confident that God's understanding of his frailty will make it possible for Him to forgive His child for his weaknesses.

Even such a sketchy account of the plot of *The Tartar Steppe* indicates the way in which the novel moves on a double track, so to speak, the literal and the allegorical. The book, by focusing on the nature and activities of a man called Giovanni Drogo, really tells of man's pilgrimage on earth, a man who, like other men, is engaged in earthly shallow and ultimately insignificant pursuits. It is only when our man, who happens to be called Drogo, reaches the end of his journey, that he can realize the futility of much of what he has done in his lifetime. Christians living in the Middle Ages understood and accepted the concept of life as significant in terms of an experience that tested man and prepared him for the afterlife. The Renaissance changed this perspective, secularized life, placing great value on it, stressing its worth, its beauty, the opportunities it offered for fulfillment *hic et nunc*. This in turn led to the establishment of objectives which, in time, proved to be mere fabrications, necessary to console man who found himself alone in the world.

The Tartar Steppe is, in a sense, an allegory of the condition of modern man, enduring sufferings, searching for the answers of his being, creating illusions whose sole contribution is to assert the validity and purpose of existence. This is the metaphysical context in which Drogo is placed by Buzzati: the fortress itself may be seen as life, in which the young hero is sent without any specific reason, where he is to remain for an unspecified period of time, but which has never played any useful purpose. In this context, we accept the necessity of the existence of a great challenge facing Drogo and his kind: without their illusions regarding the importance of their mission, of their dream of confronting the "enemy" some day, their *raison d'être* would cease to exist and something else would have to take its place.

It is important to stress that the formulation of certain objectives we consider appropriate, in that they respond to our desires and ambitions, should take place when we are still young and have a whole life ahead of us. We can control and redirect our energies and persist in our quest because time is on our side: Little do we suspect that time has a way of passing faster and faster than we realized or anticipated. To be sure, we may well become aware of this and attempt to reorder our priorities. The fact that our perceptions of our limitations and mistakes may even lead us to conclude that we have spent too much time and energy in the pursuit of questionable goals is admirable.

But what of the years we have consumed in the process? Buzzati attempts to shed some light upon this rather universal aspect of the human condition by action and reflection. One of the objectives of the first half of the novel is to show us how Drogo is slowly, and inextricably, trapped by circumstances and his decreasing willpower, into his condition. He has the opportunity to speak with the tailor of the fortress, Prosdocimo, who constantly discusses his impending departure, and with his assistant (who turns out to be his older brother) who warns him not to be fooled by the promises of the commanding officer, Colonel Filimore, of challenges soon to present themselves. He also has the opportunity of reflecting about what the future realistically can offer him. He takes his chances, and plays the game even with odds stacked against him. Together with the members of the garrison and his peers, Drogo blunders into accepting life that is to be spent in the fortress fooling himself into thinking that somehow he can master his own destiny. Ironically enough, he is aware of the consequences of his choice, but he is drugged (and here the reader may discover the intimations of this condition in the hero's name, Drogo) by the illusion that that precious commodity that is Time is on his side. Habit is ultimately the element that persuades him to continue: keep a bird in a cage long enough, and he will probably end by accepting it as the place where he must stay. Life in the fortress becomes a sort of sequence of rituals that enables Drogo to be comfortable and secure—even though the price he must ultimately pay proves to be inordinately high.

The setting of the novel helps create the right mood for Drogo's inevitable downfall: the impersonal, chilling architecture of the fort, the vagueness of its geographic location, the lack of specific details regarding the kind of enemy (called simply the "Tartars") threatening Drogo's motherland, the indefinite time of the action, all serve to pinpoint and define the major themes of the novel, and its universality. Suspense is achieved by sudden apparitions (horses? men?) as the story progresses toward its resolution. Silence is what reflection and introspection require; but silence also increases the awareness of our solitude when we try to come up with complex, and perhaps insoluble problems. Silence is the realization that there is no one with us when we suffer and need companionship, comfort. The slightest noise we hear may reach us with unexpected, frightening force, perhaps foreboding impending disasters. In the loneliness of silence, human ambitions become trite matters, inconsequential in every way: Drogo's promotion from second lieutenant (when the story begins), to major (when it ends), becomes the ultimate insult of a wasted life.

There is a special irony in *The Tartar Steppe* that Buzzati's other novels lack: even a life of discipline, honor, obedience to, and respect for the code (in this case, the military), yes, even a life completely dedicated to service to one's country, fails totally to bring the desired sense of happiness and fulfillment. This constitutes a stunning blow, the coup de grâce, to the bourgeois vision of life which predicates happiness based on a system of values so strictly accepted and cherished by Drogo, who does not hesitate to sacrifice even love of a woman in order to live by the code. Time, whose flight Drogo had hoped to stall, has passed irreversibly; nothing will buy it back, not the promotions or honors, not the sacrifices made, not the examplary way in which all duties have been discharged—and the suffering of the end is somehow made bearable by the consciousness that it means no more sufferings, and as such death is welcomed.

A fate of loneliness emerges as an inescapable fact of life: human beings are likened to "stones speaking a foreign tongue." Like people jailed for life, with no hope for parole, simply because they live, Buzzati isolates his characters in a milieu that reminds one of Thomas Mann's *The Magic Mountain*. While they are conscious of their condition, they accept with a sort of masochistic resignation the dehumanized routinization of their existence, and give up hope that anything other than what discipline and duty have made daily habits will ever touch their lives.

The Tartar Steppe, together with *Bàrnabo delle montagne*, is choice Buzzati. By and large, the promises of his early novels, with few exceptions, have remained unfulfilled. His connections with such writers as Poe, Chamisso, Wells, Kafka, and Camus, in the near-unanimous opinions of Italian critics—from De Michelis to Falqui, from Cecchi to Milano—have failed to materialize into something more than a mere superficial resemblance. While the "presence" of such masters in Buzzati's work is undeniable, one must agree with Renato Bertacchini's remark that the novelist has passively accepted, rather than assimilated their "lesson." In Kafka, the theme *is* the hero of the novel, suffering is never superimposed on either character or action, because it is an inseparable part of both: time itself, so conscientiously recorded by Buzzati and so nostalgically felt by his characters, has no limits, no boundaries in Kafka. Buzzati's sensibility, his almost inevitable propensity toward allegorical fables, do indeed give occasional birth to terrifying moments. But the overall effect is frequently damaged by a superimposed religious acceptance of life's disappointments. And, as Gian-Paolo Biasin notes, "a moral judgment is implied in his images, but the element that comes to the fore and focuses the attention of the reader is mainly the magical one." Anguish, terror, sadness, fear, in fine, become too frequently treated according to a formula that is dictated by specific requirements of the medium in which the stories appeared.

5

Carlo Levi: The Essayist as Novelist

There are two questions a student of Italian letters must ask himself vis-à-vis Carlo Levi: first, is he, and to what extent if he is, a novelist; second, is his place in contemporary literature to be determined by his fiction or by his nonfiction? Italian critics are not always very helpful here, and it is not surprising that Giorgio Pullini, in his informative and valuable study of the postwar Italian novel chooses to discuss not *L'orologio* (1950; *The Watch*, N.Y., 1951), Levi's only novel, but *Cristo si è fermato a Eboli* (1945; *Christ Stopped at Eboli*, N.Y., 1947), the work that catapulted its author to international prominence a few months after its appearance in the book stalls. The confusion may turn out to be less justified than expected once we realize that Carlo Levi belongs to that rare breed of literary artists who can successfully write essays that read like novels, a novel that reads like an essay, and a body of work that is at once autobiography, fiction, history, sociology, anthropology, and last but not least, poetry. And that is a rare accomplishment indeed.

Unlike most writers, Carlo Levi came to writing, and to fame, through an unusual route. Born in Turin, on November 29, 1902, Levi had originally planned to pursue a career in medicine. He entered the University at the age of seventeen, and received his degree six years later. Even before finishing his secondary studies, he was drawn to politics. In 1918 he met Piero Gobetti, a young, dynamic, and brilliant person of liberal political convictions articulated in articles published in a biweekly sheet entitled *Energie nuove* [New energies]. In 1922, Levi became Gobetti's closest collaborator in a newly founded magazine, *La rivoluzione liberale* [The liberal revolution]. With each year, Levi's involvement in politics increased: a distasteful, violent act he witnessed while serving his tour of duty in the armed forces radicalized him even further. In 1929 Levi, together with the Rosselli brothers, living in exile in Paris, founded the movement "Giustizia e Libertà" ("Justice and Freedom"). Shortly before completing his medical degree, he turned to painting as a hobby. A painting he submitted to the commission of the Venice Art Festival was accepted and shown in a special section reserved to promising young artists. Some years later, Levi, now Doctor Levi, decided to leave medicine and devote his creative talent to painting.

In 1934, he was arrested and jailed for several months because of his "subversive" activity. Some time later, arrested again together with more than eighty persons, he was sentenced to the *confino* (political exile) in the desolate towns of Grassano and Galliano in the southern region of Lucania, the setting of his future *Christ Stopped at Eboli*. Released some months later, Levi traveled constantly so as to avoid close police surveillance and lived in France. He soon returned to his country, played an active role in the Italian Underground, and was arrested shortly before the end of World War II. In the summer of 1944, Levi became the editor of the Florentine newspaper *La nazione del popolo*; a year later, he left for Rome to take up the editorship of the Roman newspaper *L'Italia libera*, the official organ of the "Partito d'Azione." In the summer of 1946, the party was disbanded, but Levi's interest in politics continued unabated. In 1963 in honor of the contribution he had made to Italian artistic and political life, he was elected independent senator in the list of the Communist party. Before his death in 1975 he published *Paura della libertà* (1945; *Fear of Freedom*, N.Y., 1950); *Le Parole sono pietre* (1955; *Words are Stones*, N.Y., 1958) winner of the coveted Viareggio Prize; *Il futuro ha un cuore antico* [The future has an ancient heart] (1956), an account of his travel to the Soviet Union; *La doppia notte dei tigli* (1959; *The Linden Tree*, N.Y., 1962), an incisive report on Germany, based on his journey there, and, in 1964, *Tutto il miele è finito* [All the honey is finished], a poetic portrait of the island of Sardegna he visited on two different occasions.

Christ Stopped at Eboli, written between December 1943 and July 1944, has long been considered Levi's masterpiece and, in the opinion of several critics, his only book. Perhaps there is considerable truth in the assertion of Carlo Muscetta that the book is less the story of Levi's encounter with the South, long neglected and exploited, than this image as mirrored in the eyes and hearts of the poor *meridionali* (Southerners). But the book goes beyond the personal and becomes, thanks to Levi's sensitive and compassionate attitude, a noble attempt to understand, indeed penetrate the essence of life in the South, explaining how the traditional inflexibility, ignorance, and passiveness of the *meridionali* are the direct results of constant manipulation, oppression, and exploitation at the hands of the government, the Church, and the landowners. Life in the hamlets and farms of the *Mezzogiorno* (South) is one with little joy and much resignation: the system is beyond repair, and there is nothing the peasants can do politically to reverse the tragic course of their lives. What is unusual about the book is the deep affection for the poor, the empathy for their lot; every page is made to talk the truth of the miseries of the South in a language that manages to convey the despair of the peasants, abandoned even by the dim hope that those in power will ever come to their assistance. Even religious hope has abandoned them: "Christ," as one of the local sayings goes, "Never came to Galliano. He stopped at Eboli."

The structure of the book is unusual: there are reflections and observations of life in the South and elsewhere, as there are many short, effectively described episodes, along with masterfully written vignettes of people. The result is an absorbing human tableau, painted with striking colors (pastels are not Levi's forte), and written in a language which is always controlled and exact, never pretentious or learned. Levi's link with the great narrative tradition of the nineteenth century, and more exactly, and not surprisingly, with the great novels of the master of "*verismo,*" Giovanni Verga, is both natural and clear.

L'orologio appeared in 1950. Among the comments it evoked from the critics, one of the most pertinent is that of Luigi Russo, posed as a question. "Why the title of the book?" he wrote. "It is superfluous to decipher the symbol: [the novel] is entitled *The Watch* but it could easily have been entitled *The Bowels of Rome*, or the *Diasphora of the New People of Israel*, or the *Miseries of a Great Civilization in Ruin*, or *The Last Days of Democratic Pompeii*. All these are intellectual titles, which the writer's good taste would reject, but equally intellectualistic, because of its symbolism, is the title *The Watch*."

Why the watch? We frequently look at our watches in our daily living to check the time; the watch reminds us that time passes by and, in so doing, becomes part of our conscience, a reminder of our obligations and commitments. It is important to notice that the narrator of the story has a dream as the book opens, a dream that will turn out to be prophetic: his timepiece falls and it breaks. Much to the chagrin of the narrator, for whom it has great sentimental value, it cannot be repaired. "It was a very beautiful watch with a double case of the best make: an Omega chronometer that did not miss a second. It had been given to me by my father years and years ago on graduation day, as is the custom. . . . Watches such as mine," the narrator continues, "have a story of their own, a family and paternal history. One rarely buys them for one's own use. They are almost always a gift, and an important gift, from father, grandfather or uncle on an important occasion at the most decisive moment of life, when a young man enters the world, acquires his autonomy, detaches himself from his past, from the uncertain security of the tepid family clan to start making his own personal time."

In view of the prominence given to the watch, we assume or suspect that it is really a metaphor for time passing by, carrying away with it lost opportunities to work together for the common good. Our intuition proves to be correct when, later in the novel, Levi writes:

> As for the watch, it might symbolize many things. First of all, it was a curved, round, closed object like an Indian *Mandala*, and what's more, it was an astrological object divided into twelve parts, like the twelve signs of the zodiac. He [Marino] added, parenthetically, that the number thirteen, which does not appear on a watch and is considered an ill omen, actually brings bad luck (and he supposed I knew) only in countries inhabited by people who will never develop. Furthermore, a watch is a jewel, a precious object, and the watch, in essence, has now established itself scientifically, securely and without any possibility of doubt. . . . To lose a watch means to be outside of one's own true time, to lose oneself. I had lost mine in

a dream, and then found it again, but inside another time-piece, an alarm clock. Also, it was broken.

During the three days during which the story unfolds, we are always with the hero-narrator of the novel, we are given the privilege of witnessing, one is tempted here to say "participate" in, the events of that fateful year. The autobiographical dimension of "Don Carlo," as he is affectionately called by his friends and associates, is but a thin screen for the personality of Levi himself: he is an intellectual very much engagé in the sociopolitical and moral reconstruction of his country, an articulate idealistic journalist-editor of a newspaper printed under the greatest of difficulties in post–World War II Italy, a keen ideologue who perceives that an important turning point in the history of his country has been reached. Two themes are now joined: the political situation has deteriorated to the point that the hope for a better and more democratic Italy has been dashed with the fall of the government headed by Ferruccio Parri, and the "personal" story of the protagonist, who achieves a keener and wider perspective of the situation of his country, possible after the death of his uncle. The meaning of time, the perception of the necessity for thoughtful action, temporarily lost when the watch was accidentally broken, is regained once Don Carlo inherits a watch from his uncle Luca.

The Watch is probably one of the most intelligent "non-novels" of Italy in the forties and fifties. The characterization "non-novel" may be appropriate in view of the almost total absence of a plot —a fact that justifies the definition of Carlo Muscetta in these words: "[*The Watch*] is not a tale; it is an ingenious literary machine whose finality is not to measure time but to fight a quixotic war against time or even against historicism."

The book's structure is quite similar to that of *Christ Stopped At Eboli*. Like Levi's famous essay, *The Watch* is impressive in its re-creation of a certain climate not through the unfolding of a story, but through the unusual technique of a narrative made up of a series of vignettes describing the protagonist's encounters with a wide assortment of people: newspapermen, landladies, traffickers, politicians, ministers, black marketeers, servants, and, in the last section of the book, gypsy cabdrivers and even brigands. Indeed, the last fourth of the novel, describing the narrator's incredible one hundred and fifty-mile journey from Rome to Naples, where his uncle Luca is dying, is among the finest written by Levi. In Naples, Don Carlo speaks briefly on the telephone with his uncle, who asks him to delay his visit until the following morning, so that both will be less fatigued and thus enjoy the pleasure of being together again. But when Don Carlo arrives, sad news awaits him: his uncle has just passed away, leaving him a beautiful watch, "a gold watch, a doctor's watch, with a hand that counts the seconds, a splendid old Omega, in every way like the one my father had given me." The cycle is now complete, and Don Carlo goes back to Rome in the official car of an old personal friend who is a minister of the government.

Writing about *Christ Stopped at Eboli*, Giovanni Fallaschi asks: "Is it a novel? Is it a journalistic reportage? Is it a book of memoirs? A diary? Is it a sociological essay?" These questions could be raised, though to a lesser degree, about *The Watch*. And the reader may do well to keep the various levels in which Levi's themes are developed separate. The result might well be an absorbing view of how an intellectual understood, as an astute observer and participant in the historical process, the events of the immediate post–World War II months in Italy. Particularly central, in this respect, is the attention given to the Italian Underground movement, and how much hope many people had put into it, and what meaning it had for those working for a better, freer Italy:

> The question now was whether that extraordinary movement called the Resistance would actually develop further, remolding the shape of the country, or would be pushed back into historical memory, disavowed as active reality, be relegated at best, to the depths of the individual conscience, like a spiritual experience without visible fruits, filled only with the promise of a distant future. In these days the movement's strength was being tested, and not only in terms of sheer impulse, motivation, numbers and influence, not in terms of its capacity and ability. . . . It was one of those times when everyone's destiny hung uncertain, when the ablest politicians assess the forces in the field and prepare clever moves in a complicated game of chess, a game they are doomed anyhow to lose, since the only

way to win it would be to find a word, a true word capable of creating new forces, of overturning the chessboard and transforming the game into a living thing. Would the word be found?

It is often said that a writer has but one story to tell: certainly this holds true for Carlo Levi. Much like *Christ Stopped at Eboli*, *The Watch* is largely based on the author's experiences; both books show a wide interest in history, politics, and sociology; both books reveal what is probably one of Levi's most solid achievements—his ability to take a long view of certain cultural-political-economic patterns (which lead him to what cannot be described in any other term but contempt toward the landowners) and, at the same time, the creation of a large number of characters from most walks of life whose role in his books is of short duration. Levi's great gift is well served by his artistry as a painter and the humanistic quality of his mind. The problem is that in fiction, and the novel in particular, characters must be developed, their roles constantly enriched by symbolism, thus broadening the relevance of the artist's vision. This generally eludes Levi, despite some notable visual successes, such as the depiction of Giuseppe Biscaglia, known as the king of Poggioreale. Extremely wealthy, powerful, in every way feared and respected by politicians and the people, despite the mysterious way in which he has amassed his fortune, he becomes an unforgettable figure in a book so crowded with intellectuals.

In the last analysis, *The Watch* is a strange blend of historical, autobiographical, and ideological elements, skillfully woven into a tapestry that is at once unusual and insightful. A cursory glance at the literary scene of the post–World War II years would reveal the rather massive number of novels that were inspired by the long period of Fascist tyranny, or by the destruction and pain brought about by the war. Yet, none deals with the climate of confusion and uncertainty that generated many of the political compromises that led to today's chaotic situation. "Historical reality," wrote Emilio Cecchi when the novel was published, "assumes the fluctuating mask of a larva." The ultimate purpose of *The Watch* is to record, study and put into perspective the historical factors responsible for the lack of substantial progress in the long-delayed restructuring of Italian society. Hence the rather substantial part of the book given over to discussions and

analyses central to the author's purpose. An illustration of this
tendency is the passage explaining the nature of the two main
classes into which Italy finds itself divided: the *"Contadini"* and
the *"Luigini:"*

Who are the Contadini? First of all they are the peasants, of
course, those of the South and also of the North, almost all
of them, with their civilization that lies outside of time and
the course of history, with their closeness to living, their kinship to animals, to the forces of nature and the land, to their
pagan and prepagan gods and saints; with all their patience
and all their wrath. . . . But the Contadini are not only the
peasants. . . . Of course there are the barons, too. . . . I said
'barons'; the real ones, with castles on the tops of the mountains—the peasant barons. . . . Then there are the industrialists, the contractors, the technicians, most of them in small and
medium industries but some of them in big business as well.
. . . And also the agrarians, even the rich landowners. . . .
And the workers too. I don't mean those who are corrupted
and join with their masters in the petty affairs of their regions.
. . . But all the others, the great mass of workers who are educated in the creative rhythm of the factory, its voluntary discipline, the value they exist in. . . . Contadini, too, are artisans,
doctors, mathematicians, painters, women—true women, not
the imitation. Finally . . . *we* are Contadini. I don't mean
the three of us, but those who used to be called by that odious word 'intellectuals.' . . . And who, then, are the Luigini?
They're the others. The great, endless, formless, amoeba-like
majority of the petty bourgeoisie with all its species and sub-
species and variations, with all their miseries, inferiority com-
plexes, morality and immorality, misdirected ambitions and
idolatrous fears. They're the ones who submit and command,
love and hate the hierarchy, and serve and reign. They're the
bureaucratic mob, employees of the state and the banks, model
clerks, the military, the magistrates, lawyers, the police, college
graduates, errand boys, students and parasites. They are the
Luigini. The priests too [are Luigini] . . . then there are the industrialists and businessmen who keep going on the multimil-
lions of the state, and also the workers who stand by them and
the landowners and peasants of the same sort. . . . There are

the politicians, the organizers of all sorts and shades. . . . Beware . . . because the Luigini are the majority. Democratically, vote for vote, they're the winners. . . . [They] have the numbers, they have the state, the church, the parties, the political language, the army, the courts and the press. The Contadini have none of them. They don't know that they exist, that they have any common interest.

These insights, now offered almost three decades ago, commend Levi to the reader of today and tomorrow. But the intellectual challenge of the book is only part of the reason why it will continue to be read in the future. It not only gives an absorbing picture of post–World War II Italian politics, and offers an accurate diagnosis of the fracture in Italian society, but it anticipates the "death" of the novel as we knew it up until the mid-forties:

"What sort of novel do you want after Auschwitz and Buchenwald? Did you see the photographs of women weeping as they buried pieces of soap made from the bodies of their husbands and their sons? . . . There you are! Your *tranche de vie*—a piece of soap? . . .

"A piece of soap," he continued, without giving us a chance to interrupt him, "that we must bury with tears. A piece of soap that is the body and soul of man. That's the result of the Faustian action. That's the conclusion, the destination of your novels and your abstract reasoning."

It would be several more years before Italy, Europe, and numerous other nations would realize and understand the significance of this statement.

6

Carlo Emilio Gadda: The Experimental Novel

"L'abito non fa il monaco," so goes an old Italian adage: "Looks can be deceiving." Indeed they can: one of the most conventional-looking persons who could be seen, whenever he made one of his rare appearances in Roman cafés or literary gatherings, was a man who, at an age when most people are enjoying retirement, was regarded as the unofficial leader and idol of the literary avantgarde in his country, a novelist whose work, by nearly unanimous critical consensus, had earned him a place in his literature comparable to that occupied in Anglo-American letters by James Joyce. Gadda was his name—Carlo Emilio Gadda, to be precise —Milanese by birth (November 14, 1893), but European by interest and outlook, maverick author of poems, critical essays, several novels, and a precious journal: engineer by necessity not by choice, a man who, by virtue of his literary work, was destined to be talked about far more than actually read (let alone understood!), admired more than appreciated, a not too uncommon fate of many uncommon artists. An exceedingly private person, he led a secluded life to the point of giving the impression of being unfriendly, if not a recluse. "Stately and courtly," notes his English translator William Weaver, "he [lived] in a lower-middle-class apartment in Rome, where the yelling of children, the clatter of dishes, and the laundry hanging on the balconies contrast[ed] violently with the cloistral austerity, the shy solitude of the writer's quarters." Ironically, it was only in the last years of his life that Gadda became known to a large audience, even though he had been writing since the twenties, and his work had received a number of prestigious prizes, including the Viareggio (1953), and the International Editors Prize at Formentor, in 1963.

Much of what Gadda wrote has a Leonardian quality about it: begun at a given time, put away for months or even years, extensively rewritten and enlarged, often published in parts, but never really "finished." Typical of this unorthodox procedure, as we shall see, are his major works, *La cognizione del dolore* (*Acquainted with Grief*, N.Y., 1969), published in parts and in volumes in 1938–41, 1963, and 1970, and *Quer pasticciaccio brutto de via Merulana* (*That Awful Mess on Via Merulana*, N.Y., 1965), also published in three different versions in 1946–47, 1953, and 1957.

A number of biographical events contributed substantially to molding Gadda's character. The first was the irresponsible decision his father made in 1899 to build a country home ("una fottuta e strampalata casa di campagna," as Gadda was to dub it) at Longrine al Segrino, in the lovely, verdant Brianza region of Lombardy—a house that literally drained much of the family's limited financial resources until its sale, in 1936, after Gadda's mother passed away. The second was the long, bitter months he spent at the Celle Lager, in Hannover, Germany (from October 1917 to the end of 1918) as a prisoner of war. The third was the death of his beloved brother Enrico, a twenty-one-year-old flier whose aircraft was brought down by Austrian flak barely a few weeks before the Armistice.

Back home, at the war's end, Gadda returned to school to complete his education interrupted by the war. In 1920, he achieved his degree in electrical engineering and found a job that took him to Sardinia. From 1922 to 1924, he worked in Argentina; back in Italy, he accepted an assignment that enabled him to spend much of his time in several European countries, thus satisfying his intense wish to travel. He was first published in the press of that bold, sophisticated Florentine "little magazine" *Solaria*, and his writings attracted the notice of what would eventually become a wide range of critics that included Giacomo Devoto and Gianfranco Contini, with their impeccable credentials of university professors of philology, newspaper critics like Enrico Falqui and Pietro Pancrazi, novelists and poets Alberto Moravia, Nobel laureate Eugenio Montale, and the late Pier-Paolo Pasolini, poet and film maker and possibly one of Gadda's most acute interpreters and "disciples."

Unlike most Italian writers, usually schooled in the humanities, Gadda was a scientist: his mind was trained in the exacting disciplines of mathematics, physics, chemistry—hence his propensity, particularly in his early books, toward accuracy of details, precision and solidity of structure. But Gadda was a maverick, from whom one cannot expect the ordinary. His interests as reflected in his writings make that clear: a wide and deep acquaintance with philosophy (in which he nearly took a degree)—especially Leibniz, Spinoza, Kant; classical and modern historians (Caesar, Tacitus, Michelet); a familiarity with Italian, Continental European, and American poets (Ariosto, Belli, Villon, Shakespeare, Whitman) and the writers of the so-called "Lombard Group," Manzoni, Porta, the penologist Beccaria, the Verri brothers, the historian Carlo Cattaneo; and, finally, his broad, almost encyclopedic knowledge. A man with a mind trained to be intellectually rigorous, he could confess: "Il pasticcio e il disordine mi annientano" ("mess and disorder defeat me"). Compulsive for order, structure, and competence, he suffered more than usual because of the inefficiency, the incompetence, the superficiality with which he met, as a soldier, a scientist, and a man, and the ensuing frustration burst time and again into explosions that reverberate in many pages of his many books.

Like most other intellectuals, Gadda came to perceive the meaning of being a child of one's own era, witnessing and living the dramatic political and social changes that altered so radically the quality of contemporary existence. His dreams clashed with the facts; his ideals became shattered by reality, and his own ideology frequently became contradictory and confused by his aspirations and by what appeared to be necessary restrictions on personal freedom imposed by the new regime. It must be pointed out here, as Guido Baldi and, after him, Robert S. Dombroski have done, that Gadda is essentially conservative—at times even reactionary by today's standards—and that his position in politics is by no means consistent, not to say contradictory. Yet, by 1918, Gadda began to perceive the sham of official values, often mere devices to suppress the legitimate aspirations of decent men everywhere. War itself, at first welcomed as a chance to assert his own individuality and power, as well as a means to achieve for his country what peace had not, revealed its ugliness when Gadda was informed of his brother's death. And at that moment, war became a sad painful experience in his life, causing pain not even the passing of time could easily assuage.

The inefficiency of the governmental bureaucracy and leadership, particularly visible in the manner in which it conducted the war, the irresponsibility of the industrial complex, busily trying to make as large a profit as possible, the stupidity of the military hierarchy, the dreadful training and illiteracy of the troops—all these, and other factors, turned Gadda into a man who only with extraordinary difficulty could contain his impatience and utter dissatisfaction. His slow transformation into a man grown weary of life, disenchanted with his youthful idealism, gradually drawn into a metaphysical mess without escape, may be read in a diary, *Giornale di guerra e di prigionia* [Journal of the war and of (my) imprisonment] (1953, revised 1965) parts of which are unfortunately lost. The portrait that emerges from the book is that of a man unusually sensitive and unusually arrogant, afflicted by many traumas, terrified by the prospect of being thrown back into a "mediocre life," feeling useless (partly because of his own decision of not identifying with a society he cannot respect), left on the margins of society and history: "My life is a complete detour, a waste of marvelous faculties."

The end of World War I, and Gadda's reentry into civilian life, did not materially affect his situation. If anything, we find him reacting with more bitterness and scorn toward a society unwilling to make room for all those who fought so gallantly to make the Italian dream of total unification and independence come true, only to be pushed aside, left without employment, publicly insulted. "The reality of these years," comments Gadda, "is shitty." Italy finds itself on the threshold of fascism: "My life is useless, it's like that of an automaton who has survived himself, and who performs a few material gestures, without either love or faith." In the course of a few years, Gadda had moved from a patriotic, nationalist proponent of war to one of complete contempt for his country's political structure—a stance that was to harden gradually during the dictatorship of Mussolini. In short, Gadda withdrew as much as life permitted him into a tower from which he could manage to launch his poisonous arrows at the stupidities of human behavior, the banalities of existence, the fraudulent schemes of politics and of social conventions. His traumas, his neuroses, his painful sense of dislocation, added to what seems to have been a life unusually marked by the absence of affection and tenderness, may in fact have been the elements that spurred Gadda to create that artful linguistic *pastiche* that distinguishes his literary work, as we shall see later.

In 1940, he felt the need to transfer his residence to Florence, following the example of one of his favorite writers, Alessandro Manzoni, in order "to learn the [Italian] language," and hoping to take advantage of the city's magnificent libraries. He wrote for several newspapers, and a selection of his pieces was brought out in 1943, with the title *Gli anni* [The years], reissued by Einaudi of Turin in 1964 as *Le meraviglie d'Italia* [The marvels of Italy]. During the last war, Gadda, privately a staunch critic and satirizer of fascism, found himself in difficulties; without a job, under suspicion for his political views, he experienced hunger and deprivation. At the end of the war, he resumed his journalistic activities; from 1950 until 1954 he worked in the cultural division of the Italian Radio and Television (RAI). The last years of his life were spent writing new works (*Eros e Priapo: Da furore a cenere* [Eros and Priapus: from frenzy to ashes], 1967), collecting his critical essays (*I viaggi la morte* [Travels, death], 1958), revising his novels and short stories previously published, such as his *Giornale di guerra e di prigionia* (1953, revised 1965) and *La meccanica* [Mechanics] (1970). He died on May 21, 1973.

Much if not indeed all of Gadda's literary production seems to pivot around the idea of striving to present a portrait, through fiction on the one hand and the more frankly autobiographical work on the other hand, of a tormented, confused era. This ambitious goal is less impressive per se than for the expressive instrument Gadda laboriously created to express his world: a language that is unusually open to dialects and rich enough to be deservedly defined as "baroque," a challenging, delightful *pastiche* that is a constant source of discovery of meanings.

Gadda's first published book, *La Madonna dei filosofi* [The philosopher's Madonna] (1931), is a collection of short stories in which the personal elements play a large role. *Il castello di Udine* [The castle of Udine] (1934), a three-part volume that includes autobiographical pages, a section entitled "Crociera mediterranea" [Mediterranean cruise], an account of a voyage that provides the author with numerous insights into the travelers and the many ports of call, and a section made up of several shorter pieces. And, finally, a short story, "La fidanzata di Elio" [Elio's fiancée], steeped in life and society of Milan.

L'Adalgisa (1944) reaffirms Gadda's serious commitment of leaving to posterity an accurate, philosophically justified portrait of a society undergoing a period of social, political, cultural upheaval that eventually made possible the rise of fascism and its temporary success in much of Europe. It is a collection of ten short stories, or "*disegni*" ("sketches"), the main of which is the one that gives the book its title. (In 1955, together with *La Madonna dei filosofi* and *Il castello di Udine*, *L'Adalgisa* becomes the third part of *I sogni la folgore* [The dreams, the thunderbolt].) Published in a limited edition of 1,000 copies, *L'Adalgisa* is a diverting, acute, and revealing foray into the lives of a number of distinguished, and not so distinguished, Milanese families, and their idiosyncrasies, the way they bring up their children, their tastes, their concepts of what life is—in short, their values. In the hands of Gadda, a writer whose sarcasm, irony, and humor are difficult to match, the resulting tableau is nothing less than scathing. But Gadda's eye is simply not satisfied to remain fixed exclusively on the middle and upper bourgeoisie. Following a tradition which counts such poets as Giuseppe Parini, Carlo Porta, and others, he zeroes in on the "lower" class, what the Roman poet Giuseppe Gioacchino Belli called *la povera gente* ("the poor people"), and much of the vitality of the "sketches" is achieved through the unusually expert manner in which Gadda blends (and here perhaps is the best illustration of the extent to which he felt the influence of another famous Milanese writer, Alessandro Manzoni) history and poetry. The result is not only a highly amusing book, but a valuable source of information about the festas and customs on Milan in the 1800s, right down to foods, traditions, amusements, clothing, and so forth, enriched with other fascinating tidbits of Italian life at the turn of the century. The different "designs," thanks to the author's subtle strategy of mentioning or referring to the same names of families throughout the volume, become a sort of episodic novel which begins (appropriately enough) with the bankruptcy of a "Domestic agency," called "Confidenza," and the "Bank of Milan." The woman who turns out to be a kind of protagonist of the book (and after whom the work is titled) is Adalgisa. An opera singer, once married to Signor Carlo Biandronni, an accountant no longer living, she had striven to climb the social ladder so as to earn the respect and affection of her late husband's family. But this is the past, and in this sense the story of the heroine is precisely about the past, the lost opportunities for happiness that are too real and believable not to be recognized as Gadda's own.

It would be difficult to call *Quer pasticciaccio brutto de via Merulana* (*That Awful Mess on Via Merulana*) a novel in the traditional sense, hardly surprising in the light of the unorthodox nature of Gadda's literary production. Consisting of five "episodes," more or less tied together, *Quer pasticciaccio* was originally written in the last months of World War II, and published in serial form between 1946 and 1947, in the Florentine magazine *Letteratura* (numbers 26–29 and 31), with publication in book form announced to take place shortly thereafter. The difficulties in which *Letteratura* found itself caused a drastic delay of original plans. The book was put aside, as Gadda's new commitments as freelance journalist and, later on, as writer and consultant for the Italian Radio and Television, took up his time. In 1953, with the encouragement of Livio Garzanti, of the publishing house by the same name, Gadda began the long labor of revision and rewriting that the book required. Published in 1957, it ws an immediate critical and popular success.

The setting of *Quer pasticciaccio* is Rome, the time is 1927. Both are deliberate choices, dictated by the author's strategy. Rome is the capital of Italy, a bureaucratic city (in this sense, similar to Washington, D.C.), "the center of Italy," observes Robert Bongiorno, "Babel, where all tongues come together and blend into a hopeless confusion." To live in Rome can be particularly difficult, for it means to live a mediocre existence in the shadow of the remains of a splendid, glorious era of power, political prestige, and cultural greatness of long, long ago. The year 1927 is also crucial in that it marks the moment when Italy, for the previous five years led by Benito Mussolini, has already witnessed the disappearance of some of her most articulate and influential adversaries of fascism by murder or prison terms: Socialist leader Giacomo Matteotti murdered (1924); Antonio Gramsci and Palmiro Togliatti, arrested; others driven to, or preparing for the bitter road of exile. The government is busy displaying the first visible progress of its "law and order" policy: beggars are disappearing from the streets; trains are beginning to run on time; labor unrest is over, since unions have been abolished and strikes have been declared illegal; the people are back to work, and the nation is now cleaner and prouder than it has been in many a year; crimes and suicides, as well as other acts of violence and antisocial behavior, have been sharply reduced, judging from newspapers accounts. Of course, the papers have been instructed not to give prominence to criminal acts, and suicides may be reported only as "accidents."

The novel, divided in ten chapters, begins in a casual way, at via Merulana, No. 219, Building A—called the "Gold Palace" because of its affluent tenants. On February 20, 1927, Dr. Francesco Ingravallo, a thirty-five-year-old police inspector known to his friends and relatives as Don Ciccio, is the luncheon guest of his friends, Remo and Liliana Balducci. Less than a month later, on March 14, a thief, wearing a green scarf, enters the apartment of a neighbor of the Balduccis, Signora Menegazzi, a widow, and forces her at gunpoint to hand him her precious jewels plus a substantial amount of cash. An investigation is launched at once, and Don Ciccio finds a streetcar ticket stub on the floor, where it had inadvertently fallen when the thief had pulled out his gun. A streetcar conductor remembers a young man wearing a green scarf as having been aboard on the day of the robbery. Three days later, on March 17, Don Ciccio, still deeply involved in his investigation, is informed that his friend Liliana Balducci has been found dead in her apartment, her throat slashed. Her body has been found by her cousin, Giuliano Valdarena, a young engineer employed by the Standard Oil Company, who had come to say goodbye to Liliana on the eve of his departure for Genoa, where he had been reassigned by his company.

The next three chapters (3, 4, and 5) deal with the investigation of the two crimes. A number of factors, such as Giuliano's being the only male of the family and as such a rather favorite person in Liliana's eyes (she has no children of her own) and his carefree life-style, make him a prime suspect. His ironclad alibi, however, eliminates him from at least a direct connection with the crime. Liliana's husband, Remo, was actually away from Rome on the day of the crime: upon returning home, he notices the disappearance of a box containing his wife's jewels. Chapter 6 tells us how the green scarf has been found by the police of Marino, a nearby town, thanks to the cooperation of Zamira, a prostitute and a madame. A new character is introduced: Ines Cionini, a prostitute once employed in Zamira's bordello, and formerly a resident of Torraccio, in the vicinity of Rome, the hamlet of the streetcar ticket found by Don Ciccio in Balducci's apartment. Her deposition (chapter 7) make feasible the development of a new theory, linking the theft and the murder. In the next chapter, various leads bring *brigadiere* Pestalozzi, who has been in charge of one of the phases of the investigation, to Zamira's house and finds Lavinia, still another girl with connections with the former madame, wearing a large topaz ring lent her a couple of days earlier by her cousin Camilla. At last, the stolen jewels are found in a chamber pot, hidden under some walnuts in Camilla's house. The investigation continues: Ascanio Lanciani, who occasionally runs a roast-pork sandwich stand, and who is the brother of Diomede, Ines Cionini's boyfriend, is arrested. As the book comes to the end, Don Ciccio is about to check out yet another suspect, Assuntina (or Tina) Crocchiani, Signora Balducci's former maid, who left Rome to assist her dying father. But Assuntina denies any direct or indirect part in the crime and, with her shouts of denial, the story ends.

If it is true that no synopsis of a serious literary work succeeds in giving the reader more than a fleeting hint of its significance as an effort to shed light upon the human condition, this is even more genuinely true in the case of *Quer pasticciaccio*, on the surface a book about two of the most pedestrian, ordinary crimes one can think of. If such are the appearances, we must take a second look to begin to see what Gadda's novel is about.

The first question that comes to mind is why Gadda, an unusually serious writer, should have turned to writing what in Italy is known as a *"giallo,"* a detective novel usually printed with yellow (*"giallo"*) covers. Robert S. Dombroski speculates that *Quer pasticciaccio*, completed in the mid-forties, with its satirical depiction of certain aspects of life under fascism, would make Gadda reach an audience far larger than the small number of devotees who had followed his career during the previous two decades or so, and help him to become, after years of poverty, financially successful. If this is an acceptable hypothesis, it is puzzling why Gadda, once the review *Letteratura* went bankrupt, should not have explored other possibilities to bring out his book, and waited nearly ten years before seeing it into print, substantially revised. So much for the practical side of the question. But surely Gadda, an astute writer and student of the art of fiction, was also moved by other considerations in his decision to write under the guise of a detective novel what could well be his major work. My hunch is that he must have realized how perfectly the conventions of that genre suited his ambition to give shape and meaning to his view of the world, even at the cost of defying those very conventions he was supposed to embrace and accept.

Quer pasticciaccio is a novel almost bent in breaking all precedents: it is the only work of its kind to have been written by an important, and possibly major artist of our time; it has no real "hero," an inconclusive ending (since the perpetrator of the crimes is not apprehended), and is written in an unusual combination of dialects and "literary" Italian. If on the surface at any rate, the classical pattern of the detective novel is respected, it soon becomes clear to the reader that Gadda is far less interested in pursuing the criminal who must be delivered into the hands of justice, than he is in the murdered woman, in the complicated web of relationships (of an implicit lesbian kind) that could have possibly generated the motivation for the murder. Insofar as the events are fabricated by Gadda's imagination, the novel is a sort of game of deceit, in which the investigator is presented as a skillful problem-solver, and as such, gratifies the reader's yearning for reassurance and order. But in failing to bring the feelings into a comprehensible structure, the novelist is clearly addressing himself to the impossibility for him to "pursue," as Olga Ragusa underscores, "an overall linear development in which events are related to one another consecutively and logically." In our time, a novelist can no longer be expected to play God, and the reader will have to accept the task of making sense out of the experience presented to him. We may suspect at first that this is another clever trick of the trade: as readers, we know that every event, word, or action included in the book has its justification in the author's strategy. This time, however, the strategy proves to be of a negative sort, as it were—not to illuminate and to make us understand, but to obfuscate and leave us as puzzled as we have been all along. The end of the novel merely confirms what we may have suspected—to make its "point" the story must remain unfinished, just as the mystery of life, at least for Gadda and those who see things as he does, is a puzzle only death can end, if not resolve.

When viewed from this perspective, the question of the language of the novel, consonant as it is with its theme, becomes clearer. Let us note at once that there are several dialects used in *Quer pasticciaccio*, chiefly the Roman, the Molisan (from the Molise region), the Neapolitan, the Venetian, and the "standard," official Italian, which Gadda ranks as a dialect sui generis.

The first problem posed by the use of dialects is one of communication. Since literature is ultimately a sophisticated vehicle through which the artist transmits his or her feelings and ideas about life, it is natural that the writer wishing to reach as wide an audience as possible, must rely on the concept of a national language. It is generally conceded that dialects are a kind of "corruption" of the national tongue, a corruption in which geography (and its ensuing cultural provincialism and isolation), in addition to economic and political factors, plays a strong role. It is also a fact that an increasing social mobility, a national system of education, and the increased penetration of the media into everyday occurrences of even the most isolated hamlets have largely contributed to the steady erosion of the strength, vitality, and need for dialects. How to make the most felicitous use of dialects, with their unique tone, resonance, and vibrancy has always proved to be a challenging task for Italian writers. Experiments of all sorts have been made, with varying degrees of success, ranging all the way from texts completely composed in dialect (Goldoni, Belli, Porta, Di Giacomo are the first names that come immediately to mind) to novels in which dialects are integrated in the story (Fogazzaro) retaining their spelling and structure, to the more difficult transformation of the dialects into a language that has all the appearances of standard Italian but "sounds" and is structured like a dialect, a feat fully accomplished by Giovanni Verga.

In the light of these observations, and conscious of the risks involved in using dialects in a novel, one wonders what motivated Gadda to make dialects an integral and substantial part of his narrative's language. At first, it was thought that his decision was motivated by his possible acceptance of the poetics of post–World War II neorealism, which emphasized a natural, "spoken," as opposed to a traditional, literary idiom. But Gadda himself, in an interview eventually published, along with others on the same topic, in book form (*Inchiesta sul Neorealismo*, edited by Carlo Bo, 1951) categorically denied that such was his intention, and went on to say: "It is all well and good to tell me that a volley of machine gun fire is reality. But what I expect from the novel is that behind those seven ounces of lead there be some tragic tension, some consecution at work, a mystery, perhaps the reason for the fact, or the absence of reasons. . . . The fact by itself, is but the dead body of reality, the—pardon the expression—fecal residue of history. I would therefore want the poetics of neorealism to be extended to include a nouminous [*sic*] dimension." (Trans. by Olga Ragusa.) The statement clearly points to directions other than those primarily concerned with a mimetic representation of reality.

Other theories present themselves: one, advanced by a number of critics, sees dialects, expertly mingled with the precise, technical language Gadda liberally draws from the sciences, as a form of protest against the national language as a symbol of the cultural and political establishment: "The linguistic polemic," writes Cesare Segre in his volume *Lingua stile e società*," coincides in [Gadda's] work with a polemic against Milanese society (the industrial and commercial middle class), Roman society, the literary society, [which] suffer blows whose violence is accentuated by Gadda's stylistic *outrance*." Segre's position finds support in Gadda's own confession about the nature of writing which he sees as a kind of "vengeance" for the injuries fate inflicts upon men, himself first among them: "My storytelling often manifests the resentful person who speaks while withholding his wrath, his indignation." Obviously, his style must reflect his condition: hence, the outpouring of words, the convolution of his prose, the verbal pyrotechnics that have become the distinguishing trademark of his writing. His lack of faith in reality is magnificently reflected in his lack of faith in language; his inability to seize reality is mirrored in the puzzling, inconclusive ending of the novel.

What emerges from *Quer pasticciaccio*, as Angelo Guglielmi has underscored, is an unusual attempt not so much to interpret reality, as to construct it, to demystify things by freeing them from meanings. "Gadda's merit," he continues, "is to have precipitated the situation of Italian narrative, freeing it from all academic delays, and starting it, irreversibly, toward freer and more open forms." To present the world as it is, without didactic intentions, would seem the best an artist can achieve in our time. In this sense, the use of dialects—often so different from one another as to be, for all practical purposes, nothing less than different languages—conveys the sense of alienation pervading the writings of Gadda, particularly esteemed by the generation of new Italian novelists. Similarly, the open-ended structure of his work, its freedom from many conventions, its numerous original innovations, have broken the barriers of naturalism and linked the Italian novel with the most solid and respected writers of Europe's avant-garde, from Musil to Joyce, from Beckett to Robbe-Grillet.

That *Quer pasticciaccio* is a stylistic *tour de force* few, I am certain, would be ready to deny. In every way brilliantly conceived and brilliantly executed, it succeeds in giving life to a story that never took place without moving the reader, making him feel the shock of recognition. By contrast, *La cognizione del dolore* (*Acquainted with Grief*), as a book that, despite its difficulty, touches deeply the most private areas of our feelings. It is at once a novel and an autobiographical essay, "one of the few books of [Italian] contemporary fiction," as Adriano Seroni suggests, "worthy of being defined of European caliber." In a larger sense it, too, is about the mess of our lives, as is *Quer pasticciaccio*; it, too, is a novel in which a murder (also unresolved) takes place. But it is, above everything else, a book about "pain," the grief experienced by a strange character, who lives in a strange country, a hero who could be the author, not the author-as-the investigator of *Quer pasticciaccio*, but a human being who suffers and whose anguish is what makes our identification with him, and our empathy with his situation possible.

The setting of *Quer pasticciaccio* was Rome, and the references to that city were both numerous and detailed. *Acquainted with Grief*, on the other hand, is set in South America, in a country called Maradagàl. There is no need to check the location of such a place because it exists only in the imagination of the novelist.

Like many of Gadda's books, *La cognizione del dolore* has a long and complicated publishing history, having appeared in parts before being issued as a book. It was first serialized in the review *Letteratura* (Nos. 7–10, 13, 14, and 17) between 1938 and 1941; then, appeared as a book, in 1963, accompanied by a lengthy introduction by Gianfranco Contini, and by a fictitious dialogue between the author and his publisher regarding the "recovery" of the manuscript. The novel, further enriched by two chapters (originally composed in 1941 and revised in 1960), appeared in the final edition in 1970, at last apparently completed. Two long sections of the work were originally part of *L'Adalgisa* (1944). However, the numerous notes that were published when the work was serialized were almost totally eliminated in the 1963 and 1970 editions. Two more sections included were part of a collection of short stories entitled *Novelle dal ducato in fiamme* (1953; [Stories from the duchy aflame] (1953) and *I racconti. Accoppiamenti giudiziosi* [Short stories. Wise matchings] (1963).

The title *Acquainted with Grief* is the first, and most important clue of the author's intention—not, as the English mistakenly suggests, "acquainted" with grief, but the process of experiencing and learning what pain is all about. The purpose of the novel is what the title implies; through incidents, real or imagined, we will discover and understand not only Gadda's suffering, but how his pain derives from and is hurled back to society itself.

In many ways, *La cognizione del dolore*, begun long before *Quer pasticciaccio*, but taken up here because of its appearance in its definitive edition several years after *That Awful Mess*, represents the culmination of Gadda's long, complex, difficult literary career, as well as a refining of and a refocusing on the main themes of his books. To point out the autobiographical character of the book should not be misinterpreted as yet another attempt to write about incidents of a personal nature. What concerns Gadda is not merely to trace, from the beginning, the elements that shaped his existence, but to retrieve the historical, psychological, philosophical factors that transformed radically both the character and quality of contemporary Italian (and, by extension, European) society. The art of fiction, for Gadda, must be not a pastime, but an instrument of knowledge, illuminating the intricate byways of life, the mystery of what Cesare Pavese called "the business of living."

Long before commencing work on *La cognizione del dolore*, Gadda had revealed, in his *Giornale di guerra e di prigionia* [Journal of the war and of (my) imprisonment], the great, unfulfilled needs of his life, and his anguish: "I have had no love, or anything. . . . I shall die like a dog, in ten, thirty years; without a family, without ever having enjoyed along the painful journey [of life] the presence of my mother, my dear brothers. . . . I have suffered everything, poverty, humiliation, illness, weakness, impotence of body and mind, fear of ridicule, to end up at Caporetto, in the end of ends." "My life," he noted again, "is a total derailment, a waste of marvelous faculties." An unsatisfactory home life, incompetent, stupid, narrow-minded teachers, an inflexible social structure, a rigid and repressive upbringing are the flesh and blood of the sufferings experienced by the young Gadda during his critical formative years. If this sounds like a catalogue of grievances against society, the impression must be further enlarged: his situation was made ever worse by another unnecessary burden, which in the book appears as that "fucking" house that caused further economic sacrifices.

Dubbing the novel autobiographical is indeed justifiable, it we accept the premise that all works of fiction are indeed more or less drawn from their author's life. But in *La cognizione*, Gadda adroitly uses not only his personal experiences as the basis of the plot, but his deepest emotions, the complex web of his neuroses that explode in a frontal, savage ideological critique of the false idols of contemporary existence. In short, the autobiographical references are too obvious to escape notice: for example, the hero of the book, Gonzalo, like Gadda, is an engineer, a war veteran (never mind which war), whose brother died in the service; his physique is modeled on Gadda's; he lives in a sprawling villa (the country house that consumed so large a share of the Gadda family's limited resources); Gonzalo, too, suffers from a long-repressed anger, which is about to explode. "Gadda," remarks Citati in a perceptive essay on the novel, "shares Gonzalo's tears and remorses, protests and curses with him, seems prisoner of all his passions. However, he distances himself intimately from his character: he does not feel sorry for him, does not forgive him anything; he judges him, and, through him, comes to know and to represent lucidly his life."

The time of the story is between 1925 and 1933. Maradagàl, bordering on the Cordillera, has just ended a war with neighboring Parapagàl a year earlier. Now both states are enjoying a modest economic recovery. Near the city of Pastrufazio, on the slopes of the Cordillera, in what had been a fashionable villa, in a state of decline, live the members of the Pirobutirro family: the Señora, now a widow, and her heavy-built, forty-one-year-old son Gonzalo Pirobutirro d'Eltino, an engineer.

As the story opens, on the hot day of August 28, the Señora is shown going to the cemetery to place fresh flowers on the family tomb; it is a calm, serene scene that gives no inkling of the end of the story, all violence and blood. The family doctor is summoned to the villa by Gonzalo, for a medical checkup. Gonzalo does not enjoy a good reputation in town: he is temperamental, cruel (one of his *peones*, José, claims that he has "all seven mortal sins in his gut"), a true misanthrope, stingy and cruel to his aging, sickly mother. The doctor's visit to the house, his conversation first with the servant Battistina and then with Don Gonzalo, take up a large part of the first part of the book, which serves to begin unraveling the situation at the core of the hero's problem.

The difficulty of the times, charged with all sorts of dangers, and the rapidly rising rate of crimes, make it wise for anyone with the necessary means to seek the protection of the "Nistitúos provinciales de vigilancia para la noche" ("Neighborhood Night Patrol Organization"). Gonzalo is offered that protection, but turns it down, while his neighbor the Cavaliere Trabatta, accepts it at once, fearing that his house will again be raided by thieves. One night, Bruno and Gildo, Trabatta's security men, alarmed by strange noises coming from Gonzalo's house, decide to check the situation there. Gonzalo's mother is found on her bed, critically stabbed by a mysterious intruder. Before dying, she exonerates her son from any part in the whole affair. The investigation now turns to other possible culprits, especially one Gaetano Palumbo, the assumed name of Pedro Mahogones, a night watchman.

Again, this "detective novel," too, lacks a conclusive end: we do not know, with any degree of certainty, just who murdered Gonzalo's mother, nor what his motivation might have been, and this point seems not to trouble the novelist. The thin plot may not satisfy a conventional reader trained to expect a resolution of a story, but it is most assuredly sufficient to allow Gadda to give vent to his highly charged emotions, his ravings and rantings (much like some of the Shakespearian tragedies, particularly *King Lear*, with which it has some points in common), his utter contempt for the bourgeois values his characters placidly accept— the war, for example, which bleeds unnecessarily nations which (in *La cognizione del dolore*) cannot enjoy the fruits of what is assuredly a hollow victory. The expectations of Don Gonzalo's mother are equally bourgeois, and therefore fraudulent and ridiculous—the paternalistic attitude toward the *peones* and the working class; all rituals, such as the house in the country; the retinue of servants no longer justifiable, in view of the family's economic decline.

These problems, however difficult or insurmountable as they prove to be, hardly conceal a far more devastating "malaise," which Gadda calls *"il male oscuro"* ("obscure sickness"), deeply embedded in the darkest recesses of the sensitivity of Gonzalo, a projection of his very creator: his neuroses, presented in the form of his insistence that the stone wall protecting his property has been built by his neighbor in a way calculated to rob him of a considerable slice of his land, or his paranoic fear that the *peones* want to harm him physically, or destroy his "nest," usually a symbol of the security, love, and protection his own parents, too busy pursuing the goals of money, prestige, and success, denied him during his childhood.

At this point, the reader may wonder whether Gadda is really offering a part of his life disguised as fiction, a self-portrait of his agonies. There is little question that certain childhood events had a powerful impact upon Gadda, to the point of causing him sufferings unrelieved through the last years of his life, his pain, the *"male oscuro,"* is transformed into a controlling image of the sense of alienation that has become a pervasive quality of contemporary existence. It is understandable why Gonzalo, returning from the war, should want to make his family house a safe refuge from the cruelties and stupidities of the world. Yet, for all his good intentions, Gonzalo and his mother, living under the same roof, remain incapable of communicating with, and understanding each other: his anger at his dead father, responsible for so much of their economic plight, can be vented only by throwing his picture on the floor and stamping on it.

In the expert hand of Gadda, Gonzalo and his mother are transformed from principal characters into archetypes, "Mother" and "Son," living symbols of the sham of the values of the social class to which they belong, typified by their attachment to material things—the villa, their jewels, their property—their attitude toward the *peones*, their emphasis on social decorum, prestige, lineage, charity to worthy causes, their insistence on a façade of respectability, and last, but not least, the foolish agricultural experiments that caused yet another loss in the ledger of the family's business. Like in Tozzi's novel *Il podere* [The farm], Gonzalo is angry with his life, aware of the numerous sacrifices imposed upon him by his late father's incompetence and mismanagement, and resorts to persecuting and threatening his mother in what must be understood as a rejection of his ties with his family. Gonzalo, a victim of his unexplainable malaise, is built up as a potentially tragic figure, eternally fighting the present because he is unable to comprehend his past. The future will not redeem him, and the present is to be wasted in a total indictment of any human activity, be it political, intellectual, emotional, economic, religious. There is no safety, no hope, no design for tomorrow: the world has been torn asunder, the only thing one can expect is the lightning of the gods that will put an end to all this misery.

Yet, for all the allusions historical and literary, whether to Caesar or Shakespeare, Gadda's "hero," like Moravia's heroes, will not attain tragedy. There is no real nobility in his soul, no depth, no possibility of greatness. He is a man torn by his acute awareness that life's greatest gift, love, has passed him by, and that somehow he will never be touched by it; a man wounded by the lack of parental tenderness; a man who cannot, and will not, make peace with himself and the world. There is little he can do in his circumstances besides letting anger be the rhythm of his life, rise over the grotesque, ridiculous, insignificant personage he is, intent only at shouting at the world, condemning rich and poor alike, the middle class of his native Lombardy (praised in Gadda's earlier *Il castello di Udine* for its great gift of stability and "its tradition of refined gentleness") and the new rich that have taken its place.

What emerges is a word of inauthenticity, of passion and violence left unchecked by love, of political vacuum, where everything is reduced to its lowest common denominator, where even the mother's death (left unexplained in the first version of the book) followed by a near stampede of the peasants into the villa, loses its tragic connotations—the vulgarity of those rushing into the villa is no different, in many ways, from that of its occupants. The mother's precious jewels, so eagerly disparaged and yet wanted by her son, are stolen; her body, almost lifeless, its head stained by blood, is found, covered by a blanket, by those who, under pretext of a decent concern for a human being, now confront the chilling sight. Like Gonzalo, Gadda, too, feels guilty, angry, and devastated. Life is difficult, our existence filled with insoluble problems, strained by the heavy burden of the past. Here, perhaps, the courage to address oneself to the dilemmas and the ensuing neuroses, in a language which, with all its convolutions, is fresh and full of vitality, is Gadda's originality. Precisely by virtue of the originality of his approach, and the steadfastness of his purpose, his work deserves to be read and studied by all serious readers of the novel as an art form.

7

Cesare Pavese: Symbols, Myths, and the Novel

August 27, 1950. It could have been a day like any other in late summer: hot, sultry, lazy. Traditionally, most Italians are on vacation then, or getting ready to return to work at the factories, at the offices, at the stores. What made that day different and tragic, at least for the intellectual community, was the news that earlier that morning the body of Cesare Pavese, age forty-two, essayist, poet, novelist, translator and editor-in-chief of the prestigious Giulio Einaudi Publishing Company, had been found dead, on the bed of Room 43 of the modest Hotel Roma in Turin. Cause of death: an overdose of sleeping pills.

The news was all the more bewildering in view of the popular and critical sucess Pavese had been enjoying during the months prior to his suicide. In 1948, he had received the Salento Prize for his *Prima che il gallo canti* [Before the cock crows]; in 1950, he was awarded the prestigious Strega Prize for *La bella estate* (*The Beautiful Summer*), originally written in 1940 but brought out in 1949, and his latest novel, *La luna e i falò* (*The Moon and the Bonfires*, N.Y., 1953) had been greeted with lavish praise by the critics and the readers who had begun to appreciate the beauty and significance of his work. It was not clear then, as it was to be a few months later when his diary, *Il mestiere di vivere* (1952; *The Burning Brand: Diaries 1935–1950*, N.Y., 1961) appeared that his death far from due to a momentary state of depression represented the culmination of a long, complex, emotional and intellectual preparation that had begun during his youth for the one act that he had come to value for its capacity to control man's destiny. Ironically, yet understandably, his suicide sparked an intense effort to begin assessing the achievement of his art and his position in the history of Italian letters. Yet, even at this date, that question has not been satisfactorily resolved: much like Anguilla, the memorable protagonist of his last novel, *The Moon and the Bonfires*, Pavese has proved to be as slippery as an eel, as mysterious as a sphinx, as elusive as some of the mythological figures of what he considered to be his best work, *Dialoghi con Leucò* (1947; *Dialogues with Leucò*, Ann Arbor, Mich., 1965).

Cesare Pavese was born on September 9, 1908, in the small town of Santo Stefano Belbo, in the Piedmont region. His father was a minor official in the city court of Turin, his mother, Maria, came from a moderately well-to-do middle class family. His birth in the Langhe province proved to be more than a casual, insignificant matter: from his very first years, Cesare developed a deep love for the countryside, and practically every thing he wrote bears witness to his attachment to the hills, the farmlands, the places so rich in "primitive," highly symbolic meanings, the welcomed alternatives to the anonymity and alienation of modern city living.

In 1914 Pavese's father died of brain tumor, adding more grief to a family that had already suffered the loss of three children, born before Cesare, thus depriving a growing boy of a figure that plays an important role in his development. Signora Maria, from all available evidence, seems to have been a "rigid and strict" person, incapable of giving her son the warmth and understanding he needed. Quite likely, their relationship was a central element in Pavese's own frustrating sexual life, a part of his experience he objectified again and again in his fiction, as we shall see.

By 1923 Pavese had completed his middle school and entered the *liceo classico*, where he was fortunate to be assigned to Augusto Monti. Himself a writer, a learned and understanding teacher, a splendid mentor, Monti was able to challenge his students without ever losing their trust and respect, instilling in them a deep love of literature that embraced all periods, from the classical to the contemporary. In 1927, Pavese was admitted to the School of Letters and Philosophy of the University of Turin, from which he graduated in 1932, after writing a dissertation on Walt Whitman. In school, he made his first important friends: Leone Ginzburg, the Slavist; Norberto Bobbio, the philosopher; Giulio Einaudi, the future publisher with whom Pavese became associated until his death; Massimo Mila, the historian of music. Even before finishing his degree, Pavese began undertaking what was to prove to be one of his lasting contributions to Italian culture, his translations, at once faithful and felicitous of such American writers as Sinclair Lewis, Sherwood Anderson, followed later by Herman Melville, O. Henry, Theodore Dreiser, Walt Whitman, John Dos Passos, James Joyce, Gertrude Stein, William Faulkner. His activity as translator was to sustain him financially and leave an indelible mark upon his creative work as well.

In 1932, out of strict necessity and not out of conviction, Pavese joined the Fascist party, the membership card being an absolute prerequisite for most jobs, especially teaching. His translations and contributions to several literary reviews, attracted the attention and respect of several people with connections with the publishing industry. In 1934, Giulio Einaudi acquired the review *La cultura* and, after the arrest of Leone Ginzburg, asked Pavese to assume its editorship, even though it was Arrigo Cajumi who was really in charge. A year later, on May 13, the police, anxious to silence and imprison the members of the dissident political group called "Giustizia e libertà" ("Justice and Freedom") conducted a search in Pavese's apartment. They found several compromising letters by the radical agitator Altiero Spinelli (who later found political asylum in the United States) and Pavese became implicated. Along with some two hundred intellectuals and the entire staff of *La cultura*, he was brought to trial, found guilty, and sentenced to three years of political confinement in Brancaleone, a southernmost town in Calabria. The story has a strange and ironic twist: although guilty by reason of circumstances, Pavese was in fact innocent: the letters found in his apartment were addressed to a young woman, Tina, a member of the Communist party, whom he had met several years earlier and with whom he was hopelessly in love. It was Tina for whom Pavese wrote several poems of his collection *Lavorare stanca* (1936; *Hard Labor: Poems*, N.Y., 1977), identifying her only as "the woman with the hoarse voice," and it was she who changed the course of his existence. Paroled after spending less than one third of his sentence in Calabria, Pavese returned to Turin to resume his activities. A friend met him at the railroad station to prepare him and sustain him in one of his worse crises of his entire life: Tina, the woman he so deeply loved, had become engaged the day before Pavese's return home! It was a shock from which Pavese never completely recovered, and which was largely responsible for his depicting "women with a vengeance," in the words of his distinguished biographer, Davide Lajolo.

"A woman, unless she is an idiot," he wrote in his diary (August 3, 1937), "sooner or later meets a piece of human wreckage and tries to rescue him, but a woman, unless she is an idiot, sooner or later finds a sane, healthy man and makes a wreck of him. She always succeeds." "The only women worth the trouble of marrying," he noted a few weeks later (September 30), "are those a man cannot trust enough to marry. But this is the terrible thing: the art of living consists in not letting our loved ones know the pleasure it gives us to be with them, otherwise they leave us."

His intellectual activities gave him renewed hope: the publication, in 1936, of his first volume of poetry, was followed by his translations of four American novels and a marked increase in his schedule as private teacher. His first fiction—none of which was to appear until 1941—began receiving more and more of his attention. In 1942, he was promoted to the post of editor at Einaudi; one year later, he left Turin for Rome on a special assignment. Called to serve in the Italian army, he was discharged because of an asthma condition from which he had suffered for many years. War was getting closer to Turin each day: in 1943, after the fall of Mussolini and the declaration of the so-called Republic of Salò, with Mussolini again at the helm, Pavese, alarmed by the prospect of the inevitable German occupation of the city, fled to a hamlet, Serralunga of Casal Monferrato, and joined his sister Maria. At the end of World War II, he returned to Turin and to his publisher with increased responsibilities. In 1945, perhaps out of guilt feelings for his nonparticipation in the Underground, he joined the Communist party, and wrote several essays highly critical of the United States and her imperialistic-capitalistic policies. He acknowledged the debt Europe owed to America during her trying years between 1930 and 1945, years during which she was the "only gigantic theater where with greater freedom than elsewhere the drama of us all was being acted out." "In brief," he concluded "I honestly think that American culture has lost its mastery, its innocent and knowing intensity that put it in the vangauard of our intellectual world. Nor can I but remark that the loss coincides with the end, or suspension, of its fight against Fascism."

In the years that followed the end of the war, his prestige and popularity increased rapidly. By 1950, he had a distinguished production to his credit: nine short novels, most of which were completed during the last fifteen years of his life; a large number of short stories; a small, but highly original number of poems; several critical essays, noteworthy for their sensitivity and depth; a book on myths, *Dialogues with Leucò*, and a diary that remains today one of the prime documents for understanding Pavese's private and creative life. His curriculum vitae is both diversified and unusually brilliant. A translator at the age of twenty, a poet at twenty-two, a novelist shortly thereafter, he never allowed himself to stop growing, venturing into new fields of human knowledge and creativity.

On the personal side, Pavese was a loner, a man estranged from reality and life, whose very awareness of his condition contributed to the hurt he endured. Writing to his friend Tullio Pinelli, he commented: "I am one of the many decayed sons of the nineteenth century. That century was too great in thought, feeling and action; and by the laws of history, equally great must be the dejection of those who can no longer believe in its ideals and cannot resolutely find new ones. That is the way I am." "Talking to him," writes one of his closest friends and most perceptive associates, Natalia Ginzburg, in her moving tribute "Ritratto d'un amico" ("Portrait of a Friend"), "was never easy, even when he appeared gay. . . . He devised for himself over the years a system of ideas and principles, so entangled and severe as to bar him from the simplest decisions of everyday life. And the more forbidding these simple problems became the more he wanted to overcome them, tangling himself up in endlessly multiplying thoughts, tortuous and choking like a deadly plant."

No factual summary of Pavese's life however detailed can do justice to his rather complex personality. What facts omit generally are the feelings of a sensitive person, catching the contradictions, the inexplicable sides of his actions and attitudes. In some ways, Pavese had points in common with the nineteenth-century poet Giacomo Leopardi: sensitive, afflicted by a physical illness, Leopardi, unloved and not understood by his parents and family, was, for a variety of philosophical reasons, unhappy with his lot—and yet, out of his devastatingly deep unhappiness, sprung some of the most lovely, tender lyrics ever written.

Much like the poet from Recanati, Pavese remained essentially "provincial" in terms of his travels: he seldom left his native Piedmont, lived in Turin and, for a few months, in Milan and Rome (and then only for business reasons), and, with the exception of Paris, he was never abroad. Yet, what he lacked in practical experience and wide travels was more than balanced by an extraordinary culture which embraced several disciplines and literatures (Greek, Latin, Continental European, and American). At an age when most young men have little on their mind beside fun and sex, Pavese was producing translations from Lewis and Melville that were destined to become classics sui generis, even though, by his own admission, his knowledge of American slang was far from complete. Aside from his artistic creativity and his editorial work, little else received his attention and his commitment: not politics (his involvement with communism is insignificant, if not downright trivial), not personal relationships, except in rare cases.

Among his contemporaries in Italy, Elio Vittorini must certainly be singled out as the person who, by virtue of his work and interest, was his peer. Aside from their political trajectory (both were, for a while, Fascists, both turned to the left and eventually became card-carrying Communists), both dedicated themselves to what amounts to nothing less than a veritable revolution in the art of writing, whether this meant, as in Pavese's case, grafting a local dialect onto the standard literary language, or, as in Vittorini's case, developing a style that was a truly original expressive instrument of the themes closest to his sensitivity. Both strove to represent less the factual than the rhythmical, or musical, quality of the experience. Both Vittorini and Pavese eventually emerged as masters of the novel as an art form, widely admired, read, and imitated by the younger generation of writers. Along with Vittorini, Pavese devoted much of his time and talent, at least at the beginning of his career, to the study, translation, and explanation of American literature. Turning to American letters, however differently motivated, ultimately achieved a practical and a symbolic meaning for both writers, as it signified a conscious attempt to free themselves from the shackles of their native tradition and of official culture.

Much has been written, and much more remains to be said, about the "American influence" on Pavese. From our still limited perspective it is reasonable to state that the gravitation toward American letters was motivated by several factors: the award of the Nobel Prize to Sinclair Lewis in 1930 was unquestionably a stimulant to the budding interest in American culture and life. The relative virginity of the whole field was another consideration. But perhaps what captivated the new explorers at once was the freedom with which American writers made contemporary life and its vast social problems the basic substance of their work, and the manner in which they were able to mold literary language, enriching it with slang so as to make it truly capable of recapturing the reality and color of their characters and situations. "Anderson's style!" Pavese commented enthusiastically in one of his very first critical essays, "Not a crude dialect . . . but a new texture of English, entirely constructed of American idioms, a style no longer *dialect* but *language*, reworked in the mind, re-created, *poetry*. In a tale written by Anderson there is always heard an American speaker, the *living man*."

Pavese's encounter with American literature was unquestionably the single most important intellectual experience of his life: it not only enabled him to achieve a profound understanding of his own culture, it suggested to him the path to the "discovery" of what was to become his own style and the fundamental theme of his poetic world, "a contrast between city and country, between sincerity and empty pretense, between nature and petty men"— words he used in characterizing the work of Anderson.

Psychologically, suicide (or what his biographer Davide Lajolo called "the absurd vice") haunted Pavese for much of his life, receiving constant attention in his diary, from 1935 to 1950. "I am not a man for a biography," Lajolo recalls Pavese's assertion made in 1946, "The only things I shall leave are few books, in which there is all or almost all [to be known] about me." Events proved him to be right, for he led an unusually sheltered existence, monotonously bureaucratic in its routine. Like many intellectuals with creative aspirations, he worked hard at several jobs: evening school teaching, private tutoring, translating for commercial publishers, consultantships. Although he yearned for "literary glory," there is no material evidence that success went to his head. On the contrary: even when he became well known and respected by his peers and the reading public, he scorned praise and remained a private, simple person. His diary confirms his unpretentiousness and his embarrassment about the thought of money. He lived and worked simply, trying to cope with what he called "the business of living," and writing, which he called "a métier like any other, like selling bottles or working the earth."

He was well aware of his limitations and qualities, even though, as to be expected, at the beginning of his career he had had doubts about his competence: "In my field," he wrote in one of the last entries in his diary, "I am king." He was always keenly aware of the special position of a poet writing about life: "A poet delights himself in submerging himself in a state of mind and enjoying it—that is his way of escaping tragedy. But a poet should never forget that, for him, a state of mind is less than nothing. All that counts is the poetry he will write." To the end of his life, Pavese suffered from having chosen the relative tranquility of his ivory tower to the turbulence, pressure, and responsibility of most other occupations. He conceived the whole process of writing "monotonous," and, comparing it with swimming, he wrote: "The beauty of swimming like any other of life's activities, is the monotonous recurrence of a position. To narrate is to feel in the diversity of reality a significant cadence, an unresolved cipher of mystery, the seduction of a truth always about to reveal itself and always fleeing. Monotony is a token of sincerity."

That Pavese, for a number of complicated reasons (one of which was his failure with women) suffered from a bad conscience (his lack of commitment to the cause of his country's freedom is part of it), makes a psychological interpretation of his work tempting, to say the least. And in recent years, such an approach has been made by a brilliant French Italophile, Dominique Fernandez (*L'échec de Pavese* [The check of Pavese], Paris, 1967). Speculations about Pavese's ambivalences and ambiguities, however, have led us, as Donald Heiney anticipated in his excellent study of our novelist, "to assertions that can neither be proved nor disproved and do not really throw much light on the technical aspect of his work. For the purpose of literary criticism it is perhaps more valuable to approach the problem in another way: in what form, in what precise guises, does the theme of bad conscience appear in his work?" His flaws, his feelings, his doubts are ultimately the very flesh and blood of his art. While cognizant of some of the personal events that gave birth to his vision of life, in the last analysis it is his creative production that constitutes the only legitimate yardstick by which Cesare Pavese's achievement can be measured in any responsible critical sense.

Pavese's entrance into the world of literature is marked by the publication of a slim volume of poems, *Lavorare stanca* (*Hard Labor: Poems*), a collection of some seventy-odd lyrics. Ordinarily, there is nothing particularly unusual in commencing a literary career in Italy by writing poems, for such is precisely the route taken by many future novelists—too many, in fact, to be listed here. But what is unusual, and therefore important, is that *Lavorare stanca* indicates a definite *prise de position* with respect to his predecessors and contemporaries, and at the same time presents some of the main, recurrent themes of his later novels. Pavese was deeply conscious of the importance of his lyrics, to the point of declaring in a brief essay written in 1934 and published in the second, enlarged edition of *Lavorare stanca* some nine years later, that his poetry was "among the best being written in Italy." In yet another essay with the curious title "A proposito di certe poesie non ancora scritte" [Regarding certain poems as yet unwritten], he pointed out what is one of the basic themes of his creative writing: "the adventures of an adolescent who is proud of his *paese* and imagines the city to be the same, but finds loneliness there and turns to sex and passion for comfort. This merely uproots him and increases the distance between him and both the *paese* and the city, driving him into a more tragic solitude, which is the end of adolescence." The theme of the return home pervades much of Pavese's work: "You've got to have a *paese*, even if only to have the desire to go away." "*Paese* means not to be alone, to know that in the people, the trees, the land, there is something that remains waiting for you, even when you have gone away," says the narrator of Pavese's last novel, *The Moon and the Bonfires*. Going away, of course, is also a refusal to be committed to something or someone, a cause, a woman, a country. Running away from the things that usually connect us with a kind of life we may perceive to be unattractive or even impossible to tolerate frequently proves to be a factor that leads us to further estrangement and loneliness.

Pavese's poetry is a first, but fundamental statement about his feelings toward art and life; its unpretentious language moves toward a goal of a "clear, objective and essential type of poetry," composed in an effective mixture of "veristic" and "crepuscular" style, with emphasis on the condition of clarity. He called the results of his labors *"poesia-racconto"* ("poetry-narrative"), a form which, while free from formal metrical requirements, retains its internal rhythm and power of synthesis. The subjects of his poems are drawn from life in the *paese*, its hills, its beauty and, above all, its everyday life. The first of what became an absorbing number of myths come to life is the hill, with its remarkable beauty and its mysteries. Contrasting to this is the city, with its unique landmarks and tension, and the resulting anguish and solitude. Simplicity of language detracts nothing from the directness and forcefulness of such lyrics. Intensely personal, Pavese's poetry conspicuously rejects the traditional efforts to make the self its central preoccupation. The characters who appear in such poems are largely drawn from the working class. They are common people: "peasants, prostitutes, prisoners, working women, youths," as he stated. "If there is any human figure in my poetry," so reads one of his earliest entries in his diary (November 10, 1935), "it is that of a truant running back, full of joy, to his own village, where everything is picturesque and full of color; a man who likes to work as little as he can; finding great pleasure in the simplest things, always expansive, good natured, set in his views; incapable of deep suffering; happy to follow nature and enjoy a woman, but also glad to be free and on his own; ready every morning to start life afresh. As in '*Mari del Sud*.'"

Already in his early poetry we find the theme that will eventually become one of the central motifs of his entire work—solitude —one of life's conditions that most afflicted him and which he never tired of depicting. Communication and love are two of the strongest experiences by which we establish, or reestablish, human contact, but Pavese, for emotional and psychological reasons, had difficulties in this area. "The greatest misfortune is loneliness," he observed, "Work is an equivalent to prayer, since ideally it puts you in contact with something that will not take advantage of you. The whole problem of life, then, is this: how to break out of one's loneliness, how to communicate with others. This explains the persistence of marriage, fatherhood, friendship, since they might bring happiness! But why it should be better to be in communication with another than to be alone, is a mystery." Here, Pavese's ambivalence is quite clear: *thinking* that love, friendship, concern, commitment (social or political) will bridge the gap that keeps us isolated does not mean that he was ready then, or throughout his life, or capable of experiencing them: "We are frightened of being alone," comments Deola in the poem "Ritorno di Deola" ("Deola's Return"), "but we want to be alone."

Although Pavese continued writing poetry until the last months of his life, by the late thirties his need to "narrate in [verse] form" was satisfied. He no longer felt challenged by the difficulties of his chosen medium to the point, as he wrote in the opening pages of his diary, that "I am no longer troubled to seek for deeper poetic discoveries, as though it were merely a question of applying a skillful technique to a state of mind. Instead, I was making a poetic farce of my poetic vocation." "So far," he concluded, "I have confined myself, as if by caprice, to poetry in verse. Why do I never attempt a different genre? There is only one answer, inadequate as it may be. It is not out of caprice, but from cultural consideration: sentiment, and now habit, that I cannot get out of that vein, and the crazy idea of changing form to renovate the substance would seem to me shabby and amateurish." Yet, these doubts, however carefully worded as they are, strongly point to Pavese's decision to turn to fiction.

"If I have truly lived these four years of poetry," he continued on October 15 of the same year, "so much the better: that cannot but help me towards greater incontestability and a better sense of expression. . . . I must not forget how much at a loss I felt before 'Mari del Sud,' and how, as I went along I grasped an understanding of my world that I had created. . . . Now that I have exhausted that vein, I am too worn-out, too circumscribed, to be still strong enough to throw myself with high hopes into making a new excavation." "It really seems to me that my technique has become automatic," he wrote two days later, "so that, without deliberately thinking about it, my ideas now come out in the form of images, as if in obedience to that fanciful law I mentioned on the 10th. And I am very much afraid that this means it is time to change the tune, or at least the instrument. . . . My formula for the future is discovered: if once I tormented my mind to create a blending of my lyrical forms . . . the result was 'Mari del Sud,' with all the works that followed it; now I must find the secret of fusing the fantastic, trenchant vein of *Lavorare stanca* with that of the *pornoteca*: slapstick, realistically declaimed to its public. And, beyond all doubt, that will mean prose."

The passage from poetry to fiction was far less abrupt than it was believed, or as Pavese himself had indicated. As early as 1928, he wasy trying his hand at fiction, writing stories most of which were to appear only after his death. But it was only in the summer of 1936 that his efforts began reaching the promising stage with the completion of "Terra d'esilio" ("Land of Exile"), the first of some sixty short stories he wrote in his lifetime. Toward the end of 1938, now working for Einaudi in Turin, Pavese began *Il carcere* (1948; *The Political Prisoner*, London, 1955), the first of nine novels he was to write, all fairly brief (running an average of one hundred printed pages), generally completed within a three-month period, and all uniformly divided into short chapters. The shift in genre, however, did in no way diminish Pavese's seriousness of approach and high creative consciousness. IIe brought to the art of fiction thc samc carc hc had given to poetry. Indeed, he regarded fiction as a logical extension of what he had tried to do in poetry, namely to poetize prose, without (and this is what separates him from the school of the *"prosa d'arte"* of the teens and twenties) losing the story, the events of a novel. In this sense, his concern with writing a poetic novel was shared by Elio Vittorini, whose *Conversazione in Sicilia* (1941; *In Sicily*, N.Y., 1949) signaled an important new direction in the history of the genre.

One of the most striking aspects of Pavese's novels, poetry, and nonfiction, is that they were all conceived, in his own words, as integral parts of a "monolith," all, whatever their artistic merit or deficiencies, connected to each other in subtle, symbolic ways. Much like other great writers he admired enormously—Mann, Proust, Pirandello, and Beckett—Pavese built a circular "world," in which every part is at once its beginning and its end. "I feel sure," Pavese declared in a radio interview (February 6, 1946) whose text was included in the omnibus volume *La letteratura americana e altri saggi* (1953; but not in *American Literature: Essays and Opinions*, Berkeley, 1970) with the title "L'influsso degli eventi" [The influence of events], "I feel sure of the fundamental and lasting unity of all that I have written or will write— and I am not talking of an autobiographical unity or unity of taste, which are trivialities—but of one unity of the vital interest, the monotonous obstinacy of someone who feels certain of having found his true, his eternal world on the very first day [of his writing] and can do nothing but revolve around the great monolith and takes off chunks [from it] and studies them in every possible light."

Pavese's novels are set either in the country or in the city, the two extremes, the former symbolizing innocence and beauty, the latter the prison of contemporary life. His themes are always similar and yet always different, facets of the same stone their creator never tired of polishing and holding to the light. The people summoned by Pavese's imagination to recite a role whose end, death, is their only certainty, constitute an odd lot indeed: men and women drawn from the middle class, boring and bored professionals, teachers and students, disillusioned intellectuals, shopkeepers, peasants, seamstresses, fashion models, would-be-artists, prostitutes, workingmen from the blue-collar sector—people frequently spineless and at times dead to feelings, uninteresting and even banal, all seeking to cope in a world where little happens, where existence, as Pavese once wrote about himself, is an escape "from the damnation of daily sadness." Among them, the figures of the adolescent, the wanderer, and the unemployed seem to receive special attention of the novelist, perhaps because he sees in the first the symbol of hope, in the second the symbol of the man searching with diminishing hope, and in the third the person who no longer has a constructive place in society, to which he has become a burden and a threat.

The space in which such characters live is limited to the street, the cafés, or the inn, where they can drink their wine and talk about things, "places" as Fernandez remarks, "where we can go anytime, metaphors of a possibility without limit." "Pavese's hero," adds Fernandez, "is ready for all possible experiences because he is touched by none of them, and because he is certain of being retrieved by his myths and his deep nature at any time he wishes." A few friends, maybe a woman, a few excursions to the hills to dance, and sometimes a few discussions about the past, their love affairs, their feelings. fill the existence of Pavese's characters: more often than not, they share a reluctance, or perhaps an unwillingness, or incapacity to connect with other human beings. They live a life without fire, with little if any emotions or deep commitments, lost birds in unfriendly skies, true antiheroes in a world with no possibility of tragedy. Stability, tranquility, and peace are clearly denied to them. The world being what it is, it is problematic to sink roots, however vital that is; solid relationships are rare, evasion common, genuine love almost unknown.

In some ways, Pavese's characters resemble Albert Camus's Meursault (of *L'Etranger* [*The Stranger*]), or some of Jean-Paul. Sartre's existential characters. What impresses us is how frequently they are, really or symbolically, "strangers," away from their home for a variety of reasons—in political confinement, like Stefano (*Il carcere*), in jail (Berto and Talino, *Paesi tuoi*), on vacation (the unnamed narrator of *La spiaggia*, as well as his hosts, the three main characters of *Il diavolo sulle colline*), or avoiding the police (Corrado, of *La casa in collina*), or returning "home," after many many years (Anguilla, in *La luna e i falò*) —all painfully dislocated, searching for their identity, trying to make sense out of the imponderable and baffling mysteries of life. Whether by chance or design, they begin reassessing things, although seldom in a conscious manner. Almost invariably, we are told little about their past, the undramatic story of their lives, and the characters seldom memorable, facts that must not be ascribed to an artistic weakness, but to a determined, programmed intention to devalue their importance.

In a radio interview, held shortly before his death, Pavese, speaking in an objective fashion as though he were someone else, put the problem in these words:

> When Pavese begins [writing] a story, a fable, a book, it never happens to him to have in mind a socially defined milieu, a character or characters, a thesis. What he has in mind is almost always an indistinct rhythm, a play of events that more than anything are sensations and atmospheres. . . . From this comes the fact, never sufficiently noted, that Pavese does not care "to create characters." Characters are for him means not an end. Characters serve him simply to construct intellectual fables, whose theme is what takes place. . . . His tales are not descriptions but fantastic judgments of reality. . . . The char-

acters in [his] stories are all brief; they are names and types, nothing more: they are on the same plane as a tree, a storm or an air raid.

His novels also show a marked decline of the importance of plot, consonant with his views about fiction: "The art of the nineteenth century," he noted in his diary (December 21, 1949), "was centered on the development of situations (historic cycles, careers, etc.); the art of the twentieth on static essentials. In the first, the hero was not the same at the beginning of the story as he was at the end; now he remains unchanged. Childhood as a preparation for manhood (nineteenth century); childhood viewed only as such (twentieth)."

"Terra d'esilio" ("Land of Exile," a story that can be read in the volume *Festival Night*, London, 1964) revolves around Corrado, an engineer whose job has taken him to the South. In the course of his stay, he meets Otino, a young political "undesirable" who befriends him and tells him the story of his common-law wife in Turin who betrayed him and is eventually killed by another man. Two factor at least make the story less than successful: it is written too close to experience and too much attention is given to local color. *Il carcere* (*The Political Prisoner*) on the other hand, has at least the advantage of some perspective Pavese could bring to his own painful experience.

The novel was completed in five months (November 27, 1938– April 16, 1939), but it was not to appear in print until almost a decade later. The novel's protagonist, Stefano, is also an engineer and like the author a political prisoner in a remote southern village of Italy. The setting is, in at least one way, symbolic: it evokes loneliness, and a sense of dislocation that pervades so much of Pavese's fiction. The mood of the story is similarly remote, detached: there is a marked lack of concern about a certain segment of the population, which is made to feel inferior, unworthy of understanding and help, and thus alienated—thus reflecting obliquely, the traditional historical stance of fascism toward the *Mezzogiorno*.

Pavese himself, unlike another intellectual from Turin, Carlo Levi, also a political prisoner in Lucania, is hardly interested in the whole range of social, economic, and human problems of the South. He is ready, however, to accept and use, for his own fictional purposes, the solitude that stems from Stefano's refusal to come to terms with the condition of the villagers, absorbed as he is in his own existential problems. This helps making *The Political Prisoner* a sort of severe, unsparing account of the author's situation and a reflection upon it, achieved primarily through Stefano's relationship with two women who cross his path: Concia, a servant girl who embodies the sexual, almost primitive force that cannot be bent, much less tamed (and emerges as the "she-goat" of Pavese's early poems), desirable but unattainable, ever-present in his dreams but amazingly elusive; and Elena, a mature, understanding woman, who is the landlady's daughter, who embodies maternal love, and actually encourages him to look at her as his *"mammina,"* reassuring, understanding, of course, but also potentially castrating. When Elena does indeed take on that role, Stefano proceeds to end a relationship with which he never felt comfortable. The confusion besetting him bears close similarity to Pavese's who, as his diary shows, was aware that no meaningful human relationship can exist in a vacuum: indeed, friendships and understanding can pierce and eventually knock down the walls that imprison man. Yet, particularly during his youth, Pavese stubbornly regarded solitude as a sign of self-sufficiency and saw love (unconsciously perhaps) as a threat in that it implies opening, and giving oneself to others, accepting the risks as well as the benefits. The natural need of love, however, clashes with the fear that it might actually increase his dependency on someone and becomes a nightmarish paradox defying solution.

The main point of *Il carcere* is the discovery that the world is always a "jail" (in the Pavesian sense, at least), a metaphor which, as Donald Heiney perceptively notes, is "the very immensity of a world in which the individual feels himself in some elusive way an exile, longing to establish contact with other men yet cut off from them by mysterious and invisible walls." On every front, Stefano behaves in a way that is alienating and ultimately destructive: he uses Elena's body (although it is Concia he really wants), indirectly and directly making his relationship with his mistress oedipal; he refuses to make any connection with the local folk and tells Giannino (the only person whom he befriends) about his affair with Elena, who unable and unwilling to continue a relationship seriously tainted, vanishes. The final pages of the book acquire a new meaning through the implicit symbolism of the actions and words spoken by the characters. Thus, through a trusted friend, Pierino, Stefano sends a message to Giannino, who has been arrested for "carnal offenses." "Tell him," Stefano asks Pierino, "that it is much more satisfying to leave jail than political confinement. Beyond the bars [of a jail], the whole world is beautiful, while life in political jail is like the other life, except a little dirtier."

At the center of the novel, there is a problem that has to do with the idea and the reality of solitude, on the one hand, and of liberty, on the other. Given the facts of man's condition, is it possible to be at the same time genuinely free and happy? Is not mankind ultimately condemned to endure the loneliness of togetherness? It is no shock that those whom we love by necessity restrict our freedom: but would we prefer being alone, without commitments, or obligations, or concerns? Stefano makes his choice, and must ultimately pay the price for it. He rejects Elena because he has her, and wants Concia (who has been the mistress of Spano, a "foul old man" as he discovers) because she eludes him. He plays the game as best as he can—avoiding at all costs any action that might hurt him, however accidentally—and shuts out every pleasure and every emotion. Love, therefore, is unacceptable since, in an indirect way, it poses the danger of dependence, just as solidarity (political or human) is to be shunned because it presents practical dangers, as Stefano knows all too well, having already spent some time in a conventional jail. When Giannino is arrested, on a charge of "carnal pleasure," Stefano severs his relationship with him. Similarly, when he receives a note from a political prisoner just arrived, he proceeds to burn the message at once, lest that should cause difficulties with the authorities, and instructs Barbariccia (who has acted as the go-between) not to bring him any more messages. Soon thereafter, Stefano receives the official notifications of a reprieve. He sees Elena for the last time, proposes that she visit him that night (she does not), and leaves the next afternoon for the North, "home."

Some of Pavese's most informed critics, Armanda Guiducci among them, have called *The Political Prisoner* "ambitious, ambiguous, desperately and narcissistically literary; all told, inferior to its ambition." It is a harsh assessment, with which the present writer generally agrees. Its imperfections, ranging all the way from the shallow manner in which the excessively numerous characters of the novel are depicted, to the unclear political stance of Stefano, to the unfelicitous choice of a third person narrative form (inappropriate in the light of such a highly personal story), all these and other flaws do not take away the reasons of its significance. In its sketching out, for the first time, the condition of man as prisoner of life, Pavese succeeded both in translating through literature some of his experiences into universal symbols, and in creating what is possibly one of the most vital metaphors of his entire novelistic output. Without its being a "masterpiece" (as Franco Mollia claims the book to be), *The Political Prisoner* occupies a prominent place in our understanding of Pavese. In his very first book, he was able to perceive with great clarity the heavy price man must be prepared to pay when, threatened from without—emotionally or politically—he wishes to retain his identity: that price was solitude, withdrawal in time and space from the turmoil of existence.

Pavese's second novel, *Paesi tuoi* (*The Harvesters*, London, 1961) belongs to the other side of his interest: the *paese*, sex and violence. Written between June 3 and August 16, 1939, published two years later, the book's title derives from an old, widely known Italian adage, *"Donne e buoi dai paesi tuoi,"* or "Pick your wife and your oxen from the people and places you know and trust." When Pavese sat down to compose his novel, he already had behind him considerable experience with American literature, as a translator and commentator, and his critical perception of the problems of the novel was increasingly sharper.

The novella was received with mixed feelings by the critics, who objected to the violent nature of the story and its rough, ungrammatical, unliterary style. The history of Italian literature, particularly in the last century, is replete with examples of works (by such writers as Giovanni Verga, Federigo Tozzi, Italo Svevo, and Alberto Moravia) whose grammatical "impurities" have earned them a hostile critical reception. Almost inevitably, doing violence to language, however irreproachable one's reasons may be, carries a price and censure few writers can afford, but must be prepared, to pay. However, Pavese must have believed the risk worth taking. His reading of certain American novelists, particularly Sherwood Anderson, James Cain, John Steinbeck, had persuaded him that no serious writer could avoid the labor of experimenting with language and technique. A few months after completing his second novel, we find this entry (December 12, 1939) in his diary: "The story of an artist is the successive improvement upon the technique employed in his previous work, with a fresh creation that imposes a more complex aesthetic law."

How effectively Pavese applied his concepts to the art of the novel can be measured in *Paesi tuoi*. This time the story is set in the author's native region, Piedmont, and is narrated by its protagonist, Berto. As the book opens, we find Berto, who has decided to accompany Talino, a fellow inmate with whom he has shared his cell for about a month, setting off for his destination, Monticello, a hamlet in Piedmont. Both men have been released from jail, where they have served time, the former on a minor count, the latter on a count of arson. In a sense, the story begins where *The Political Prisoner* had left off. Berto's decision to join Talino springs from his desire to reconnect with life. Both men long for "home," and home in a normal context means the love and security of family life and affection, loyal friends, and roots: both men look forward to a new beginning, a new life. But their expectations are soon dashed: we, as readers, steeped in a tradition in which the "*campagna*," (countryside or farm) is supposed to be an idyllic place of beauty and tranquility, a healthy antidote to the pressure and alienating ways of urban living, are suddenly brought to confront not a place of peace, but of strife and conflict, not a spot where gentle love reigns supreme, but where violent, bloody lust prevails.

At first, Berto is content with his situation: working for Vinverra, the owner of the farm, is not easy as a rule, but Berto's special skill as a mechanic gives him a special status not enjoyed by the farmhands. Moreover, courting the town's girls and Gisella, Talino's beautiful, sensuous sister, makes life considerably more interesting—until, that is, several potentially ominous signs begin to surface. The most dreadful of these is that it was Gisella's squealing to the police that sent her brother to jail for arson, arson motivated by his jealousy of Ernesto del Prato, who had set his eyes on Gisella, herself victim of her brother's incestuous love. The scar on her womb, which Berto had been told to be the result of an accident while working in the fields, is in reality the permanent reminder of an abortion undergone when she was fourteen. Berto is considerably frightened by this confession, and advises Gisella to be careful not to irritate or provoke her brother in any way, an advice that does not stop the tragedy from running its course. One day, during the harvest, and quite unexpectedly, Talino, angered by a trivial act, kills his sister by thrusting his pitchfork into her throat and then flees. A few hours later, despite the modest medical care Gisella has received, she dies. The hunt for the murderer begins, unaided by the traditional lack of co-operation Italian families observe during police investigations of this particular type of crime. Deeply grieved by Gisella's death, and now aware of the fact that the *paese*, where he had hoped to find peace, is a no better or safer place than the city, Berto leaves for his "home," in Turin.

If Pavese's first novel was marred by a pervasive intellectualism in subject and treatment, *Paesi tuoi* represents an intriguing, radical change in the author's direction. For one thing, there are no intellectuals in the book. But, what is even more pivotal in terms of the gradual growth of Pavese as an artist, the construction of the novel is such that the events narrated and the characters created may be seen both as what they are *and* as symbols of a universal condition. Thus, the fact that Berto is a mechanic has its importance in the story itself but also underscores the conflict between two kinds of society, the city folks and the farmers. People in the city are closer to machines, to mechanisms; people who live in the *campagna* are closer to primordial feelings and to nature. The elements play a significant role in the lives of the *contadini*: too much sun, or too much rain, can ruin a harvest; too much wind may damage it; and certain insects can destroy it. Traditions are stronger in the country than in the city, where they are frequently turned into "festivals" whose only value is commercial, and whose object therefore is generating business and thus improving the economy. The setting of the novel, its characters and plot, required a language consonant with, and capable of expressing its passions, needs, fears.

Pavese was quite conscious of the impact the style of his novel would have, particularly his subtle blending of Piedmontese and the standard, literary language. In his diary he noted (December 4, 1939):

My language is very different from a naturalistic impression-ism. I did not write an imitation of Berto—the only one who says anything—but translating his meditations, his wonder-ment, his raillery, as he would have expressed them himself, *had he spoken Italian*. I introduced errors of syntax only to in-dicate occasions when his own spirit grew scornful, involved or tedious. I wanted to show, not how Berto would write had he forced himself to speak Italian (that would have been dialectic impressionism) but what his own words would be, had they been changed into Italian by some new Pentacost. In short, his thoughts. [This passage is actually quoted directly by Pavese from a letter he had written to his friend Pinelli.]

The narrative sections of the book are no less successful, par-ticularly in conjuring up the tense, terse atmosphere ready for the powerful drama that is about to explode: the intense heat that gen-erates both sweat and lust; the smell of the animals on the farm; the sounds of the crickets and the birds; the scent and taste of the fruits, particularly the apple's (with its sexual and biblical refer-ence), and their connection with Gisella, depicted as "made of fruit." The gesture, actions, and words of Talino's father, Vin-verra, a tough, crude, earthy authoritarian who does not hesitate giving Gisella a good thrashing, and his son's personality (added to his incestuous relation and his pent-up anger) all contribute to a terse, ugly climate of personal relationships that will ultimately lead to the bloody murder of Gisella, a tragedy which, in the words of another critic of Pavese, Elio Gioanola, is described as breaking out like "a furious summer storm whose water is quickly soaked up by the parched earth."

Apart from the new thematic interests of its author, *The Har-vesters* breaks new ground in the gradual "sexualization" of the landscape: the hill is time and again called, or compared to, a woman's breast, and the bushes on its top are seen as the nipple. The interest in myth, dating back to the thirties, and to such ethnological studies as James G. Frazer's *The Golden Bough*, begins to yield its first results in Pavese's second novel, in which realism harmoniously coexists with symbolism. Hence the in-creasing importance of the many rituals associated with country life, ranging all the way from the daily tilling of the soil to the harvests held in different times of the year, presented as rituals that are more than merely interesting bits of folklore that add color to the tale, but elements that add a new dimension to the story. In short, The *Harvesters* offers Pavese's first sustained attempt to enrich a story by mythicizing its events much as Dante had sought to do when he expressed his journey in allegorical terms.

The question of symbols and myth was one that occupied Pavese's attention and study for much of his productive life. Thus, for example, referring to "the 'breast' in *Paesi tuoi*—a true epithet expressing the sexual reality of that countryside," he added: "No longer an *allegorical symbol*, but an *imaginative symbol*—an additional means of expressing the 'fantasy,' the story." Several years later (on Feb. 20, 1946) he wrote in his diary:

> We are convinced that myths are a language, a means of expression; not arbitrary, but pregnant with symbols that, like all languages, have a special significance which can be expressed in no other way. When we introduce a proper name, an action, some legendary marvel, we are expressing, between the lines, and in a syllable or two, something comprehensive, all-embracing; the pith and marrow of a reality that will vitalize and nourish a whole living structure of passion, a complex conception of human existence.

In *The Harvesters*, Pavese is quite successful in depicting the *campagna* in a manner that serves the development of the tense, erotic, and basically primitive plot. We learn to see and hear and smell the land, the trees, the animals. We feel the almost unbearable heat, we appreciate the coolness of the water, we almost experience what it means to go barefoot, or to be bothered by flies, or to taste the dust of country roads. In short, the country is discovered by Pavese. Only in his later novels, however, will he make full and appropriate use of the myths and symbols so richly stored in the *campagna* in a more genuinely "unliterary" (or spontaneous) representation of his world view.

Originally entitled "La tenda" ("The curtain"), *La bella estate* (*The Beautiful Summer*) published in English in London in 1955, with *The Political Prisoner*, was written between March 2 and May 6, 1940. It originally appeared in Italy in 1949, in an omnibus volume bearing the same title (together with *Il diavolo sulle colline* and *Tra donne sole*), and was warmly received. *The Beautiful Summer* (the title is not without irony), is the first of Pavese's novels to deal with the petit bourgeoisie and the first to be told by its heroine. It is also the first to be set not in the desolate Calabrian hamlet of *Il carcere*, or the fields and hills of the Langhe region, but in a city, Turin, and more precisely in the quarters and studios of artists and bohemians. It is not difficult to appreciate why such places should have a certain magnetism for a girl who, like the protagonist-narrator, comes from the *paese* to the city, and is lured by a place that offers the anonymity and freedom often necessary to control one's own life. The name of the girl is Ginia: she is just sixteen years old, and works as a seamstress. The theme of the book, and the substance of the story, is her initiation into life.

In Turin, Ginia shares a flat with her unmarried brother, Severino, an electrician by profession. Her best friends are Rosa, a worker at the factory, and, a bit later, Amelia, a sophisticated model who spends much of her free time at the cafés. Through her, Ginia is introduced to the world of so-called artists and would-be intellectuals: Barbetta ("Little Beard"), an artist who sketches her face; Guido, a mediocre painter, and Rodriguez, whose association with artists is a means to bolster his own ego. But no matter: Ginia, at first shocked, and even dismayed, that her friend Amelia poses in the nude, soon realizes that this need not degrade her body or her as a person. Like Alberto Moravia's Carla, of *Gli indifferenti* (*The Time of Indifference*), Ginia thinks that her affair with Guido, with whom she has fallen in love, will drastically change the course of her life, a belief that soon proves to be totally mistaken. The other shock comes when Amelia confesses that she is a lesbian and that she contracted syphilis when she had an affair with another woman. Disappointed by her experiences, Ginia nevertheless gains some understanding of the mediocre, self-indulgent world in which she, too, will be doomed to live. Yet, she accepts this fact, and asks Amelia to lead her in future days.

It has frequently been noted that Pavese's novels are largely autobiographical, but such is not the case of *The Beautiful Summer*, which is a commendable effort to re-create a world that was largely alien to our novelist, and yet one to which he was strangely attracted. Seen from another vantage point, the book revolves around what has emerged as Pavese's special interests: the theme of love and sex, the sexual experience as the principal element in the transition to maturity; the themes of city life, work, and friendship; and, of course, the rather pitiless examination of bourgeois values. In *The Beautiful Summer*, Pavese enters the world of women, reporting their conversations, their ways of thinking, their fears and aspirations—a tall order indeed. The shift in setting, from the *campagna* to the city, is accompanied by other changes: violence, so pervasive in *The Harvesters*, gives way to apathy; lust to bourgeois "love"; primitive instincts and mythicized passions turn into superficial sentiments. If there is something horrifying about the cruelty and violence of *The Harvesters*, there cannot be anything but contempt toward the hollow and dissolute existence portrayed in *The Beautiful Summer*.

Is the novel successful? The answer, as always, is bound to vary from reader to reader: Armanda Guiducci, one of Pavese's sensitive readers, praises the "extraordinary index of the writer's stunning capacity to identify himself with the feminine psyche." If it is quite true that Pavese's heroine Ginia is well drawn, it is also true that the major weakness of the novel is in the limitations of her character, which lacks depth and sensitivity. The action, or what there is of it, is slow-moving if not downright dull. As for the ambience, it is too pervasively fraudulent to be completely convincing. And the male characters prove, once again, to be far more weakly portrayed than their female counterparts.

The book raises another problem: as an intellectual, Pavese had no trouble "knowing" how people like himself behaved. But all his life he was challenged by "the others": the workers, farmers, outcasts, derelicts of society, servants, pseudo-artists. Much of his fiction is about them, and how they try to break the wall of solitude, how they attempt to communicate, and establish a bond, with other human beings, how they reach out for that happiness, or contentment that eluded him with a frightening regularity. How to bridge the enormous intellectual gap between them and Pavese, and how to make them interesting, articulate, and problematic, without robbing them of their independence, remained one of the great obstacles our novelist had to confront and did not always completely overcome.

The Beautiful Summer ends on a note of pathos: there is tacit acknowledgment that things did not turn out quite as Ginia would have wished, and appropriately enough, the story, which began in the summertime, ends in the winter. The warmth, the brightness of the sun, the sensuous garments worn in the summertime, give way to the cold of the winter, a season that forces people to take refuge in their homes, and turn inward, after the promises of the summer. For many people, summer is carefree living, vitality, hope—but, in Pavese's third novel, hopes are dashed and Ginia's acceptance of being led by Amelia (at the end of her short-lived affair with Guido) is in itself a symbolic surrender of her freedom and individuality, her acceptance of a corrupt life she had always hoped to avoid.

In some respects, *La spiaggia* (*The Beach*, N.Y., 1968) continues, in a different direction, the "mood" of the previous novel, but without resolving artistically the thematic and stylistic problems of *The Beautiful Summer*. There is evidence that Pavese himself was not very happy with it. One wonders why should a writer of the sensitivity of Pavese allow the publication of a work he himself acknowledged was "not a chip from the monolith?" The answer is simple, and surprising as well: the editor of the literary magazine *Lettere d'oggi* requested a contribution from Pavese which he, as a loyal friend, could not refuse. Written between November 6, 1940, and January 18, 1941, the work was serialized in *Lettere d'oggi* and appeared in book form, in a very limited edition, under the magazine's imprint. Only in 1956, six years after Pavese's death, did *La spiaggia* become widely available in book form.

The structure of the novel, with the exception of a short section at the beginning of the book is, like the story it tells, fairly linear. Doro, a friend of the anonymous thirty-five-year-old professor-narrator, is married to a tomboy-type girl, Clelia. At first, the narrator resents their marriage (he refuses their invitation to their wedding), but makes up with them and agrees to be their guest one summer, at their little villa on the Genovese Riviera, a plan postponed for purely personal reasons. The unexpected visit by Doro startles the narrator: the two friends decide to go to the country, the Langhe region, for a bit of fun in what turns out to be a sort of excursion into the past. They indulge in a little drinking and singing, and their escapade culminates in an incident in which a flower pot, accidentally pushed by an irate person annoyed by their loudness, barely misses their heads!

The purpose of what at first may seem to be a purposeless diversion is less a Proustian attempt to recover the past than a way to dramatize how the friendship of two men has been changed by their new condition: the duties and obligations of marriage have indeed altered the delicate balance of feelings and commitment that once existed. The choice of summer is similarly part of the overall strategy of the novel: what better time than summer to engage in an attempt to reassess one's own life in a period of vacation, when the weather itself seems to encourage men and women to disrobe, exposing their bodies to the light of truth? On the other hand, vacations relax people, distract them, and the light of the sun blurs their vision, altering their perceptions, even inviting them to look at life from an unusual, not to say exceptional, vantage point. Doro and Clelia understand, and indeed accept this reality—he indulging in little escapades from marital fidelity, she allowing Guido, a well-to-do young man, to court her. One day, while sunning himself at the beach, the narrator meets one of his former students, Berti, who wants someone in whom to confide. A sensitive, shy person, Berti is vacationing and, in a sense, trying to learn about life and people, particularly the narrator and his small circle, and is attracted to Clelia and the young Ginetta.

Nothing much happens in the book: indeed, we are kept waiting, in vain, page after page, for a surprise, for the introduction of a new element that might inject a touch of vitality into a sagging tale. The dull pace of *The Beach*, of course, is planned: what its author intended to write was a sort of commentary on the values and relationships of his middle-class characters. The sand of the beach is gray, and is a major factor in the sameness of the landscape. The affluent vacationers spend much of their time sunning their bodies, facing (or should one say staring?) at "the empty sea," incapable of appreciating the beauty of nature surrounding them, indulging in empty conversations. Even their friendships are based on the casual coincidence of the same vacation spa. In all this, there is a hint of Fitzgerald. The decadent scenes in Pavese's portrayal of boring and bored characters might well have been created by Alberto Moravia. The ending finally provides the one surprise one almost wishes might have come sooner: Clelia is expecting a child, and Doro looks forward to his new role as a father. Their relationship finally gives signs of maturity. The narrator himself, accompanied by his former pupil Berti, leaves for Turin, and with that the book comes to the end.

The parenthesis of the summer is concluded: everyone returns home, including the narrator who will once again take up his role of "professor," hopefully a little more mature. But it is only at the end that we perceive that the book is, among other things, a study of what makes marriage work, seen from the perspective of an intellectual who, like Pavese himself, remains skeptical, ambivalent, ungenerous, and envious of his best friend's attachment to his wife. The question the book raises, if only indirectly, is one that recurs time and again in Pavese's fiction: How can man break through the walls of his loneliness? How can he communicate to other human beings his fears and trepidations? Can he experience some kind of joy (one hesitates to use the word "love" from a world so consistently lacking in love as Pavese's) in his relationship with a woman? Is there any way, other than artistic creativity, which allows man to give of himself to others generously and freely? The answer would have to wait for Pavese's last novels.

Il compagno (*The Comrade*, London, 1959) was written between October 4 and December 22, 1946, five years after *La spiaggia*—five long, hard, painful years during which war raged all over Europe and elsewhere as well. Reading Pavese's diary one is shocked to find but a few, casual references to a war that not only destroyed hundreds of cities and killed millions of people on the battlefields and in the concentration camps, including some of his best friends, among them Leone Ginzburg and Giaime Pintor. Between 1941 and 1946, Pavese lived in Turin and Rome, where he had been sent by Giulio Einaudi to lay the foundations for a gradual expansion of the activities of his publishing house. For a few months during that period Pavese took refuge in the hamlet of Serralunga, in the hills of Piedmont, with his sister Maria, avoiding the danger of being arrested by the police for his political views. While the bombs were relentlessly falling on the industrial targets of Turin and other cities, Pavese read and studied, taking no part in the underground activities that were intensifying. He was to suffer from his uninvolvement, and be criticized by many of his intellectual friends, including his future biographer (and future member of the Chamber of Representatives), Davide Lajolo.

The book's title, with its strong Marxist allusions, should not mislead the reader into thinking that *The Comrade* is either a tract or an opinionated tale. In point of fact it is hardly a political novel, although it is fair to characterize it as a tale that follows carefully the gradual political awareness of its main character. The name of the hero of the book is Pablo: "They called me Pablo because I played the guitar," an opening strongly reminiscent of Melville's *Moby Dick*, which Pavese had felicitously translated into Italian a few years earlier. Briefly stated, the story of the book, narrated by Pablo, a young man who works in his family's salt and tobacco shop, pivots at first on Pablo's relationship with Linda, the girl friend of his best friend Amelio, bedridden (perhaps permanently) after a serious motorcycle accident. Pablo's relationship with Linda, a well-known seamstress and a strikingly independent woman insofar as her private life is concerned, troubles him considerably as he feels guilty of betraying his best friend, who happens to be a fine young man, a positive character whose role, as is frequently the case in Pavese's novels, is doomed to remain marginal. The encounter with Linda has a large part in Pablo's life: for one thing, he is introduced to the group of seedy entertainers who form the entourage of a small-time, yet wealthy impresario (Lubiani) with whom Linda has an affair. Deeply hurt by the affair, no longer willing to continue leading a purposeless existence, Pablo decides to leave for Rome, accompanied by his friend Carletto, in search of a new, meaningful life.

Rome offers him new friendships, a new girl (Ginia), and, what is more important, a new political consciousness. "I worked during the day, and read in the evening." Slowly, guided by his new friends, he begins to discover new and forbidden literature on fascism, Marxism, and socialism. He also begins to understand the necessity of actively fighting, not merely opposing, fascism, a cancer that must be eliminated if man is to be free again: the politics it advocates can only result in a system of life based on a continuing exploitation of the working class at the hands of the bourgeoisie and the landowners. The destruction of such a repressive system must therefore become the ultimate commitment of the working class. At the same time, there must be an effort to develop leaders from within the working class: "To trust those who study," says Pablo, "we must study." "One should study," he remarks, "so as to do without those [others] who study. So as not to get screwed by them." What Pablo is insisting on is a culture that is relevant to the needs of the people, training them not only for a job, but for an understanding of political issues and of the governing structure.

In Rome, Pablo finds himself a job in a bicycle shop, is introduced to the Underground and to some of its most respected leaders, such as Scarpa, veteran of the Spanish civil war, and his friends. He becomes politically involved, his activities come to the attention of the police, and he is arrested. After several weeks in jail, he is released for lack of evidence and ordered back to Turin and to a period of police surveillance.

The problem of the novel seems to spring, on the one hand, from its having been written in order to acknowledge its author's belief in the soundness and worth of the Communist program, and, on the other hand, as a substitute for an experience and a genuinely personal (and not merely intellectual) commitment Pavese, for a variety of complex reasons having to do with his personality, was unable to make. As a result, the unevenness of the second part of the book, despite some excellent pages depicting Pablo's Roman sojourn, is due to the obvious and unexplained lack of motivation of Pablo's political position, now anti-Fascist. But the "political" theme was an important one in Pavese's work, and he returned to it, this time with greater sensitivity and precision, in *La casa in collina*, written a few months later.

Both *La casa in collina* (*The House on the Hill*, N.Y., 1968, the sixth novel) and *La luna e i falò* are, in the writer's opinion, the best novels Pavese produced, beautiful and extremely touching works indeed. Composed between September 1947 and February 1948, *La casa in collina* was published, appropriately enough, with *Il carcere* (*The Political Prisoner*), in 1948 in an omnibus volume, *Prima che il gallo canti* [Before the cock crows]. The title is an allusion to Peter's betrayal preannounced by Christ, that before the cock crowed three times Peter will have betrayed Christ. As often the case with Pavese, the genesis of *The House on the Hill* goes back to several short stories, particularly "La famiglia" ("The Family"), which can be read in the anthology *Summer Storm* (London, 1966), and "Il fuggiasco" [The fugitive], written respectively in 1941 and 1944. The novel was written out of Pavese's innermost and most troubled feeling: it tells, with unusual clarity and perception, a great deal about the distanced and uninvolved role Pavese chose to play during the war. Its hero, as Davide Lajolo observes in his biography of our subject, is "the character into which Pavese poured the most of himself." Because the author achieved a perfect blend of autobiography and fiction, and because he was, at last, truly honest about himself, the resulting book is not only one of the best tales to have been inspired by the Resistance, but a deeply personal statement about the futility of any war, and the destruction, chaos, and misery it brings to mankind—a judgment lived, not just spoken or intellectualized, by the protagonist of the story.

The title of the book itself is symbolic: the house on the hill, where the protagonist lives in a rented room, is a safe place, away from Turin, target of constant air bombings in the final months of World War II, but it is also a convenient place to which he can withdraw and avoid reponsibilities and commitment. Like so many other Pavesian characters, Corrado is an intellectual, a *liceo* professor, with a special fondness for the hills with which he associates his childhood happiness. Again, he is depicted as unable to establish meaningful relations with anyone: not with Elvira, the daughter of the landlady of the house where he has taken a room; not with Cate, a young woman whom he meets in a tavern (she is a war refugee), and with whom many years before he had had an affair; not with her offspring, Dino, whose father is unknown but might well be Corrado himself. Much has happened since Cate disappeared from his life: she has matured emotionally and politically, has become a fierce anti-Fascist, has had a child, Dino. Corrado, on the other hand, has become even more cautious, uncommitted, and estranged, apparently satisfied with looking at life from the sidelines.

The story begins with a remarkably straightforward statement by the narrator-protagonist: "I should say—as I begin this story of a long illusion—that blame for what happened to me cannot be laid to the war. On the contrary, the war, I am certain, might still save me. . . . All the war did was to remove my last scruple about keeping to myself, about consuming the years and my heart alone. . . . The war had made it legitimate to turn in on oneself and live from day to day without regretting lost opportunities."

What follows is the frank study of how Corrado tries to achieve some sort of perspective on his "extreme scruples" about being apart from the others during the war, avoiding death or physical harm without changing much and yet never feeling good about his own survival. The fact that Pavese chose to publish the novel with his earlier *Il carcere* (*The Political Prisoner*) must be viewed as part of his strategy of showing the manner in which the heroes of the two stories deal with their lifelong efforts to come to grips with themselves and their rapport with the world. Thus, the titles themselves are symbolic: whereas in his first period of writing Pavese used the metaphor of jail to express his conviction that it is impossible to free ourselves from our fate, in his mature productive years he acknowledged the incapacity or impossibility for him to take a hand in the process of history. There is ample justification to support the widely held belief that Pavese's novels were written out of his guilt feelings rooted in his sexual and political life. Yet, in his best novels, *his* bad conscience becomes *our* bad conscience, certainly insofar as politics are concerned. The forty-year-old Corrado, safe in his ivory tower at first, and in his family's house later, tries to explain his unwillingness to accept an active role in the war, possibly with the Underground, in these words:

"It was as if I had been waiting for the war a long time and had been counting on it, a war so vast and unprecedented that one could easily go home to the hills, crouch down, and let it rage in the skies above the cities. Things were happening now that justified a mere keeping alive without complaining. That species of dull rancor that hemmed in my youth found a refuge and a horizon in the war." "Blood and fire: here the experience of the war," observes perceptively Fernandez, "is substituted to the experience of woman and love. . . . *The House on the Hill* is the novel which sets the historical necessity of participating in the political and military action, of enlisting in the ranks of the Resistance, against the mythical necessity of living in the hills."

As in many of his earlier novels, Pavese makes of the contrast between the city and the country one of the central motifs of his book. Turin (where some of the action is set) is presented as the place where one constantly feels the terror of the war in every way, particularly through the air raids whose mission is the destruction of the factories. The hills, and more specifically the room where he lives, allow him to view the spectacle of the war in relative safety. City and country become the two diametrically opposed loci of his experience. The hills now seem to symbolize the regularity of nature, while the city represents the upheavals, uncertainties, and unpredictability of life itself. Corrado's feeble attempt to make some sort of life for himself evaporates suddenly, one day in early spring when Cate, along with a number of partisans, is arrested while he watches the whole scene, petrified by fear, from the relative safety of a large tree. After Cate's arrest, Corrado leaves Dino to his fate (although still a youngster, he apparently joins the Resistance), and he will never see Cate or Dino again. He then wanders restlessly from one hill to another, witnessing the death and destruction caused by the continuous clashes between the Underground and the Fascists and Nazis. The war has changed the once peaceful country into a hell of fire and blood. For a while, he finds refuge in a seminary. But the fear of being found, compounded by his guilt feeling for his nonparticipation in the struggle against fascism, persuade him to make his way home in what is a symbolic journey through memory of the innocence and happiness of his childhood. Protected by his mother and his sister, Corrado finds safety but not peace. The last chapter is a fitting epilogue for the book: Corrado has been home for six months now, but the horror of the war and what it means not only to him, but to Cate, Dino, to his friends and family, as well as the enemy, haunts him every day of his life. We know, of course, that he may be safe, but in many ways he is as good as dead: he will never learn to be a father, or a husband, or a brother to other people. His selfishness, his egocentricity, his cowardice have spared his life, but they have robbed it of any significance. His incapacity for becoming involved has killed most of his decent feelings. He is left wondering about the war, life and death, humanity and inhumanity, cruelty and compassion:

> Looking at certain dead is humiliating. They are no longer other people's affairs: one doesn't seem to have happened there by chance. One has the impression that the same fate that threw these bodies to the ground holds us nailed to the spot to see them, to fill our eyes with the sight. It's not fear, not our usual cowardice. One feels humiliated because one understands—touching it with one's eyes—that we might be in their place ourselves: there would be no difference, and if we live

we owe it to this dirtied corpse. That is why every war is a civil war; every fallen man resembles one who remains and calls him to account.

Throughout the story, Corrado, much like Pavese himself, has lived accepting everything, including his own solitude: "The courage of being alone as if nobody else were alive, thinking only of what you do and thus accept oneself and the others." Yet, such indifference toward life ultimately leads Corrado to realize that "living by accident is not living, and I wonder if I have really escaped."

The book ends in a philosophic meditation about the experience Corrado has gone through: "Now that I've seen what civil war is, I know that everybody, if one day it should end, ought to ask himself: 'And what shall we make of the fallen? Why are they dead?' I wouldn't know what to say. Not now, at any rate. Nor does it seem to me that the others know. Perhaps only the dead know, and only for them is the war really over."

In his diary, under October 7, 1948, Pavese wrote: "On the 4th of October, *Diavolo sulle colline* was finished. It has the air of something big. It is a new language; dialectic, written with an atmosphere of culture and introducing 'student discussion.' For the first time you have really set up symbols. You have revitalized *La spiaggia* putting into it young men who make discoveries, the liveliness of debates, mythical reality." Pavese's story (translated as *The Devil in the Hills*, N.Y., 1959) is probably the most difficult and intellectually intricate of his novels. It is a cool portrait of bourgeois decadence, emptiness, and boredom, as well as an incisive treatment of one of the most painful themes of Pavese's work—man's incapacity to communicate with other human beings and the resulting estrangement from reality. All this is set, once again, in a manner calculated to bring out the dichotomy of farm and city. The main characters are all young, and men: the narrator, his friend Pieretto, both law students, and Oreste, a medical student. All three spend much of their time meandering in the streets of Turin or in the nearby hills in what is an attempt to evade their responsibilities as students. One night they meet Poli, a wealthy young man, and join him in his frequent escapades with his mistress, an aging woman by the name of Rosalba. Poli is hardly satisfied with his existence: in fact, he is nauseated by his constant escape into sex, liquor, and drugs in his search for whatever meaning life may have. One day Rosalba, sensing that their relationship has run its course, shoots him and nearly kills him. Poli's father, hastily summoned by Oreste, wishing to avoid a scandal, uses his influence to have the whole incident dismissed as an accident, and places Rosalba in a convent.

The action now shifts to a small village in Piedmont, to the country house of Oreste's family, by whom the narrator and Pieretto have been invited to spend the rest of the summer, and the occasion affords them the opportunity to come into a closer contact with the earth. Indeed, much of the descriptions of nature, and of the activities of the three friends, becomes part and parcel of Pavese's determination to build into the work a number of symbolic myths, that *give* intellectual *substance* to the story.

The three friends decide to pay a call on Poli, who is convalescing in a nearby town. Much to their shock, they find him living with an attractive, young woman, Gabriella, his estranged wife who has returned home to help him recover. The group resumes a rather dissolute life, which concludes a short love affair between Oreste and Gabriella, with Poli aware of, but unconcerned with their relation. The book ends with Poli shown being driven in his car to the city's clinic, facing impending death by tuberculosis.

In a letter to his teacher and mentor, Augusto Monti, Pavese remarked that the novel was meant to be "a youthful hymn of discovery of nature and society: everything seems beautiful to the three boys, and only little by little, each in his own way, do they establish contact with the sordidness of a 'futile' world—a certain bourgeois world that does nothing, believes in nothing, [a world] which I see no reason to hide under a veil."

As in some of his earlier novels, what is portrayed in *The Devil in the Hills* is yet another treatment of the theme of the "return": this time it is not the protagonist-narrator who is "going home," but his friend Oreste, accompanied by Pieretto and the narrator. Moreover, their experience seeks to recapture something of the mythical dimension of the country, with its magnetic power. What was to be a discovery of the earth, turns out to be a confrontation between the "civiltà contadina" and the "civiltà cittadina"—the former raw and violent, but basically healthy, the latter sophisticated but thoroughly decadent and corrupted by vice, drugs, and an absence of a sense of purpose. The book, with its attempts to reach down to the symbolism of its themes, is also about the evasion of responsibility displayed by the three young friends and the metaphorical illness of Poli and Gabriella. "As in [Thomas Mann's] *The Magic Mountain*," writes Gianni Venturi, "the illness is not merely physical, so in the story of Poli and Gabriella the vice of the former and [his] relationship with the latter alludes to hidden truths, that is to say the impossibility of retrieving the sense of life without cherishing the sense of death."

As is often the case with Pavese, the story unfolds in the summertime, and this makes possible an uninhibited exposure of the naked bodies of the three friends to the sun, basking in its heat in what is presented as a ritual, a "vice" sui generis. When the narrator asks Poli whether "cocaine could add to the peace of the soul" he answers "that everyone takes some kind of drug, from wine to sleeping pills, from nudism to the cruelty of the hunt. 'What has nudism to do with it?' Oh yes, it was part of the picture: people go naked into company to brutalize themselves and defy convention."

The search for meaning in this apparently incoherent world becomes more intense when the action moves to the Greppo hill, and after a highly symbolic thunderstorm: "You could hear the almost solid mass of water falling and rumbling. I imagined the steaming and running landscape, our cleft boiling over, roots laid bare, the most private cracks in the earth penetrated and violated." But the search ultimately proves to be fruitless: the devil is in the hills, and there cannot be any peace. Man is his easy prey, victim of the havoc he brings to his soul, who must surrender to his "destiny." His only hope is to be spared the tragic end of Poli and the sufferings of an implacable, savage, unforgiving Nature.

Tra donne sole (*Among Women Only*, N.Y., 1959) is told in the first person, is set in Turin's world of haute couture, and has an almost complete cast of women. What attracted Pavese to such a world has not, to my knowledge, been satisfactorily explained. If our reading of Pavese is correct, our novelist preferred situations that did not require much action (as *Il carcere*, *La bella estate*, *La spiaggia*, and *Il diavolo sulle colline* indicate), and where time is of no immediate consequence. In this sense, the choice of the world of haute couture was felicitous, in that it is frequented by the affluent upper middle class, with ample money to spend and an equally ample time to waste, untouched by the pressures of earning a living. Moreover, clothing is connected with the way one looks, with his or her appearance as it were, and we know how important it is for the bourgeoisie to dress "properly," just as we are aware of how Pavese felt about appearance and substance.

As in *The Devil in the Hills*, Pavese thought highly of his eighth novel. In his diary (April 17, 1949), he noted:

> Discovered today that *Tra donne sole* is a great novel; that the experience of being engulfed in the false, tragic world of high society is broad and incongruous, and blends well with Clelia's wistful memories. Starting from her search for a childish, *wistful* world that no longer exists, she discovers the grotesque, sordid tragedy of those women of Turin as it is, of her own realized dream. Her discovery of herself, and the emptiness of her world, which saves her ("I've got everything I wanted").

The central character of this novella is Clelia Oitana, an exceedingly capable and mature businesswoman, of humble origin, who has just arrived from Rome to speed up the construction of her own boutique. The arrival at her hotel takes place with the removal on a stretcher of a woman (Rosetta Mola) who has tried, unsuccessfully, to take her own life. The nature of Clelia's interests brings her into contact with the "woman's world" of Turin, as well as the well-to-do friends and prospective clients. Here is one of the problems besetting the protagonist: her social origin makes difficult, not to say impossible, her being accepted by the affluent bourgeoisie whose values she does not respect. At one point, she admits she respects prostitutes, although she is not always sensitive to the hardships of those who, like herself, have had a tough struggle to gain a certain position in society.

Much of the story revolves, then, around four women: Clelia, ambitious, torn by her past and present love affairs; Momina, a hard, cynical, abrasive woman who is one of Pavese's most profoundly existential characters, who experiences nausea toward so much of what she does, and is ultimately fed up with life itself;

Rosetta, a sensitive, weak, tormented creature controlled by Momina; and Nene, the thirty-year-old companion of a mediocre painter, Loris, who has preserved, despite her situation, an unusual degree of naïveté and shyness. In all cases, there is a strange, but stubborn rejection of a meaningful relation that could have eased the women's pain of living: thus, for example, Clelia is unwilling to engage herself in a serious relationship with Becuccio, the architect who is supervising the remodeling of her shop, or Guido, her lover of some years earlier. Success proves not to be the key to happiness either, and here Pavese touches deeply on his experience as an esteemed editor and a respected, successful novelist. Through Clelia's meditations, he remarks: "This was all my past intolerable and yet so different, so dead, I had told myself so many times in those years—and later, too, as I thought it over, that the aim of my life was really to be a success, to become somebody and one day return to these alleys where I had been a child."

"To be somebody," or "To be something," two yearnings expressed in *The House on the Hill*, prove to be illusions, like much that life seems to offer, or that man wants to achieve. And *Among Women Only* becomes the story of the particular condition in which women, bearing the burden of discrimination, stereotyping, and male chauvinism, have to resolve their dream of what life ought to be for them.

Perhaps the salient features of this unusual novel are to be found in the struggle Clelia fights to enter the world of the well-to-do, decadent middle class (her prospective clientele), her stubborn self-confidence in business matters matched by a marked confusion when it comes to her feelings, and the way in which Pavese focuses on the particular manner in which the heroines of the story deal with their conditions. The book opens with a suicide *manqué*, and closes with the death of the same person, Rosetta, whose death is given away by the scratching of a cat. Her suicide (which she is almost goaded to commit by Momina) represents the price one may well have to pay when, unable to live a lonely existence, one perceives the fact that life is simply unbearable, too ugly to be endured for long. Clelia, a businesswoman, can accept the compromises one must make to retain one's sanity. Not so in Rosetta's case: and for her, death becomes the liberating factor from the loneliness and sadness of existence.

If it is true that only exceptionally do literary critics find themselves in agreement in their assessment of literary texts, the proverbial exception to the rule is Pavese's last novel, *La luna e i falò* (*The Moon and the Bonfires*, N.Y., 1953). Written feverishly in less than two months' time (September 18–November 9, 1949), it was published in April 1950, about four months before Pavese's suicide. Not without some flaws, and though it lacks the sensitivity toward human sufferings shown in *The House on the Hill, The Moon and the Bonfires* is unquestionably an impressive, hauntingly poetic novel. But the virtues of the book are to be found not only in the story it tells, or in the superb handling of its characters and motifs, but in the masterful manner in which so many of Pavese's themes are brought together, and how his poetics are lucidly translated into practice. Thus, for example, Pavese's deep feelings for the country—especially the hills of the Langhe region—his love for his native Piedmont, its rites, its mores and myths, are fused with the motif of the return "home." This time, however, the protagonist comes back from a faraway, almost fablelike land, America, where he has lived for many years in what is, essentially, a forced exile because of lack of work in his own country. The prolonged stay and the distance add an extra perspective to the experience, and the feeling of being "home" once more is both deeper and more complex.

The protagonist of the novel is a forty-year-old man, known only by his nickname of Anguilla ("Eel") who recently returned from California. He is now wealthy, thanks to his thrift and his work, and has settled in Genoa where he operates a small business. As often as possible, he comes "home," to his town in the Langhe hills. His *paese* is in his blood: he cannot forget it, nor can he live without it. His travels, his long period away from his native town, have taught him a great deal, for he has led a varied existence, experiencing new values. Although he has achieved considerable success, he knows that going back to his *paese* is essential if he is to understand the meaning of what has happened to him. Moreover, he really does not know where he was born, nor does he know his parents, as he was raised by someone else. And so he comes as a stranger, as someone who actually never lived there, who is eager to put together the pieces of his life, his boyhood, his years in America, and the present, and, eventually, the time of the Italian Resistance during World War II. For the time being, he has to acknowledge that "The faces, the voices and the hands that were supposed to touch me and recognize me were no longer there."

The question posed indirectly by the novel is fundamental to Pavese's world: "Can we go home again?" Thomas Wolfe answered it in the negative. And no wonder: we can stand on familiar ground and find our bearings, remember the past, and recapture many lovely or sad memories. But time has passed. We have lived and experienced much: we have been hurt by life and, if we are fortunate, we have been blessed by some happiness. As time passes, people change and are molded by life, and find the values that will guide them in their adult years. Coming back to a place left long ago, particularly when still young, makes our understanding of places and people left long ago more difficult. Yet, this is also what gives Anguilla some sort of perspective: having lived away for so many years is what ultimately enables him to understand so much of what would otherwise have remained an enigma for him. And so Anguilla finds himself "home" (but a "home" he never really knew) after many years spent abroad, in a country he could never call his own, uprooted by necessity from what was the closest thing to a family he could have, happy to return if, for no other reason, because it is comforting "to know that in the people, in the trees, the land, there is something that remains waiting for you, even when you have gone away." The quest for his roots begins with a frank admission. "There is a reason why I came back to this place, here and not to Canelli, or Barbaresco, or Alba. I wasn't born here that's almost certain; where I was born, I don't know; there isn't any house or piece of earth around here, any bones that belong to me so I could say: 'here is what I was before I was born.'"

The story itself is constructed as a relived, remembered experience. Memories of a life full of events and doings, both in Anguilla's native town and abroad, become the elements he tries to sort out in his search for his roots and his identity. Padrino and Virgilia, his foster parents, are no longer at the Gaminella farm, now rented to Valino, a surly type who resembles Talino (of *The Harvesters*), and his crippled son Cinto, befriended by Anguilla and Nuto. The three play the central roles of the story, while the women occupy a less central position. Anguilla, who narrates the story, is, as often is the case with Pavese, largely passive. Nuto, on the other hand, although not a principal figure in the events narrated, assumes the part of the guide into the past and the commentator on many of the special characteristics, particularly the rites and symbols, of country life. His friendship with Anguilla goes way back to their boyhood, and, while many years have passed, he has retained his respect, affection, and loyalty. He becomes now a sort of guide, or historian of the town's events during the last twenty years. This is, in a sense, an extension of the role of mentor he played during Anguilla's boyhood, when he encouraged him to study a musical instrument and read books so as to widen his knowledge of the world. Unlike Anguilla, he remained in his *paese*, growing and participating, if only in a limited manner, in the events of his country in the closing months of the war. A cordial, peaceful man, who abhors violence, he has nevertheless taken part in at least one violent incident. Basically an optimist, he truly believes in man's ability to change, to some degree, his life, thus emerging as one of Pavese's few positive characters. He is a carpenter now and as such an artist sui generis. Once a gifted clarinet player, he hung his instrument on the wall when his father passed away, an act that suggests his seriousness and his realization that he could never support himself with his music, which gave him so much joy and fun. It is Nuto, finally, who explains the meaning of the element of nature in a rural civilization, and how the symbols of the kind we normally associate with the *campagna* are parts of the structure that, to a considerable degree, shapes the beliefs and the actions of the peasants.

We have seen how, in his previous novels, Pavese sought, with sporadic and uneven results, to achieve a fusion of the realistic and symbolic elements of his fiction. Generally, his failure is probably to be ascribed to the intellectual nature of his characters, or to unwarranted or inappropriate superimposition of symbolism on personages and events. In *The Moon and the Bonfires* these difficulties have been resolved, thanks first of all to the natural way the characters speak (a kind of Piedmontese "Italianized," as it were), and their capacity to sustain a symbolic significance appropriate to their real, lived experience of the earth. It is through his understanding of the myths and symbols that Anguilla will ultimately come to grips with the meaning of life.

In his efforts to find the pieces of his past, and fit them into the puzzle of his existence, some of the main events of Anguilla's boyhood are reviewed: his brief stint as a servant and, later on, as a laborer at La Mora, Sor Matteo's farm; his first attachment and sexual attraction to Matteo's two elder daughters by previous marriage, Irene and Silvia, tall and beautiful, the first blond, the second black-haired, and the awe he felt for Matteo's youngest daughter, Santina, whose fate unfolds in the closing pages of the book in what ranks as a tragic end. The women's wealth and beauty in no way bring them happiness: Irene dies after having been brutally beaten by her husband Arturo, a mediocre man who has squandered her dowry; Silvia leads a promiscuous life and becomes pregnant. Her father, unable to bear the shame of the event, dies after a stroke, while Silvia dies after an abortion, having "filled her bed with blood," uttering the word "Papa" just before passing away. An even more tragic fate awaits the youngest of the sisters, Santa, called by her endearing diminutive Santina, and remembered by Anguilla all dressed in silk at Irene's wedding, when she was barely six years old. During the war, she betrays first the Fascists, then the Partisans, by whom she is eventually captured. As she attempts to escape, she is killed by a rapid short burst of submachine-gun fire in an incident remarkable for its economy and effectiveness of details. Still clad in her white dress, her body is covered with branches over which gasoline is poured and set afire by two men who loved her, Baracca and Nuto, in a scene that is presented as a frighteningly impressive ritual: her ashes will fertilize the earth.

The theme of violence is realized dramatically through the events of another character, the farmer Valino. In a moment when he can no longer control his anger, he mortally beats his sister-in-law Rosina, threatens to kill Cinto, who runs away, and finally sets fire to the haystacks, the stalls, and the farmhouse (the old grandmother, unable to move, is burned to death), and then hangs himself in the vineyard. After his death, Anguilla and Nuto agree to assume the responsibility of raising Cinto.

Woven in the fabric of the narrative, a new theme emerges with extraordinary force. Three chapters (3, 11, and 21) are devoted to Anguilla's American experience. It is a tribute to Pavese that, although he had never set foot on these shores, he so convincingly captured the spirit of a life so different from that of his native country. But what is also remarkable is the manner in

which an imaginary experience—one that was exclusively intellectual—is made so real and so much a part of the story itself. As
Gian-Paolo Biasin perceptively notes, the three chapters "em-
phasize the fundamental difference between America and Piedmont, between valleys and hills, between artificiality and nature,
between chaos and custom; and yet, in their similarity they em-
phasize the fundamental analogies between Anguilla and Santa,
between terror and death." The story, set in 1948, or approximately the time of its true composition, stretches back some
twenty years, a date that coincides almost exactly with the beginning of Pavese's intense and fruitful experience with American
literature when, as he wrote in one of his post–World War II
essays printed in *La letterature americana e altri saggi* (regrettably
not included in the English translation *American Literature:
Essays and Opinions*), he saw America as "something serious and
precious," a country that was free, unhampered by traditions,
whose "culture enabled us to see our drama unfolding as though
on a gigantic stage."

The rejection of America by Pavese the intellectual is made to
coincide with that of Anguilla of *The Moon and the Bonfires*,
private emotions becoming part and parcel of the world of art.
Two ways of life, and two different worlds are placed squarely before the reader. The contrast between Piedmont and the almost
endless landscape of California (where Anguilla lived and worked)
could hardly have been more sharply and effectively dramatized.
An alienating land, bare as the moon, "there is nothing, it's like
the moon," Anguilla remarks at one point, with no real women
and no wine, plenty of sex but no love, America is depicted as
an illusory heaven ultimately to be rejected. Despite the opportunity it offers to hardworking individuals to make money so that
they might go back to their *paese* and enjoy their mature years,
it actually increases their rootlessness once they have returned.
The moon of the title takes on a double meaning—the sterility
of America and the magic, awesome power that influences so
much life in Piedmont—and mirrors the novelist's own ambivalence toward a nation whose generosity could give to so many
people a chance for a life of dignity and work, and whose power,
with its atomic bombs, could threaten the future of the world—a
conflict that haunts young and mature people alike today, almost
thirty years after Pavese's suicide.

8

Elio Vittorini: The Poetization of Ideology

For more than thirty years, from the 1930s to 1966, when he died after an heroic struggle against cancer, the star of Elio Vittorini was among the brightest and most promising in the Italian literary firmament. For years, every book he published was an event not to be missed, certain to be followed by spirited discussions about the achievement of his new novel, and the particular direction Vittorini was promising for a truly contemporary work of the creative imagination striving to depict man's condition. His imaginative, sensitive, poetic mind remained receptive to the end to the changes of technique he perceived would make his novels not just mirrors of life in our hectic era, but living testimonials to an artist's search for "truth." His good friend and collaborator, Italo Calvino, once identified the elements of such a novel in these words: "Its mythical form is the journey, its stylistic form is the dialogue, its conceptual form is the Utopia."

Life, as Vittorini conceived it, was precisely this: a journey to a better understanding through a dialogue with his readers in the pursuit of a dream of freedom, justice, and peace without which life would be intolerable and even absurd. In this respect, Vittorini sides with those writers who, with considerable justification, hold that everything one does, to be truly meaningful, must be an inseparable part of the human and creative self, a reflection of the growth of the total being. In Vittorini's case, this was true whether he was working with a construction gang building a bridge in the Veneto region, correcting proofs for a newspaper, writing criticism or fiction, translating, fighting as a member of the Underground during World War II, editing the socio-political cultural sheet *Il Politecnico* (1945–47), making important or even controversial decisions (such as rejecting Lampedusa's *The Leopard* because of its backward ideological position and its awkwardly archaic structure) as a senior editor of Mondadori Publishing Company, or running for political office. In this respect, Vittorini was an intellectual on the order of Jean-Paul Sartre: a person highly conscious of his position in society, a privileged citizen who, precisely because of his privileges, has a special responsibility toward his craft and toward history. The state of the world could, and did, make changes in his strategy necessary: but Vittorini hung on to his fundamental belief in the dignity and worth of the individual, in the ability of man to recognize and fight against evil and work together with other men for a better world.

He was, despite his deceptively simple personality, a complex man and an equally complex artist. Measured by the usual standards, his literary output is hardly impressive: a small number of short stories, eight novels and novellas (two of which were published posthumously), a travelogue of Sardinia, an absorbing volume entitled *Diario in pubblico* [Public diary] (1957, 2d ed. augmented, 1970), in which he collected the bulk of his articles, reviews, notes and comments on a broad variety of cultural, political, and literary matters (all previously published in reviews and newspapers), sections of his novels not included in the final version—and, finally, clarifications of his ideas written shortly prior to publication of the diary. Nonetheless, as Donald Heiney has suggested in his study of Vittorini, our novelist will probably be remembered "primarily [as] the author of one novel. But he is that kind of one-book author, like Rabelais and Cervantes, who adds a new artistic dimension to the history of literature."

As is almost invariable in the case of great and influential writers, there is in Vittorini's total literary work an exceptional degree of thematic coherence and a similarly fascinating and equally erratic progression toward "his" book. Whatever Vittorini wrote, and however the reader may wish to label it—allegories, fables, realistic, or symbolic tales perhaps, written in a highly imaginative and poetic style—should be regarded as parts of an intriguing work in progress cut short by his death. And here is the rub: despite their achievements, none of Vittorini's books, with the exception of *Il garofano rosso* (1948; *The Red Carnation*, N.Y., 1952), the one work he all but completely rejected when it was published in book form, can claim to be what Warren Beach would have called "the well-made novel."

Part of Vittorini's difficulties may be traceable to his constant dissatisfaction with practically every book he wrote, subjecting it to furious revisions, eliminating chapters or episodes. Nowhere can this be seen more clearly than in *Le donne di Messina* (*The Women of Messina*, N.Y., 1973). Begun in 1946, published with the title *Lo zio Agrippa passa in treno* [Uncle Agrippa goes by on a train] in serial form in the review *La rassegna d'Italia* between 1946 and 1949, revised some fourteen times and published in book form in 1949, and then completely rewritten and published in 1964! Hence the dilemmas of technique and form, the inevitable dissatisfaction with the finished product. "I have never aspired to write books," he once noted, "I have always sought to write *the* book. . . . I write because I believe there is 'one' truth to be said; and if I turn from one thing to another it is not because I see 'other' truths that can also be said, or because I have 'more' or 'something else' to say, but because it seems to me that something constantly changing in the truth requires that the way of expressing it be constantly renewed."

To this end he indeed dedicated the better part of his creative efforts, but not in a regular, "disciplined" manner. It is, in fact, the astonishing diversity of his activities (translations, editorial work, creative writing, and so forth) that led one of his critics to comment how "his way of reasoning . . . is like a small jungle: to confirm, to consolidate an idea that has just struck him, Vittorini loses himself in other arguments, at first parallel and similar, then always more disparate, always less probable, finally opposed to one another." "I envy," Vittorini wrote another time, almost as though he were in effect answering his critics, "those writers who have the capacity to remain interested in their own work while pestilences and war are raging in the world. . . . A big public event can unfortunately distract me and cause a change of interests in my own work just as, no more no less, can a personal happy event or a misfortune. Thus the outburst of the Spanish Civil War, in July of 1936, made me suddenly indifferent to the developments of the story [*Erica*] on which I had been working for six months in a row."

Like traditional novelists, say Moravia or Pratolini, Vittorini draws from reality the subjects for his books: unlike them, how-ever, he is less interested in telling a "good story" than he is in recapturing deep and universal feelings about life. Everyday events are magically transformed into a timeless, "mythical" real-ity, far more real and effective than reality itself, stripped of its banalities, but where even commonplaces become poetry. It is unquestionably true that, when compared to his contemporaries, his range, both in terms of situations and themes, is considerably more limited and much more special. For him, the main prob-lem with which he struggled during much of his creative years was to find a suitable language to objectify his vision of the world, which in his particular case meant to translate his ideology into poetry.

To be sure, in all his books after *Conversazione in Sicilia* (1941; *In Sicily*, N.Y., 1949)—which, as we shall see, is a turn-ing point in his development as an artist—he presents a world that has a fragile, though vital, connection with the "real" world we know, but is far more deeply connected with the world of our dreams, hopes, and aspirations. Justice, freedom, communion, peace—human and political concepts—are what his stories are all about. To accomplish his objective, Vittorini's books transport the reader into a no-man's-land, where people feel intensely and suffer, to be sure, but don't work or play or make love. It is not for nothing that his finest tales take place in a mythical Sicily (*Conversazione in Sicilia*) or on a train, as in *The Women of Messina* and *La Garibaldina* (1956; *La Garibaldina*, N.Y., 1973), or anywhere in postwar Italy (but is it really Italy?) as in *Il Sempione strizza l'occhio al Fréjus* (1947; *The Twilight of the Elephant*, N.Y., 1973) rather than in the realistic cities in which the action of *Il garofano rosso* (1948; *The Red Carnation*, N.Y., 1952) and *Uomini e no* [Men and nonmen] (1945) is set.

Vittorini was born in Syracuse, Sicily, in 1908. His father was an employee of the State Railroad and, being a southerner and a worker, he wished his son to be a white-collar worker. Elio and his three brothers traveled daily to a nearby town where they completed their elementary schooling. The author was then en-rolled in a technical school to learn accountancy. He did not succeed in winning the diploma however, realizing at the age of seventeen what he had long suspected: that studies did not suit him, and that it was better to give them up once and for all.

Using his father's railroad pass, he traveled frequently, sometimes leaving his home for weeks at a time. One day, in 1924, he left —for the fourth time in three years—with his mind made up not to return. He had left for the "Continent," hoping to begin there a new life away from home.

He settled in Gorizia, a small city in the extreme northeastern part of Italy. The years there proved to be very important for him: his job as a construction worker revealed to him a whole different world from that of the petit bourgeoisie into which he was born: most of the characters that were to people his fiction would come from the working class and, more often than not, would be the dispossessed, the exploited, the poor. But this discovery might have been less significant had it not gradually been accompanied by an intense and vital discovery of a whole nucleus of writers (mostly novelists, but some poets as well) who were either in the avant-garde of Continental European letters or from a world quite different (and in this sense ripe for a true discovery at the human and cultural level) from his own: Italo Svevo, Eugenio Montale, Stendhal, Proust, Mallarmé, Defoe, Kipling, Stevenson, Mansfield. It is important to stress here that, much like Moravia, Vittorini was an autodidact: and if this process of educating oneself is not without its share of pitfalls, it has at least the distinct advantage of bypassing the whole backward bourgeois educational scheme that only rarely encourages a periodic reassessment of the worth of its writers, particularly of the so-called sacred cows. It should come as no surprise therefore, if the very first piece collected in *Diario in pubblico*, entitled "Maestri cercando" [Looking for masters], should focus on the necessity to search for something better (more responsive, that is, to the contemporary sensibility) than Carducci, Pascoli, d'Annunzio, and Croce, then the solid and respected pillars of modern Italian literature and philosophy.

By 1930, he was ready for the next move—Florence, in those years the cultural capital of Italy. A few months earlier, he had published his first essay in *Solaria*, the Florentine review which, under the editorship of its founder, Alberto Carocci, dedicated its best efforts to translating and commenting on the finest narrative and poetry being produced on both sides of the Atlantic. *Solaria* opened its doors to Vittorini, and won him over completely: "I became *solariano*," he wrote in *Diario in pubblico*, "and *solari-*

ano was a word that in the literary circles of those days meant to be anti-Fascist, European, internationalist, antitraditionalist." For some years, he worked as proofreader for the newspaper *La nazione* and, with the help of a co-worker, he began learning English, practicing his skill on *Robinson Crusoe*.

In 1931 he published his first book, *Piccola borghesia* [Petit bourgeoisie], a slim collection of eight short stories. They are exercises of sorts, competent tales in which the author manages to transcribe in a humorous, slightly ironical style, the monotonous life of middle-class bureaucrats. Shortly afterward, Vittorini decided to earn his bread through intellectual activities. In 1933, the first of his translations of three novels by D. H. Lawrence was published by Mondadori, and three years later Vittorini's second book, *Viaggio in Sardegna*, a curious work that is not the travelogue it may seem from the title, appeared. The setting itself is especially central. As we shall see, the best of Vittorini's future fiction is deliberately set in places undisturbed by bourgeois civilization, chosen not for their color but for their stark simplicity, their primordial quality that encourages the effort of recovering something precious and long lost with a maximum degree of effectiveness and a minimum degree of distraction.

Two books seem to have left an indelible impression upon his sensibility: *A Thousand and One Nights*, with its Oriental charm, and Daniel Defoe's *Robinson Crusoe*, a novel that *in nuce* prefigures so much of Vittorini's own work, with flights to semideserted places, his desire to regain touch with Nature, and begin all over the human discovery of the world, and of man's place and meaning in it. From his very first book—*Viaggio in Sardegna*—to his last completed novel—*Le donne di Messina*—we witness a voyage of one sort or another, either to an island which is "like a boyhood" (and therefore replete with a sense of magic discovery) or to a place where man, with other men and women dislocated by the war, may begin anew a life of fellowship and trust, as in *The Women of Messina*. It was only in the early thirties that the importance of his early reading began to make itself manifest.

In the meantime—early in 1932—his first novel, *Il garofano rosso* (*The Red Carnation*, N.Y., 1952) began to take shape. By 1933 the novel was well under way. As the book was half finished, and as is customary in many European and Latin American countries, installments of the story began appearing in magazine form, in *Solaria*. But Vittorini's handling of certain aspects of the story, and his candid, graphic language, met with serious objections of the censor who decided that its language and content clearly were contrary to "morals and good customs," and ordered the sixth issue of the magazine withdrawn from circulation, even though it had already reached its subscribers. Quite a similar fate awaited the work, when the manuscript was submitted for publication in book form. Although many of the passages to which the censor had originally objected had either been rewritten or deleted, and other changes made in the novel to preserve its integrity, permission to publish was flatly denied.

In 1945, with the war over and the Fascists out of power, Vittorini's publisher saw no reason why the novel could not appear, and appear it did in 1948. In view of the fact that some thirteen years had elapsed between the original writing of the novel and its publication in book form, Vittorini felt obliged to discuss his own changed attitude toward his work, and its particular position in the context of his literary production. The discussion took the form of a lengthy essay which ranks as a major pronouncement on the art of the novel, the author's poetics, the special historical circumstances in which *The Red Carnation* was written, and its position in the author's work, and as such it is a compelling statement that calls for scrutiny.

But let us first turn our attention to the novel itself. The story it tells is seemingly pedestrian: Alessio Mainardi is in love with a fellow student, Giovanna, from whom he receives a red carnation. He tells of his love to his friend Tarquinio who, in turn, boasts of an affair with a more mature, somewhat mysterious woman, Zobeida, who, if not a prostitute, is "a lady of easy virtue," and is involved in a narcotics ring. Tarquinio, who is not exactly a good and generous friend, proceeds to seduce Giovanna, presenting his bloodstained handkerchief as evidence of his sexual prowess, while Alessio becomes involved in Zobeida's life. Intermingled with the narrative are several letters by Alessio's friend Tarquinio and sections of the hero's diary. Nothing much happens as the story unfolds. Alessio fails his courses and begins preparing himself for the October make-up examinations, but he is still not promoted. At that time he learns from Tarquinio himself of Giovanna's affair with him, and the book comes to an end.

The novel, which belongs to the tradition of middlebrow European fiction, could normally be dismissed as trite, were it not for certain aspects that make it a much better and interesting book than it might appear at first reading. For one thing, the underlying two-headed theme of sexual and idealistic love is linked with the violence of fascism: there is the blood-stained handkerchief boldly shown by Tarquinio as proof of his virility, and the anger shown by Alessio when he cries out to his friend: "I wish you were another Matteotti, and I would make you understand!" His words reflect the temptation of translating sexual frustration into positions on the extreme sides of the political spectrum.

Another interesting side of the novel is in its hints that the regime has the acquiescent, if indirect, support of the liberal middle class: Alessio's father is a businessman, formerly a socialist, who, in his son's eyes, has saved himself at the expense of his workers. The air echoes with familiar names, events, and contemporary political movements: Matteotti's murder, Rosa Luxemburg, fascism and socialism, Lenin, and, ever-present in the background, Mussolini himself. The restlessness of the students and young intellectuals and their "ambivalent" political attitude (as Vittorini rightly defines it) are persuasively dramatized. The theme of politics gradually proves to be, in Vittorini's later fiction, progressively more pervasive, urgent, and deeply felt, always connected with a tireless search for a better, less repressive, fairer sociopolitical order. And it is when seen in retrospect, as it were, that *The Red Carnation*, for all its apparent confusion (or, at the very least, its ambiguity) most decisively marks the transition between its author's first and second (or more mature) period. A change in a writer's way of looking at the world, and his view of life, by necessity calls for a change of style and structure. Such a change, to be sure, did not occur overnight. Certain events were to hasten and encourage it. It was precisely during the first months of writing *The Red Carnation* that Vittorini took a trip to Milan:

If I ever write my autobiography, I will explain what a great importance this trip to Milan had for me. I came back enamored of places and names, of the world itself, as I had never been except in my childhood. This state of mind had not come of itself; I had sought it out. Yet it came in an extraordinary way, after a period of five or six years during which it seemed to me that only as a child had I had spontaneous relations with the maternal things of the earth. It came at a time when I looked only to the past, when I wrote with my eyes to the rear.

The Red Carnation had cost him "cold sweats of study." When confronted with the book as it was taking shape, he discovered its "technical mistakes," the incoherence and immaturity of its point of view, and, above all, his own inability to identify himself with the characters he had created or with the book's view of the world. "The power of contact, the passion I had recaptured in March '33 had little by little worked its way into every aspect of my environment, and now I could 'feel passion' for political events as well. I felt that the wrongs of fascism against others now offended me personally." Vittorini's changed attitudes toward a world he had more or less accepted lessened his belief in his manner of writing. While engaged in writing his novel, he also began to feel uneasy and unhappy with the fundamental vehicle of expression of a writer, the kind of language that was available to the contemporary Italian novelist working within his tradition.

Such a language constituted a century-old tradition that every novelist, Italian or otherwise, could bring up to date. One could bring to it those variations suggested by his sensibility as a writer . . . but in practice he had to respect its structure and no one could be called a novelist unless he did so. [Such a language] was excellent to gather the explicit facts of a reality, and to connect them with each other explicitly; to show them, explicitly, in their conflicts, but today it is inadequate for a type of representation in which someone wishes to express a total sentiment or a total idea, an idea that might synthesize the hopes and sufferings of men in general, all the more if [they were] secret.

This problem obsessed him and continued during the months following the completion of *The Red Carnation*, right to the next novella, *Erica e i suoi fratelli* (published in English in the volume *The Twilight of the Elephant and Other Novels: A Vittorini Omnibus*, N.Y., 1973). He wrote the tale between January and July 1936, interrupting it because of external circumstances ("I envy those writers who have the capacity of remaining interested in their own work while pestilences and wars are ravaging the world"). He put aside the manuscript and forgot about its existence, until 1953 when it was found by his late son Giusto in a trunk packed with personal papers left with his family for over a decade. One year later it was published in the Roman review *Nuovi argomenti*, accompanied by a letter by the author addressed to the editors, Moravia and Carocci. In a note appended to the novella, Vittorini once again told why he had been both unwilling and unable to finish the work, even when the manuscript had been retrieved:

> The manner in which I have been accustomed to write from *Conversazione* on, is not exactly the same in which the present story is told. Today I have become used to refer to my characters' feelings and thoughts only through their exterior manifestations. . . . It no longer comes natural for me to write that such and such character "felt" that, or that "he thought" that. . . . But when I wrote this book it was still natural for me (as it had been in *Piccola borghesia*, or in *Sardegna*, or in *Il garofano rosso*) to say directly what one felt and what one thought. The book is, in fact, replete with "she thought," "she felt," "she used to think."

Traditional in structure, *Erica* is clearly Vittorini's first work not genuinely autobiographical, the first experience of handling the theme of poverty in a world of cruelty and hypocrisy. The story revolves around the experiences of a fourteen-year-old girl left in charge of her younger brother and sister by her mother, who leaves town to join her husband working in a distant locality. Erica shows her maturity and good sense by assuming the role of a mother, and the three manage well as long as they can subsist on the few provisions of *pasta*, coal, beans, and oil left by their parents. Even when she is under the pressure of repeated offers of help from her neighbors Erica insists on living her own life. One day, however, when her provisions are exhausted, she realizes that she has reached an impasse. She becomes a prostitute, for it is the only thing she can do without feeling that she is begging others to help her. Her decision is readily accepted by her neighbors: "Indeed just because she was little more than a child, and because they had witnessed the long agony which debouched in this misfortune they were silent more than ever . . . in a certain sense, they also felt grateful to Erica for having freed them of their preoccupation about what she should do." Despite the numerous wounds she suffers—wounds that only time and affection can heal—she is proud of the fact that she can continue to take care of her little family and face life with courage and serenity.

This novella is left unfinished at the point when the young girl, in Vittorini's intention, was supposed to enter the world and find a partial solution to her problems. Written in a simple style, defined by Sergio Pautasso as almost "a watershed between the [artistic] experience of his youth and his maturity," the novella is particularly notable for the depth with which the author explores complex feelings and social situations, reducing them to understatements in order to heighten their effect. The importance of *Erica* is clearly thematic rather than purely stylistic, to be sure. And while we are not quite at the threshold of that special richly symbolic language capable of expressing basic, profound truths about life, we begin to sense that both the texture and the substance of the narrative are indeed something different from *The Red Carnation*. The theme and preoccupations of *Erica* may well betray something nineteenth-centuryish about them (that no doubt reminds us of Dickens, Zola, and the work of many Italian *veristi*), and the language is more lyrical, more delicate, less restrained by realistic considerations. In fact, we might even speak of two tones, that of Erica and that of the objective narrator-observer. Of the two, it is the former's that stands out: it is a language of the kind of writing Vittorini always preferred, the language of poetry, childlike in its simplicity, rich in its evocative power, capable of expressing what really matters in a human discourse—feelings, states of mind, in short, the "truth" about ourselves. The kind of book *Erica* turns out to be made this possible: after all, it is a kind of fable (in its original meaning) within which unfolds the story of its heroine.

Erica is raised in a city, in the gloomy years of the depression following "a war," haunted by the fear of being abandoned in the woods (or the jungle of the unknown) by her parents, just like in the fairy tales, that, for most of her girlhood, constitute the sole source of her knowledge about life. The fairytale turns out to be prophetic, and, for once, there will not be any possibility of being saved by Prince Charming. Her dread of tomorrow proves to be justified, as she finds herself surrounded by "witches" and "wolves," threatening her very existence. This makes the need for companionship, or camaraderie, more vital to her survival, for she needs understanding, help, and solace. But the world of Erica—our world, alas—is all too frequently selfish, insensitive, manipulative. And when people give the appearance of wanting to help her, it is exploitation they have in mind, and to this Erica will not subject herself. When she turns to prostitution as a means to survive in a cruel world and support her younger brother and sister, what we have is an implicit indictment of the injustice of the social order that breeds such a monstrous situation.

While in Moravia's fiction money is presented as an instrument of power and control, in Vittorini's *Erica* money is what buys the staples that allow us to live as well as to gain the acceptance of the bourgeois world of traders. Unfortunately, Erica herself will in a way become the victim of the same mentality, finding in "things" the companionship, security, and stability she was unable to find among living human beings, including, shockingly enough, those who belong to the working class. It is only natural that Vittorini, perfectly conscious of this condition, should channel his artistic search in a direction that would yield some of the answers to the riddle of human misery and alienation.

In retrospect, and taking into account the position of the book in the context of Vittorini's production, we realize that *Erica* contains the first fruits of a seed planted in his earlier *The Red Carnation*, a seed that eventually blossomed into the author's total identification with the aspirations of the masses. The identification was to transpire through his lyrical concern for the "doomed human race"—a race divided into "uomini e no." At the time when Vittorini was writing *Erica*, however, he was still working within the limitations of those modes of expression and structure imposed by his native literary tradition, not particularly known for its daring. It is only in scattered sections of the novel that we may find the first hints of a style soon to develop into a coherent, personal, poetic means of communication: seldom in *Erica* does an attentive reader sense that it is endowed with a magical quality of myth and fable. By the end of 1936—the great year of the

Spanish civil war and of an intensive period of translation—Vittorini was no longer interested in the facts of the day and in a realistic diction and vision. He had reached a spiritual and artistic crisis, out of which he was to produce his truly significant novels.

Conversazione in Sicilia is without doubt Vittorini's most significant book—even though he seemed to prefer the later *Il Sempione strizza l'occhio al Fréjus* (*The Twilight of the Elephant*) —his most original contribution to the novel as an art form. Better than any of the works written before or after by the novelist, it recaptures in its own cryptic form not only the spirit of the fascist tyranny in Italy, but the anguish, expectations, frustrations of modern man, fighting desperately to overcome despair. *Conversazione* is indeed a unique book: born out of hopelessness, it led its author back to hope. The writing of "his" book was taking place at a time when Vittorini had critically confronted American literature as a translator whose task was not a mere mechanical labor of changing into his native language images, thoughts and feelings of other writers, but a searching for a style that would "repeat" in Italian the stylistic quality of the original text. The exposure to a writer like Saroyan, for example, proved extremely useful to his own linguistic search, particularly in terms of the effects possible by the insistent repetition of words, or even entire sentences, at times only slightly changed by the addition of just a single word, a technique which Bruce Merry claims assumes "a liturgical, certainly a musical, function in the novel." But it was a fortunate coincidence that Vittorini's encounter with Saroyan, among others, should take place just as his own dissatisfaction with "the way" he had been writing his books with "'the way' it was then thought novels should be written" had reached a critical stage.

The intellectual experience that served as a catalyst to Vittorini's rethinking the whole question of the novel was his new, sudden, and complete love of opera, Verdi's *Traviata* first of all, as he recalls in his lengthy statement that serves as the "Introduction" to his *The Red Carnation*. What struck him, among other things, was the fact that "musical drama has the power denied to the novel, of expressing through its complexity some splendid general emotion undefinable by nature and independent of the action, the characters, and the emotions portrayed by the characters." He continued:

The novel and the opera are alike in that they are both composite things. But, while the opera is in a position to resolve its problems of scenic representation poetically, the novel is not yet in a position to solve poetically all its problems of the novelistic representation of reality. The opera can sustain and convey through music the very mental reactions of its characters. The novel has not, yet, or has no longer, the something to sustain and convey the particular elements of reality that it analyzes and presents. The opera can thus go beyond the realistic level of its events to arrive at the expression of a higher reality. But the novel, at least in the hands of the conventional realistic novelist of today, cannot, without turning into philosophy, transcend its own preoccupation with a reality of a lower order.
. . . The opera began in pure music just as the novel began in pure poetry. The opera has taken on, in its formation, a something else that is not music, just as the novel has taken on something that is not poetry. But the opera has remained music, while the novel has not remained essentially poetry. The opera has assimilated and reabsorbed into music, and reexpressed through music, all its original nonmusical elements. The opera has knitted together and the novel has split apart.

Could poetry and the novel, once a single genre, be joined again into an inseparable whole? Could the novel shed its pretensions of closely imitating reality in order to mirror and reproduce it and, without losing its credibility, be "poetic"? These were the questions facing Vittorini in the mid-thirties, as he began writing *Conversazione in Sicilia*. Only in retrospect was it to become clear how these thoughts were to lead him into new, virgin territory, and place him in a slim nucleus of experimental novelists.

He began writing *Conversazione in Sicilia* toward the end of 1937, publishing it in four installments in the Florentine review *Letteratura* between April 1938 and December of the same year. In 1941, the Florentine publishing house of Parenti brought out a limited edition of 355 copies of the novel, accompanied by a short story that gave the book its title, *Nome e lacrime* [Name and tears]. Later that year, and in 1942, Bompiani of Milan (where Vittorini had moved) published the work with its present title. The press, which had given the novel a warm reception in 1941, now attacked it, having become aware of its subtle antiestablishment stance. The censor himself could hardly remain insensitive to the novel's various implications and references, and consequently ordered it withdrawn from circulation.

For years copies of the work circulated freely among the Partisans, becoming symbolic of the intellectuals' opposition to fascism. Read in many of the Nazi-dominated countries, it reminded men of their elementary obligations to each other, the necessity of working for peace and justice; and it dramatized the great insults perpetuated by man upon mankind.

The book makes few concessions to the sort of formal structure we are accustomed to expect from a novel. Indeed, one cannot say much more than *Conversazione* is a book about a journey undertaken by the narrator-protagonist-author named Silvestro, a thirty-year-old linotype operator who works in Milan, to his native town of Syracuse, in Sicily. When read more carefully, however, we perceive that what may give the mistaken impression of being a rather loosely written, even puzzling narrative that starts off with the depiction of a "state of mind," has the calculated structure of a great symphonic work, orchestrated around a main theme and complemented by other sub-themes or motifs, such as the "dark mice" (chapter 2), the "stink" and the oranges (chapter 6), and so on. Recently, Marylin Schneider has persuasively described the musical structure of the novel in terms of the "density and organic interdependence of a four-part Baroque fugue: from its tiny word patterns to its parade of diverse characters, to its all-encompassing image of the journey, each part thrusts backwards and forwards, weaving a matrix of themes, variations, crescendos and diminuendos, movement and rest that are at once form and content."

Part 1, which serves as a prologue that sets the mood and the reason for the action that is about to unfold, begins with the description of Silvestro's state of mind, "haunted by abstract furies," paralyzed by what Sergio Pautasso called "an existential anguish," and his sudden decision to deliver a birthday card to his mother in Sicily, after having heard from his father that he has left home. During the long train trip, Silvestro meets a number of eccentric characters (notably, Moustache and No Moustache, quite obviously police spies, and the "Great Lombard," who speaks of "higher duties" mankind must accept). Part 2 begins with the protagonist's arrival in Syracuse and his meeting with his mother,

Concezione, in what is a symbolic return to the womb, and extends through their Proustian conversation about the past, and more particularly about Silvestro's father and grandfather, whose qualities and flaws are delightfully confused to the point where it is seldom clear about whom of the two they are speaking. Part 3 follows Silvestro who has decided to accompany his mother in her daily round of injections to the poor and rich alike (she supports herself through this activity), and this experience sharpens the protagonist's consciousness of the "offended world." Part 4, the central and most moving section of the book, describes Silvestro's encounter with a number of characters (Calogero, Porfirio, Ezechiele, and Colombo) all of them from the working class, who discuss with him the ways in which the "offended world" can and must be saved from further suffering by those who are conscious of "other duties" and ready to wash the woes of mankind "with live water." There is much drinking during their discussions and in Part 5, Silvestro, drunk but still in possession of his faculties, stumbles in the cemetery where the ghost of his brother Liborio, who has recently lost his life on the battlefield (a fact not yet known to the family), appears and speaks to him. When Silvestro tells his mother about his experience, she dismisses it by pointing out that he is drunk: one more day will pass before the news of Liborio's death, preannounced by the crows, flying on "unscathed through the ash high up in the sky . . . cawing, laughing," will reach the family. In a very brief epilogue, Silvestro's conversation in Sicily, which lasted three days and three nights, comes to an end. As he takes leave from his mother, he sees her washing the feet of a crying man, who is his father, with whom he does not speak.

These events, sparse and seemingly disconnected, allow the narrator-protagonist Silvestro to give vent to the "abstract furies" obsessing him at the beginning of his journey. The trip he undertakes to his native land proves to be a salutary spiritual and human experience: the people he meets (first on the train, then in his *paese*), the landscape he so deeply loves despite its rockiness and harshness that remind us of Montale's *Ossi di seppia* (1925; *Cuttle-Fish Bones*, N.Y., 1965, as part of *Selected Poems*), the thoughts that come upon him, conjure up a vision of anguish— anguish that is trepidation and sorrow for mankind for centuries abused, vilified, and exploited by a few cruel men. The voyage that began on a note of despair and hopelessness, ends with at least a hint that things will, nay, *must* change, if only man, perpetrator and victim of his mistakes, can learn from past history and chart a new route that will bring *salute* to mankind. Silvestro's journey, in short, becomes a denial of the apathy, lethargy, and indifference from which he suffered, and signals first a new resolution for becoming engaged first by recognizing the ills and injustices of the past, and second by calling for new bonds with the repressed poor—of Sicily and everywhere.

Both linguistically and structurally *Conversazione in Sicilia* marks a dramatic break with the tradition of the novel in Italy as it had been written during the previous one hundred years. The linguistic fabric of the book, for example, is made of words chosen for their simplicity and evocative power: through frequent repetitions, a melodic, almost mesmerizing effect is created, almost as though we were reading poetry rather than prose. We forget time, accept a continuity based on tone, and no longer look for a strict sequence of events, willingly accepting the symbolic dimension of the characters that appear, one by one, almost magically out of nowhere and everywhere. We accept them readily because they seem to be so very much "real," even though we are told very little about them. Even Silvestro is barely sketched out for us: we know that he is thirty years old, a lithographer working in Milan, that he is married (or is the woman his "girl"?) and that he is going home, ostensibly at the request of his father, to bring a greeting to his mother whom he has not seen for several years. And what in the hands of another writer might have well been a regional-realistic story, is turned by Vittorini's artistry into a haunting allegory of a man's, and a nation's, suffering and of the need to rekindle human hope in freedom and justice.

There are several points that demand to be clarified at this point. The first is that *Conversazione* was no mere accident, no product of fortuitous circumstances. On the contrary, it was the result of a spiritual-intellectual and political crisis that had begun several years before. Along with several intellectuals and writers, Vittorini had come to understand the moral bankruptcy of a government that had gained power thanks to revolutionary promises it could not keep without severely damaging the interests of the middle class, which together with the Church, had helped and sanctified Mussolini's ascendancy to ultimate control over the destiny of the nation.

As Vittorini's ideological consciousness increased, so did his awareness that the "one truth" he aspired to express could no longer, for practical and artistic reasons, be told using conventional structures. This eliminated the possibility of a realistic treatment, which would never receive the approval of the censor's office. Thus, the "woes of the outraged world," a theme which recurs throughout the book, together with the allusions to certain key political and historical events of the time (notably, the Abyssinian war and the Spanish civil war), are somewhat clouded by the writer who "had to express himself without actually saying it." Hence the choice of a highly symbolic, and at times hermetic form. Abstraction and realism, however, are subtly fused and balanced. And, while there is at least a semblance of action, *Conversazione* resembles less a traditional novel than a "romance" as described by Richard Chase in his valuable study of *The American Novel*:

> By contrast [with the novel] the romance, following distantly the medieval example, feels free to render reality in less volume and detail. . . . The romance can flourish without providing much intricacy of relation. The characters, probably rather two-dimensional types, will not be complexly related to each other or to society or to the past. Human beings will on the whole be shown in ideal relation—that is, they will share emotions only after they have become abstract or symbolic. . . . Character itself becomes, then, somewhat abstract and ideal. . . . The plot we may expect to be highly colored. Astonishing events may occur, and these are likely to have a symbolic or ideological, rather than a realistic, plausibility. Being less committed to the immediate rendition of reality than the novel, the romance will more freely veer toward the mythic, allegorical, and symbolistic forms.

The story of Silvestro's coming to grips with the world takes the shape of a voyage, or, better still, a Dantesque pilgrimage to Syracuse. Like Dante's *Comedy*, the book begins when its narrator-hero has reached the bottom of his despair; like Dante's pilgrim, Silvestro's understanding of what is wrong with the world will be revealed, or illuminated by his "guides" and the people with whom he comes in contact during his three-day visit. At the end of his haunting experience, having successfully connected with other human beings, he derives the strength, understanding, and hope that enable him to go back home to Milan, to his family, his friends, and his job, and face life anew. More importantly, this is accomplished in a way that infers that the salvation of the individual can and will lead the way to the redemption of a whole society that has at last recognized, and is willing to combat, the inequities of a repressive political and economic system.

The opening chapter sets the stage and mood for the novel in its portrayal of what R. W. B. Lewis felicitously calls "the loss of reality as a result of disturbances on a lower or historical level," another way of saying alienation. It is an exceptionally effective piece of narrative that deserves to be quoted in full:

> That winter I was haunted by abstract furies. I won't try to describe them, because they're not what I intend to write about. But I must mention that they were abstract furies—not heroic or even live; some sort of furies concerning the doomed human race. They had obsessed me for a long time, and I was despondent. I saw the screaming newspaper placards, and I hung my head. I would see my friends pass an hour or two with them in silence and dejection. My wife or my girl would be expecting me, but, downcast, I would meet them without exchanging a word. Meanwhile, it rained and rained as the days and months went by. My shoes were tattered and soggy with rain. There was nothing but the rain, the slaughters on the newspaper placards, water in my dilapidated shoes and my taciturn friends. My life was like a blank dream, a quiet hopelessness.
>
> That was the terrible part: the quietude of my helplessness; to believe mankind to be doomed, and yet to feel no fever to save it, but instead to nourish a desire to succumb with it.
>
> I was shaken by abstract furies, but not in my blood; I was calm, unmoved by desires, I did not care whether my girl was expecting me, whether or not I met her, glanced over the leaves of a dictionary, went out and saw my friend, or stayed at home. I was calm, as if I had not lived a day, not known what it meant to be happy; as if I had nothing to say, to affirm or deny, noth-

ing to hazard, nothing to listen to, devoid of all urge; and as if in all the years of my life I had never eaten bread, drunk wine or coffee, never been to bed with a woman, never had children, never come to blows with anyone: as if I had not thought of all such things possible; as if I had never been a man, never alive, never a baby spending my infancy in Sicily, among the prickly pears, the sulphur mines and the mountains.

But the abstract furies stirred violently within me, and I bowed my head, pondering mankind's doom; and all the while it rained and I did not exchange a word with my friend, and the rain seeped through my shoes.

Silvestro's story, of course, does not remain on the abstract level: it becomes realistic and, toward the end, even surrealistic. It has both movement (the long train ride to Sicily, the nursing rounds the protagonist makes with his mother) and stillness (as in the brief scene at the cemetery in the last pages of the book). There is the visual confrontation with poverty and despair (beginning with the sight of the men traveling to Sicily, one of whom offers Silvestro an orange for sale and, when he politely refuses it, eats the orange himself, "as though he were swallowing curses"), and the articulation, first by the "Great Lombard" and then by Ezekiel, of the devastating effect social and economic injustice has had on mankind. The Great Lombard speaks with these words:

"I believe that man is ripe for something else. . . . Not only for not stealing, not killing, and so on, and for being a good citizen. . . . I believe he's ripe for something else, for new and different duties, it is this that we feel, I believe, the want of other duties, other things to accomplish. Things to accomplish for the sake of our conscience in a new sense.

Ah, I think it is precisely this. . . . We feel no satisfaction in performing our duty, our duties. . . . Performing them is matter of indifference, and we feel no better for having performed them. And the reason is this: those duties are too old, too old and they have become too easy. They don't count any longer for the conscience."

His faith in humanity, his confidence in man who will ultimately begin to redeem himself of the shame of his past misdeeds, is balanced, at the end of the book, by the activism of the knife-grinder Calogero, who is looking everywhere for anything to grind: blades, knives, swords: "Haven't you a cannon to grind?" he asks Silvestro, "Knives? Scissors? D'you think that knives and scissors still exist in the world? . . . Sometimes I think that it will be enough for everyone to have their teeth and nails ground. I'd grind them into viper fangs and leopard claws."

If the Great Lombard is the moral conscience of the book, Calogero is the militant proponent of armed struggle. Ezekiel, the prophetlike personage who works in a shop located at a very high point in the village, speaks to Silvestro (who by now has become more involved in the story itself) first through Calogero who had led him there: "Tell him," he says, "that I spend my day like an ancient hermit with these papers, writing the history of the insulted world. Tell him that I suffer but I go on writing; that I wrote about all the outrages one by one, and about the outraged faces that laugh at the outrages they have inflicted and are going to inflict." With all its simplicity and directness, it is a beautiful statement, which is foreshadowed by a passage describing Silvestro's perception of just what makes one man more man than others:

> But perhaps every man is not a man; and the entire human race is not human. . . . One man laughs and another cries; both are human, the one who laughs has also been ill, is ill; yet he laughs *because* the other cries. He is a man who persecutes and massacres. . . . Not every man, then, is a man. One persecutes and another is persecuted. Kill a man, and he will be something more than a man. Similarly, a man who is sick or starving is more than a man; and more human is the human race of the starving.

If there is a problem with *Conversazione in Sicilia* it is that, whether because of the particular political situation in which the book was written, or Vittorini's ambition to endow his story with universal application, its characters at times tend to be a little too abstract and obscure, particularly in their pronouncements, rather than translate dramatically into action their noble ideals of justice, fairness, and compassion. Silvestro's mother, Concezione, is an exception: she naturally lives her goodness, and her understanding of the raw elements of life in her town—poverty and exploitation—is effectively understated. The fact that she earns her livelihood by going from house to house giving injections to the ill is never allowed to disturb her kinship with those who need her help. She is a wonderful mixture of pride and humility, of seriousness and humor. Her love of life and her candid view of sex are the sources of her strength that enables her to lead her son back to life. Her example is a fundamental factor in the changes Silvestro undergoes in the few precious days in his native town. In a sense, Concezione represents commitment, involvement, and as such she becomes the precursor if not the direct prototype of many of Vittorini's "engaged" characters.

Earlier in this chapter it has been noted how difficult it is to separate Vittorini's private life from his art. For him, art and all creative activities are the conscious offspring of his human commitments, at once indivisible and mutually sustaining. "The time which interests me," he asserted in the course of an interview, "is the one in which I am living." His growing opposition to fascism and to all forms of repression and tyranny, coupled with his utter contempt toward bourgeois values, made inevitable his decision to participate actively in the struggle of his nation against Nazism. In 1943, he joined the Italian Resistance, and out of his experience he wrote *Uomini e no* [Men and non-men], a title quite likely inspired by John Steinbeck's *Of Mice and Men*.

The novel, written between 1944 and 1945, which is to say whenever Vittorini's political activities permitted, was published shortly after the Liberation. Its links with *Conversazione in Sicilia*, both thematically and stylistically, are at once evident. Once again, the focus is on the sufferings of the exploited and persecuted—with a difference: the characters of *Uomini e no* have changed into activists. The philosophical musings of *Conversazione* have been replaced by the bullets and hand grenades of the Partisans who know that only through action can they bring change to an intolerable situation.

The one hundred and thirty-six short chapters that make up the book recount the events of a few days of the tragic months of the winter of 1944—one of the mildest winters in Milan's history. But the mildness of the weather is contrasted with the bloody action that rapidly unfolds.

The story is unusually simple: Enne 2, the hero of the book, together with a small group of Milanese workers, are committed to kill German officers of the occupation troops. Their plot will, as usual, be followed by reprisals. Several Fascists, named to a special tribunal, are given the responsibility of selecting the one hundred or more people (including women and children) who will pay with their lives for the German losses. The members of the Underground again plan a raid against the Fascists, but their mission fails, with serious loss of lives, including that of the hero of the tale, N-2.

The narrative, far from flowing in a traditional fashion, is interrupted several times by narrative passages printed in italics. There, the narrator of the story (who occasionally identifies himself with the "*Io*" ("I") of the book, evokes his childhood years in Sicily in a language that has much of the lyricism and magic of *Conversazione in Sicilia*. The critic Sergio Pautasso notes that such chapters form a block "which is not only a diversifying element, a technical artifice that characterizes moments of pause and reflection. [It also] presupposes another book, a different search of meaning to be given to one's own life, beyond the evil that offends man, but which is [also] part of man himself and [as such] indivisible from human nature."

As in *Conversazione in Sicilia*, the characters are identified primarily by monograms (as in the case of the protagonist, Enne 2, or N-2), by simple names (Selva, Berta), their status or nationality (the soldier, the German), by physical or moral characteristics (Gray Moustache, Cat's Eye, Shaved Head, Black Dog), and so on. With the exception of N-2 and Berta, very little, if indeed anything, is revealed about their past. Only through their conversations do we get to know them.

Stylistically, Vittorini relies more than ever on dialogue (narrative or descriptive passages are very rare), and experiments with the poetic effects possible through the repetition of the same phrase, only slightly changed, in a manner that recalls Gertrude Stein's famous "a rose is a rose is a rose." There is evidence that at least some of the story itself, particularly its ending, was fashioned after Ernest Hemingway's classic *For Whom the Bell Tolls*. Examples of Vittorini's technique may be found in practically every page: "'He does not have much to do with many companions.' 'Has he much to do with other companions?' 'He has nothing to do with other companions.'"

Unfortunately, it is hard to quarrel here with the objections of some of Vittorini's most severe critics, Mario Praz among them, that technique is not, in *Uomini e no*, subservient to poetry. Thus, what could have served the author well, if used with moderation, to increase the ever-mounting tension of the story, becomes something that detracts from the drama of the action, and distracts us to the point of annoyance. Indeed, after the first few chapters, the choral effect wears off and becomes another negative element which, together with the facelessness of the novel's nameless characters contributes to the general weakness of the book.

Vittorini himself was apparently not completely happy with the book (a dissatisfaction, let it be duly noted, he experienced frequently with most of the books he wrote), and retouched it several times as it went through four editions. Thus, the definitive edition (1965) of *Uomini e no*, changes the status of the *"Io"* ("I") which, in the original (1945) version was associated with the writer of the book, and his relationship with Berta. In the later version, the *"Io"* ("I") is no longer superimposed on the figure of the author—a situation that makes for a certain ambiguity when the love between N-2 and Berta is described. After all, the reader suspects from the beginning that N-2 and the author are nothing if not one and the same person. Such a technical flaw may ultimately be traceable to the vagueness or ambiguity of Vittorini's ideological position. Throughout the unfolding of the plot, it is difficult for the reader not to admire the general premises of the struggle in which N-2, Selva, and all the other Partisans are engaged ("We work," asserts Selva early in the novel, "in order that men may be happy"). But beyond this humane, reasonable statement there is little that sharply defines the ideological reasons for the struggle against fascism and nazism. We are legitimately shocked by the spectacle of seeing men being lacerated by vicious dogs set against them by the Nazis, or the ruthlessness with which women and children are regularly shot to death and left in the streets as grim reminders of the Fascists' determination to retaliate most forcefully against the guerillas. But, with Carlo Salinari, one finds it difficult, at least initially, to accept fascism "as a moral category evil," rather than as a "product of society and of one of its particular ways of organizing itself."

Some of the structural problems of the novel, as an attentive reader no doubt perceives, are intricately connected with Vittorini's undeclared ambition to shift the emphasis, firmly embedded in the tradition, from the individual to the collective, from the "*Io*" ("I") to the "*noi*" ("us"), an effort that was to culminate in his last completed novel *Le donne di Messina*. The protagonist himself, N-2, is delineated in rather general terms, and the reader is led to assume, from his general behavior and from the kind of confidence he inspires among his fellow fighters, that he is a just, brave, courageous, and deceptively simple man. In this sense, at least, he is a character closest to Vittorini himself, for whom the struggle for peace, liberty, and dignity has to be fought both individually and collectively by all "simple" men everwhere.

Thus, the discourse begun in *Conversazione in Sicilia* concerning the "insults" endured by "the doomed human race," and the depiction of the "sorrows of the outraged human race," is extended in *Uomini e no*, this time without being couched in ambiguous, symbolic, and "coded" language. It is true, of course, that the clipped, matter-of-fact style of *Uomini e no* is more consonant not merely with the demands of the story, but the changing political and historical reality: fascism and nazism and their sordid designs for a new order are being constantly resisted with bombs and sabotage, and, at long last, there is new hope for a radical reshaping of the social order. Much of Vittorini's creative as well as critical work in the last twenty years of his life reflects his vision of what society can accomplish collectively in order to realize its objectives of justice, peace, and well-being.

Il Sempione strizza l'occhio al Fréjus (literally "The Simplon winks at the Fréjus," *The Twilight of the Elephant*, N.Y., 1973), written in 1946 and published a year later, is a book written, to put it in Vittorini's own words, "*con piacere*" ("with pleasure"). Much like *Conversazione*, this book, too, seeks to recapture universal problems and feelings rather than recount a story. There is, of course, a story to be told, but it is made up of small events that do not by themselves hold our attention. *Il Sempione* is about a family, and what an unusual family it turns out to be indeed! "In our family, we are a houseful of people, and the only one who works and earns anything is my brother, Euclid. For a long time I have been out of a job. My mother's new husband was already out of work when she married him and brought him home last autumn. My sister, [Elvira,] a store clerk, was fired this summer; so along with my grandfather, we all depend on the little my brother earns at repairing bicycles for his boss who is a mechanic."

The central figure of the novella turns out to be the grandfather: a mason, in his younger days he used to be unbelievably strong. He had helped build the Simplon, the Fréjus, and, as the mother claims in what is surely a symbolic assertion, all the world's most imposing monuments: the Duomo in Milan, the Colosseum in Rome, the Great Wall of China, the Pyramids. Now he is old, tired, silent. Beloved and respected by the whole family, he is the cause of great hardship in very difficult times. A voracious eater, he consumes more than three pounds of bread every day—a mere trifle when compared to the twenty-two pounds he could eat when he worked! The family is forced, therefore, to purchase bread on the black market (bread is still rationed) and is deprived of all other necessities. The only member of the family who works is the son, and what he earns is barely sufficient to purchase the bread which, along with some chicory, picked in the nearby woods, serves to satiate their continuous hunger.

One day a man with a smutty black face (he is thereafter called Muso-di-Fumo, "Smut-Face") walks in. Grateful for the welcome extended by the family, he shares with them their poor supper. But what was ordinarily a meager meal is transformed into a sumptuous dinner when everyone agrees, without even thinking of it, to "make believe" that they are to have chicken, wine, and other delicacies. The money Smut-Face gives the father will purchase some real wine, chestnuts, and even anchovies, and the feast may be repeated all over again, without having to "make believe." The members of the family are provided with the occasion to talk about man's poverty and wretchedness, and they listen to Smut-Face talk of how he wanted to be a sorcerer. Having obtained a fife, he had found a tune. But the tune, he explains, is not yet perfect and in order to perfect it he goes every day into the woods to practice. With the perfect tune he will some day be able to enchant elephants. When he shows them the fife, they notice that a piece of red rag hangs from the end of the instrument. The music apparently is quite effective, for the grandfather, who has been a silent witness to what has been taking place before him, begins to mark time to the music with his fingers. After telling the amazed little audience how elephants die (they go to a secluded place, which man never sees, to lie down and die), the man departs. The next morning, the grandfather, who is called "the elephant," disappears into the forest, presumably to die, although the mother states that the workers will no doubt bring him back home.

While the story told by the book is both original and unique, the reader of Vittorini's work should have little trouble recognizing the connections of this novella with his previous books, particularly *Conversazione in Sicilia*. The language is still simple and repetitive, the action quite modest, and the division into thirty short chapters prevails again. The characters are few, usually identified with generic terms, or nicknames. Three stand out: among them, the mother, with her constant interventions, Smut-Face, whose smile that reveals his white gleaming teeth in a dark face, and the grandfather—biblical, majestic, and profoundly human—who seems to embody the *più uomo* ("more man") quality typifying the exploited, persecuted peasants of *Conversazione*, and is endowed with the moral wisdom of the Great Lombard. And again, the book is in essence a "conversation" about people, their condition, and their fate.

What is changed is the general climate. We are no longer in Fascist Italy, subject to the tyranny of a dictator, but in postwar Italy, with different social and political problems. But what has not changed, and indeed becomes evident through whatever action there is in the book, and through the stance and conversations of the characters, is the humanity of the *povera gente* ("poor people"), the persuasion, as Piero de Tommaso has noted, "that, differently from the corrupt ruling classes, the people are naturally disposed to entertain noble feelings and thoughts."

In *The Twilight of the Elephant*, there is more than a hint that a greater awareness of the issues of ideologies and of the various methods of struggle will inevitably help the proletariat to overcome the ruling class. Yet the novella, for all its allegory and suggestiveness, cannot be read as a political tract heralding the coming of communism. There is, of course, some naïveté in the symbol of the fife played by Smut-Face, the red flag hanging from it, and the overt declaration of a future revolution. What I find more significant is the human attitude of the author who is actually pleading for a new condition that will bring dignity to mankind. Such a condition can only mean the death of those ideologies and social divisions that are out of step with modern times.

Thus, Vittorini has great feeling for the grandfather, the old man who incarnates the accomplishments of unorganized, exploited labor. The fact that he is now old, worn out, and silent (he never speaks in the story) means little, for he can, when the real opportunity presents itself, respond to the call of history. When Smut-Face plays the fife the grandfather suddenly comes to life again and ceases being a mere spectator. Never are we allowed to forget that he built, after all, "tunnels and buildings, bridges and railroads, aqueducts, dikes, power plants, highways, and, of course, the Duomo, the Colosseum, the Wall of China and the Pyramids!" The trouble with him is that he is heavy, burdensome, and inert. No one is trying to minimize his past accomplishments. But what of the present, or what of the future? they ask. Has he, per chance, outlived his usefulness, becoming in the last years of his life an additional burden to his family?

Both *Uomini e no*, and *Il Sempione* were written in the last months of the war and the immediate postwar years, when Vittorini either through his role in the Resistance and, between 1945 and 1947, through his editorship of the leftist journal *Il Politecnico*, was actively working to change a traditional concept of culture, in its broadest forms, into a classless society under communism. Vittorini's perceptions of the role of the artist were doomed to clash with those of the party's more orthodox leaders, particularly Palmiro Togliatti, with whom Vittorini began a "dialogue" in the form of letters published in *Il Politecnico* and in the Communist review *La Rinascita*. Vittorini's liberal views, particularly with regard to the necessity for the artist to enjoy a maximum degree of autonomy, while creating something that "enriches" politics by its constant search of truth, were rejected by the Communist leadership. By 1947, the dialogue had reached an insurmountable impasse due to the irreconcilable views of the two sides, and Vittorini turned his attention to writing and other intellectual pursuits. While he remained fairly active in politics (in 1960, he was elected Council member of the city of Milan, a post from which he resigned shortly thereafter), his enthusiasm for communism diminished visibly in the last years of his life.

The political experience of 1943–45, coupled with his ambition to write an epic of Italy freed from the shackles of the past, ready to begin a radical social transformation, led Vittorini to write what was to be his most ambitious work, *Le donne di Mes-*

sina (*The Women of Messina*, N.Y., 1973), a complex and not altogether successful book that cost him "cold sweats of study." Begun in 1946, it appeared in book form in 1949 in a version that left the author sufficiently dissatisfied to hold permission to translate it into English, a translation that was eventually made from the second, definitive edition of 1964, itself some seventeen years in the making.

The sprawling tale, the longest Vittorini wrote, is quite definitely linked with his previous novels, and attempts to bring its author's search of "truth" one step further. *Conversazione in Sicilia* represents the discovery of the insults to which the human race has been subjected, and the beginning of a journey that will eventually put its despondent hero Silvestro back in touch with reality. *Uomini e no* shows the spirit of sacrifice necessary for the ultimate freedom of the people, while *The Twilight of the Elephant* dramatizes the dire need to move from certain economic-political structures, that tolerate the exploitation of the working class, to the acceptance of an ideology that will open the door to a more just and equitable enjoyment by all people of the labor of the people. *The Women of Messina* proposes to show how, after a period of conflict and destruction, mankind has within its grasp the possibility of beginning anew. The assumption, movingly articulated by the Great Lombard in *Conversazione*, was that man was ripe for something else, for "things to be done for our conscience." *The Twilight of the Elephant* looked forward to the time "when men would really be like elephants, serene like elephants. . . . But they must be free and not belong to somebody else, not from a menagerie. . . . Such a time can never have been. But perhaps it may come. And when it comes, I don't want to be alone." *The Women of Messina*, with all its flaws, represents the ultimate extension of a view of the world first sketched out in *Conversazione*: starting out from ground zero, it is a carefully and poetically worked out book that shows what the structure of society may be when certain basic premises of goodwill, tolerance, love, and dignity are accepted. This was, to be sure, Vittorini's intention back in the middle forties when he began writing his movel. The problem is that, during the period from 1952 to 1964 during which Vittorini dedicated himself to revising it, he had changed, and those changes in his political outlook had considerable impact upon the novel and its quality as a work of art.

Writing about Faulkner, in his book *The Picaresque Saint*, R. B. W. Lewis comments on John Steinbeck's *The Grapes of Wrath*, and calls it a "picaresque novel in the modern manner, an episodic long tale of encounters along the way of a harried and difficult journey—the journey of dispossessed Oklahomans toward and into the deceptively promising land of California." It is a definition that applies remarkably well to the spirit and tone of *The Women of Messina*, which tells of the search by a group of "dispossessed" Italians at the end of the last war for land on which to settle while engaged in the painful task of finding their families, separated by the misfortunes of war. The country has been defeated, much of its network of roads and railroads have been seriously damaged—that is tragic enough. Confusion and anarchy reign supreme. Yet, in the midst of so much chaos, there is one heartening note—the desire and willingness to make a new start, to piece together what the war has not destroyed, and build something more genuinely meaningful because it responds to, and emerges from, the basic human desire for peace and goodwill.

That the novel should open with the description of the breakdown of a truck on which the group of people are traveling on their way up north is no accident, but a metaphor that proves to be the controlling factor of the whole work. The truck represents, after all (at least in the context of the story), an advanced means of transportation symbolic of a fairly advanced technological stage of development: but now it has broken down, incapable of performing the task for which it was built. It must not only be repaired but completely overhauled, many of its parts taken from other vehicles so as to function again. Vittorini's perceptions as a social being and as a novelist have reached a similar impasse. Just as traditional concepts of how society is to be structured so as to live in peace and well-being, so must the novel depart radically from traditional forms if it is to depict a new society while at the same time responding to an intellectual need of the observer and the reader.

The structure of the novel, and not just its theme, reflects as closely as possible Vittorini's ideological stance. A vision of a collective society, such as he envisaged as the goal to be achieved, must be written in a "collective" manner. In this respect, Vittorini's attempt is quite similar to Verga's equally ambitious technical attempt (beginning with *I Malavoglia*) to compose a truly objective, impersonal novel that would give the illusion of "hav-[ing] grown spontaneously, like a fact of nature, without maintaining any point of contact with its author." A "collective novel" must avoid the trappings of what, for want of a better term, we may call the "bourgeois novel," with the individualism of its form and paternalism in its attitude. This means a kind of "authorless" book where the collective effort is to be channeled toward the depiction of the making of a "classless" society. Thus, the task and responsibility to tell the story is shifted from the traditional narrator (whether the same as the protagonist or an anonymous third person) to a number of other devices.

In *The Women of Messina*, Vittorini uses a variety of techniques to present the story: the first, and perhaps most innovative and original, is a so-called *Registro*, a log sheet in which the events of the community are recorded. The second, is the voice of what one could call a "commentator" on the events who occasionally offers his observations on the material in the *Registro*. Toward the middle of the book (from chapter 44 to 48) a small number of characters intervene directly to recount a slice of their experience; the last, is bits and pieces contained in the epilogue, recording the changes that have taken place since the end of the war.

Vittorini's technique is a curious mixture of different elements, and may even recall Manzoni's handling of his masterpiece *I promessi sposi* (1842; *The Betrothed*, N.Y., 1956). In that novel, Manzoni is at once the transcriber, editor, commentator, researcher, and moralist of a story he claims he has found in a manuscript of the seventeenth century. But this technique is modified by Vittorini's desire not to intrude in the telling of the story, and the comments take the form of the observations made by the characters themselves, in a way that recalls the strategy used by Vittorini in his diary, where the notes, essays, and other material published between 1929 and 1956 are frequently followed by the author's reflections prepared especially for the occasion of the appearance of the material in book form. The result is a multilevel perspective with a choral quality that is in perfect tune with the "communal" society Vittorini visualized as his Utopia.

There are three major parts in the book: the story of Uncle Agrippa, a retired railroad worker with the state railroads, who travels up and down Italy looking for his daughter Siracusa, missing from the day she left home; the love story of Siracusa and Ventura; and the story of the development of a community bound together by its needs and aspirations. It is important to note here that there are substantial differences—stylistic, thematic, and ideological—between the first and second versions of the book, and that their significance must not be underestimated. While in the original version the travels of Uncle Agrippa give the novel its particular rhythm and control its movement, in the second version the emphasis is shifted to the villagers themselves, intent on building that utopian society in miniature where differences between its members, whether due to training, profession, private wealth, or lineage no longer exist. How deeply Vittorini felt about such a society is seen in his efforts to present the various stages through which it moves, each symbolized by the wheelbarrow, the mule-drawn cart, and finally the motorized vehicle—the broken-down truck patiently restored to working order, thus making the tasks to be performed at once easier and more efficient. But this "progress" has, as anything else, its own price tag: the mechanization of work, while increasing productivity, leads to an eventual alienation of the individual from society stemming from his lack of identification with the things he makes.

Not surprisingly, Vittorini's ideological premises greatly minimize the traditional necessity of the "hero" of the tale. Nevertheless, aside from Uncle Agrippa himself, two other characters manage to emerge as central points of reference: Carlo the Bald, who appears in the opening section of the book, traveling on Uncle Agrippa's train, and Ventura or "Ugly Mut." Both had been Fascists. Now that the war is over, and fascism has been toppled from power, Carlo the Bald has shifted his allegiance to the new government, and has become a sort of informer-special agent, keeping the government briefed on the activities of the settlers. His basic mission is unchanged: he merely works for one type of government instead of another. Ventura, on the other hand, has truly repented for his past misdeeds and atrocities committed during fascism, and has become totally involved in the work of planning the structure of the new village, earning the trust and respect of his comrades through his actions. Carlo the Bald, perhaps out of his sense of guilt or out of his envy of Ventura, is unable to accept the new situation and is instrumental in the formation of an action group called the "hunters," charged with the task of tracking down anyone alleged to have committed crimes against the people under fascism, and sets them on Ventura's trail. In the original version, Ventura manages to hide for a while and contemplates the possibility of avoiding the ordeal by escaping. Terrified by the prospect of being captured sooner or later, incapable of bearing his girl's (Siracusa's) condemnation, he kills her in a stable. One half of the third part of the book consists in the reconstruction of the murder and the events that follow it—the actions of the members of the community—and how Ventura is finally shot by the "hunters." The tale ends when the author realizes that the actions he has just described have taken place in the village almost simultaneously with his writing: "we have arrived in an identical present: the village and myself. . . . And to want to continue writing would mean to continue our story in the guise of a diary."

And so the tale is finished without a "conclusive word" either about the uncle or the village. What of the town, or its people, or of their struggle against the lawful owners of the land, which they have cleared of mines, cultivating it and giving new life to it? What of the freedom of the individual citizen of the community? And what of the possibility of a society capable of leading an orderly life without the supervision and control of a merciless, bureaucratic government or an exploitative capitalistic structure? These questions are left unanswered: Vittorini is too aware that the poet may touch upon and delve into human problems and human possibilities, but man alone must try to resolve the conflicts inherent in life; he alone has the supreme potential ability to bring about any improvement in his social or spiritual life.

In the second version of the novel, however, Vittorini's extensive rewriting has radically changed the denouement of the tale and has, in a very distinct way, brought it up to date, so to speak. Since the original writing of the novel, events have changed drastically the nature of Italian, and, for that matter, European society. Thus, Ventura is no longer killed by the "hunters," simply because in what by now the reader must see as an allegory of contemporary Italian (and, in a larger sense, European) history, the old enemies of yesterday have become part of the fabric of today's society. The "hunters" themselves, formerly the valiant fighters of the Resistance during World War II, no longer have dreams different from those of "us." Life in the village has been transformed in a way that makes it pretty much indistinguishable from life in any other part of the country: commercial, crass, bitten by the bug of the profit motive of capitalistic society. Gone is the spirit of self-reliance (which reminds us of the successful Chinese policy), and gone, too, is the spirit of adventure and self-sacrifice; gone are the "hunters," who have moved on to more civilized places where they can enjoy the fruits of the "economic miracle," and with them are Red Kerchief and Toma, two of the most enthusiastic settlers of the village:

> Time passes, time has gone by—autumn, winter, March, June, August, and autumn is here again—1947, 1948, the Cold War, the Marshall Plan, a Christian Democrat government, the Berlin Airlift . . . Rita Hayworth has come and gone, and so has *The Third Man* with Orson Welles; faster planes than the Dakota fill the skies, Vespas and Lambrettas obstruct the roads; three crops of wheat have been reaped, workers in heavy industries have a new national wage scale, an attempt on the life of Togliatti has been followed by a general strike and the general strike by police repression; a new body of police, the *"Celere,"* is rough-riding over the sidewalks in jeeps, capital has flowed back from abroad, millionaires have re-opened their villas on the lakes, supermillionaires come off their Panama-registered yachts to dine in the night clubs of what used to be fishing villages, young people are dancing the samba instead of the boogiewoogie, and the beaches are crowded with girls in bikinis.

A few things are still the same as we see in the epilogue: Uncle Agrippa "is still riding the trains, just as he did in 1946." Carlo is still performing the same job of overseeing the affairs of the village, but the pattern of life there has changed so much that there is little to report to the authorities: even Ventura can no longer be considered dangerous. Although he spends a few hours a day in the fields, and has "turned out to be just the contrary of a hard nut to crack—soft, lazy, a sort of Bohemian, without any wish to get away." Today he is known just as "Teresa's husband"—Teresa being Siracusa's new name.

> When I go there and ask for him, they seem hardly to know who he is. . . . Nobody sees him every day. . . . He's gone to seed, but he doesn't know how to be a genuine peasant or how to be a nonentity. Because that's what he is, a nonentity wasting his life in a mountain village, with a wife that supports him. . . . He never thinks of improving the land. Of terracing the hillsides, and growing vines and irrigating them in the dry season, of trying out a new crop and new ways of making it flourish. Once upon a time, nobody was his equal in all these things. When he was an engineer during the war, and in the early days of the village. As long as the land was worked in common, until August of 1946, he was the guiding spirit, commanding the rest of them like an orchestra director. While now that he has only the one field that belongs to him and his wife, a vision purely his own of today and tomorrow, he floats like a half-collapsed balloon on a sea of indifference. Just the contrary of what usually happens.
>
> Of what, then is the contrary? I'm angry enough to say what I think—that he *is* the contrary. But the contrary of what? Tell me, if you can.

The concluding pages of the novel are full of irony, of an almost bitter yet inevitable acceptance of the way things have turned out: the hopes and high ideals of brotherhood, peace, and justice of the Resistance have evaporated; the strivings toward equality and a government based on the genuine consensus of the working people—the proletariat and the peasantry—have been dashed. To be sure, much has changed everywhere in the country: the rubble has been cleared away, the network of communication has been restored and improved; railroad stations, schools, churches, and public, as well as private, buildings have been rebuilt. Commerce is thriving. There is peace and many obvious signs of prosperity: the bars are crowded, the consumption of coffee and Coca-Cola (the new yardstick to measure economic well-being) has drastically shot upward. The poverty of the postwar years is now but a memory; the affluence of the "economic miracle" of the new times surrounds everyone. Things are good, to be sure. But what of the soul of mankind, what of the yearnings of yesteryear? The epilogue of the book, with its biting irony, is nothing less than Vittorini's commentary on the end of a dream. A balance sheet is unnecessary: the ways in which life has changed yield the answers to our queries.

> The land, as land, has lost its importance. The neon lights and the Motta ice cream don't conceal the reality of the situation. It's funny, isn't it, that there shouldn't be a single example of what you might call the usual and expected thing. Not even the women of Messina, who grow fat and plant grapevines. Not even Teresa, who pulls Ventura along like a wagon. She's not the Siracusa that she used to be; she's a housewife, trying to get a good price for her milk and putting up preserves for the winter.

La Garibaldina (the last full-length work completed and published by the author in book form) reads much like an extension of, or a concluding note to, *Conversazione in Sicilia* and *The Women of Messina*. Written between December 1949 and May 1950, *La Garibaldina* was originally brought out in installments in the Florentine review *Il ponte*. It is appropriate and revealing that the novella should have appeared (with two central chapters added) in the same volume with *Erica*, written fourteen years earlier, as we are thus offered a valid yardstick to measure the long road Vittorini has traveled in his poetic quest. It becomes even clearer, too, that the novelist's sense of, and feeling for, reality has increased at the same pace as his interest in depicting contemporary reality in a realistic manner has decreased.

Structurally and stylistically, *La Garibaldina*'s affinities with, and differences from, Vittorini's earlier work are evident to a careful reader. To begin, there is hardly a plot in the book, and what there is of it, is sketchy and unimpressive. The time of the action is the early part of this century, and much of the story takes place on a train, on which the passengers find themselves on their way not so much to a specific destination, but, as in *Conversa-*

zione, toward the past. The novella lacks the complex structural apparatus of *The Women of Messina* and the intense, extremely personal sensitivity of *Conversazione* (although it preserves, particularly in its baffling ending, its obscure symbolism) and the almost icy objectivity of *Uomini e no*. There are only two central figures in the novella: a *"bersagliere"* (a member of the elite corps famous for its daring exploits and its colorful plumed hat) and a woman, vivacious, assertive, articulate. The soldier is a simple young man, by the name of Innocenzo, on his way home to the town of Terranova, on a brief leave. The woman is an eccentric Signora, the Baronessa Leonilde (whose destination is also Terranova). Her past exploits (if we are to believe everything she says, would make her about one hundred years old!) include her having been a sort of camp follower during the Risorgimento, and having inspired Garibaldi himself. Whether or not her claims are true, there is no denying that her presence and her authority are extraordinary. Witness the way she dismisses the protestations of the train conductor who attempts to collect from the soldier the difference between the third-class ticket he holds and the first-class coach seat he occupies. But the Baronessa, accompanied by a large dog, Don Carlos, does more than chastise the train conductor: she hurls epithets and biting criticism at the government, institutions, past historical figures, while Innocenzo (whom she has named her orderly, and whose name she will change to Fortunato at the end of the story) serves as a semisilent, increasingly amused listener.

Ultimately, *La Garibaldina* is an effective tale less for what it says than for what it succeeds in evoking. Its style is typical of the linguistic agility we have come to expect of Vittorini, and the feeling for situations and sentiments is, as always, profound and amazing. And one can always rely on the amusing combination of encounters and confrontations as an instrument of aesthetic pleasure. There are many wonderful scenes in the book: the first meeting of the Signora with Innocenzo, their meanderings in the town after the two have gotten off the train, and the strange finale itself. What is most instructive, however, is the author's method used with considerable subtlety to fuse the real with the unreal, the present with the past, the immediate with the timeless, as in the description of the town and the impact it makes on the unsophisticated soldier:

The tolling of a bell whose tone fell suddenly, reverberating against the paving stones, reminded them both of the task they had in common, but it frightened Don Carlos who ran out of one of the alleys. They looked back at the dark town whose bronze throat had given voice. Was it one o'clock or did the sound mark a quarter after an unpredictable hour?

The town too had something that was undefinable. There were wide open doors, dark wells of emptiness, wide open windows, wells of emptiness too: and there were other doors and windows closed as if they had been blacked out for centuries upon centuries in a far distant age, before the flood.

The walls were covered with cracked dust and the northwest wind, blowing full strength, raised a yellowish clay of grit from the façades; even the houses with some sort of attempt at a style appeared shapeless with their outlines grayed, their corners rounded and their cornices nibble away. The town might have witnessed the coming of Abraham, the pilgrimage of the Three Kings, Roland's passage on his way to Roncesvalles, and Garibaldi's passing. . . . The soldier and the old woman were somehow reconciled. They stopped and decided to rest.

Things are made to speak for themselves and questions are made to contain the answer to what is being asked. And that answer, in the last analysis, is the truth of the Great Lombard of *Conversazione in Sicilia*: "I believe that man is ripe for something else. . . . Not for stealing, not killing, and so on, and for being a good citizen. . . . I believe he's ripe for something else, for new and different duties." Hence the insults in *La Garibaldina* heaped upon the train conductors who insist that the poor soldier traveling in the wrong class section pay the difference in fare; hence the heroine's magnificent rebellion and condemnation of old and useless rules, and of human folly.

People speak in this extraordinarily imaginative book frequently censuring the Baronessa's past experiences, which she so candidly discusses—including her love affair with Garibaldi himself. Houses speak also, as do ghosts. And after we are through reading the tale, and manage to find stillness again (after so much, and such astonishing *coralità*), we realize that it was not a "novel" we had been reading all along: it was a cry against despair, or a hymn to man's dignity and hope, and to the vitality, courage, and humor of a race not yet totally doomed and certainly not yet ready to surrender.

Earlier in these pages, I suggested that the various roles Vittorini played—as translator, editor, critic, *homme engagé*—make problematic an assessment based strictly on his creative writing, without taking into account the totality of his activities. Once the "wholeness" of Vittorini's work has been broken, the critical consensus has almost unanimously hailed the "man of culture" while minimizing his worth as a novelist.

A careful reading of the author's fiction is bound to reveal his strength and uniqueness: his unusual mastery of the language, coupled with an extraordinary feeling for its possibilities, can hardly be overstressed. It would be difficult to think of another contemporary Italian novelist, with the exception of, say, Cesare Pavese or Carlo E. Gadda, who can match the originality and hypnotic character of his style. Indeed, in a sense Vittorini might well be remembered for having done to prose what Ungaretti did for poetry restoring purity, meaning, and dignity to a language debased by artificiality, pompousness, and vulgarity. Better than most of his contemporaries, Vittorini has shown an uncanny ability to handle words, remaining always supremely conscious of the fact that ultimately the value of words rests on their capacity to uncover and illuminate "new" or hitherto unexplored facets of the human condition. "A word," he remarked once, "may give to a fact not-new, a new meaning." Commenting on Eugenio Montale's collection of poetry *Le occasioni* (*Occasions*), he noted: "A fact counts only when in some way, it is new for man's consciousness. Only in this circumstance is a fact truly a new fact: it enriches the [human] consciousness, if it adds a new meaning to the long chain of meanings of which such a consciousness is composed."

Words, then, are chosen carefully for their power to evoke and depict, in fablelike books, the loneliness and courage of human beings, their yearnings, their determination to work together to build a world cleansed at long last of the suffering mercilessly inflicted by men upon their fellow men. In Vittorini's hands, words become precious things, elements that allow us to keep in touch with our inner selves and the world. Words translate onto the page and in history the artist's dream: strange words at times, to be sure, highly charged with allusions and symbolic references. When he is successful, as in *Conversazione in Sicilia*, Vittorini's novels take on an extra dimension, and do indeed sound like the operas he loved so deeply, to the point of duplicating their patterns in his books. The emotions at the center of his world are strong, timeless, and universal. What makes them unusually revealing is the manner in which they are expressed through a style that Vittorini created patiently and methodically after experimenting and reflecting about his own work and that of the foreign authors he read and, at times, translated. His stylistic virtuosity is, by itself, an important element in what constitutes Vittorini's special artistry. What matters, is that his style should be so persuasively capable of projecting the hopes, and not just the despair, of life in the twentieth century.

9

Alberto Moravia: Sex, Money, and Love in the Novel

No informed observer of the Italian cultural scene can seriously deny that Alberto Moravia, recently turned seventy, remains one of the most successful, and, in some ways, attractive novelists of our time. His career has been both unusual and remarkable. He became a best-selling novelist in 1929, when, barely twenty-one, he brought out his first novel *Gli indifferenti* (*The Time of Indifference*, N.Y., 1953) previously turned down by three publishers. Ironically enough, Moravia was requested to pay for the publication of his work to the tune of 5,000 lire, no mean amount in those Depression days. Some fifty years later, Moravia finds himself in the position of dean of Italian writers, the object of numerous academic studies, and a favorite target of unfavorable criticism.

A prolific author, he boasts a publishing record second to none for its diversity and quantity: some thirty books, including a dozen novels, over ten collections of short stories, several plays (some derived from his fiction), travelogues, film scripts, and collections of critical and autobiographical essays. In addition, Moravia is an active featured writer and journalist, as well as critic (he is the film critic of the weekly *L'espresso*), coeditor, with Alberto Carocci and Enzo Siciliano, of the magazine *Nuovi argomenti*. His creative fertility has not always been appreciated by his critics, who have accused him of writing too much, of sacrificing quality for quantity, of becoming increasingly more commercial, producing books that often border on pornography, a judgment, they point out, confirmed in the early fifties when his entire work was placed in the Index of Forbidden Books prepared by the Catholic

church. As always, there is a grain of truth in all such conten-
tions, particularly with respect to his persistent concentration on
the themes of sex and money. Moravia takes his interest seriously,
however. Like Pavese and most literary artists, he accepts the
charge of being monotonous. "Good writers," he observed some
years ago, "are monotonous, like good composers. Their truth is
self-repeating. They keep rewriting the same book. That is to say,
they keep trying to perfect their expression of the one problem
they were born to understand." As we shall see, what sets Moravia
apart from other writers is his concerted effort to make of sex,
money, and love instruments of knowledge, tools that measure
the human response to life, precious indicators of man's relation
to reality in his constant search for his identity and significance
in the disconnected and alienated world of the twentieth century.

Alberto Moravia was born in Rome on November 28, 1907.
His father was a Jewish architect from Venice; his mother was
from a middle-class family of Ancona. Early in life, Alberto
showed an inclination toward humanistic studies: with the help of
a governess, he soon mastered French and a reading knowledge
of English and German. Although he was worshipped by his two
older sisters, Adriana and Elena, he must have had a lonely childhood for, as he wrote, it was not unusual for him to spend entire
afternoons recounting stories to himself, interrupting them at
suppertime, continuing them without the slightest difficulty the
next day.

The key event of his young days was an illness that was to
plague him for several years: at the age of nine, young Alberto
was struck by tuberculosis of the bone, a fact that, as he notes,
"certainly affected my sensibility in a decisive way." His illness
meant a withdrawal from the kind of life most normal children
have, and reading became, as it were, a way to compensate for
his physical pain and his loneliness. As he grew, his interest in
literature expanded. His authors were no longer drawn from his
native literature (Boccaccio, Goldoni, Manzoni, Machiavelli,
Leopardi), but from European, and later American as well: Molière, Shakespeare, Stendhal, Balzac, Flaubert, de Maupassant,
Proust, Dostoevsky, and Joyce, among others. His health continued to deteriorate: he was bedridden for months, and, at one
point, his leg was in a cast for six months and his pain became
unbearable. In 1924, a new doctor, summoned by Moravia's

mother, recommended that Alberto be sent to a sanatorium at Codivilla. His studies now hopelessly interrupted, his mother's dream of a diplomatic career for her son were shattered.

Several months later, in the fall of 1925, he was discharged from the hospital and sent to Bressanone, near Bolzano, for further care and rest. The illness had a profound effect upon him: as in the case of other sensitive writers of poor health, such as Leopardi, Rilke, and Proust, his perception of life was unusually sharpened. One of the immediate results was a thorough revulsion toward certain social institutions, such as the family and religion. "The most mistaken teachings," he observed many years later (December 29, 1965), "are those given by the family. The Italian family, however, is in most cases a temple for worship of such divinities as Prudence, Self-Interest, Ignorance, Hedonism. . . . Any school at all, even the worst, is better than the family," a statement that is corroborated by the messy family relationships portrayed in his narratives.

By the time he was eighteen, Moravia had written three novels, none of which was published, but proved to be useful preparatory exercises for an ambitious "work in progress," entitled *Gli indifferenti*, a novel that, almost overnight, became a *succès de scandale* that launched its young author into a meteoric rise in the cultural firmament. Praised by numerous serious critics, the novel hardly endeared Moravia to the Fascist authorities, which resented the stunningly cold, objective protrayal of the decadence and corruption of the bourgeoisie, the very class that had enabled Mussolini to gain power. Labeled "negative" by a government preoccupied with establishing an image of tranquility, law, and order, a nation where traditional values were deeply respected, Moravia's life became increasingly more difficult.

Many of the years that followed were spent traveling abroad, on a variety of special assignments for newspapers and periodicals. He visited London, Paris, and New York (where he held a fellowship at Columbia University), Mexico, China, and Greece, while writing several long short stories, as well as an ambitious, prolix novel (probably his worst), *Le ambizioni sbagliate* (1935; *The Wheel of Fortune*, N.Y., 1937, reissued in 1965 with the title *Mistaken Ambitions*). This time, the government actively discouraged the papers from reviewing the book. Shortly afterward, Moravia was forbidden to sign his articles except with a nom de plume. "The years between 1933, the year of Hitler's rise to power, and 1943, the year of the fall of fascism, were, from the point of view of public life, the worst of my life and even today, I cannot remember them without horror," Moravia confessed some years ago.

In 1941, Moravia married Elsa Morante, herself a writer, whom he had met five years before. The next four years were to be particularly difficult: labeled "subversive" by the authorities for the unorthodox views expressed in his work, Moravia and his wife lived in constant fear of being arrested. When Mussolini's regime collapsed, they returned to Rome, to flee south once again. They lived in Fondi, a small town in the Ciociara region, hiding for nine months in a pigsty. Out of that experience came *La ciociara* (1957; *Two Women*, N.Y., 1958, later made into a successful film starring Sofia Loren), one of few works by our subject to be directly inspired by autobiographical events.

The end of the war enabled Moravia to return to Rome, and resume his career of novelist and journalist. His novels began appearing: one of them, *La Romana* (1947; *The Woman of Rome*, N.Y., 1949) achieved a success comparable only to that of *Gli indifferenti*. Since then, Moravia's reputation has become worldwide, and his books have been translated into most major languages. Among the many awards bestowed upon his work are the Strega Prize, in 1952, and the Marzotto Prize, in 1954.

A first reading of Moravia's work may recall to mind the distinction, once made by Virginia Woolf, between types of novelists. In her lecture, "Mr. Bennett and Mrs. Brown" the noted writer divided novelists into two distinct categories, the Georgians and the Edwardians. It is to the latter group that Alberto Moravia obviously belongs, since "he does not give us a house in the hope that we may be able to deduce the human beings who live there." It is Moravia's firm belief that not only are novels "first of all about people," but that it is the writer's business to give us as complete a picture as he can of people and of what they are about. He does not subscribe to the theory that the reader is in a sense duty-bound to cooperate with the writer to the extent of supplementing, with his own fantasy, whatever has been left out due to the novelist's negligence or incompetence or lack of intuition. Moravia's greatest gift consists precisely in his ability to leave his reader with the distinct feeling that he has said all that could possibly be said about his characters, and that he has reached as deep an understanding of them as it is possible to obtain in their special circumstances.

Structurally, his work is deeply rooted in the tradition of nineteenth-century narrative. His books are marked neither by confusing techniques nor by daring stylistic experiments. In the majority of cases, the tale begins with a situation that has already reached a critical juncture. We are told something of the background of the characters, just enough to understand them and become sufficiently curious about them to want to know the nature of their situation and how it is resolved in the context of the story. Here Moravia departs from the traditional manner of handling a tale. While the nineteenth-century writer was sure of finding in objective reality the cause that held the eventual solution of his characters' "problems," Moravia gives us the instinctive feeling that such causes must be found in man's inner self. Like many of his contemporaries, Moravia believes far more firmly in the reality of man's inner feelings than in that of the external world. Because the anguish felt by his heroes is essentially metaphysical or psychological, but never physical, the situation therefore demands that it be met and resolved in new ways.

Ever since his first book, Moravia has consistently demonstrated a keen appreciation of certain philosophical ideas (coupled with an unusual deftness in using them in fiction) whose popularity is quite recent. The idea of nausea, the notions of the absurdity of life and the nothingness of existence, the chaotic quality of the modern world, could well be mistaken for gratuitous borrowing from the existentialists (whose work Moravia admires), were it not for the fact that our novelist had found "his" themes, articulating them with unusual maturity, years before the appearance of Sartre and Camus on the literary scene. He thus became, unconsciously perhaps, one of the first existentialist writers in his country. Unlike Camus and Sartre, however, Moravia arrived at his conception of life not by way of philosophical study and speculation, but through intuition. Similarly, without any attempt on his part to turn his novels into ideological works (in the manner of, say, Vittorini), he manages to fictionalize life around two prominent aspects that pervade contemporary life—sex and money—"just as it happens in times of great change and uncertainty such as ours." For him, it is not enough to know Marx and Freud intellectually: their teachings must open our emotions to new visions of what life should be, while understanding what life is; they must be acquired by our critical and creative sensitivity, lived, as it were, before they may be allowed to enter the ordered world of fiction.

There is in all this a certain amount of impatience which is reflected in Moravia's style. In a country where, by tradition, the aesthetics of language are overwhelmingly important, it is easy to understand why the critical verdict on his manner of telling should be on the negative side. His plain, realistic, almost casual prose style is hardly one that could properly be defined as poetic. There is little rhythm in his prose (although there are always isolated passages of a tenderness and beauty one would call lyrical), but there is a determination to see things clearly, with the lucidity and objectivity of a scientist. If the reader should find it difficult to become fond of Moravia because of "how" he writes, but finds himself attracted by "what" he says, then he must be reminded at this point that, as with any significant or serious writer, *what* Moravia says can only (for better or worse) be said in his particular style.

Gli indifferenti is Moravia's first novel, but not his first attempt at writing fiction. In 1925, after he had been discharged from the sanatorium at Codivilla, located in the exclusive mountain and ski resort Cortina d'Ampezzo, in the Dolomite mountains, he moved to Bressanone, near Bolzano, a few miles from the Austrian border, where he began writing in earnest. He finished two short stories: one, "La cortigiana stanca" ("The Tired Courtesan") appeared in a magazine of international pretensions, *900* [or: The twentieth century], edited by Massimo Bontempelli, and written entirely in French; the other, "Delitto al Circolo di Tennis" ("Crime at the Tennis Club"), was published some years later. Both stories anticipate the mood, themes, and vision of *Gli indifferenti*.

Reminiscing about the circumstances surrounding the writing of *The Time of Indifference*, Moravia stated:

I would find it almost impossible to say in any detail how I came upon the idea of indifference, which is the key of the book. All I can roughly say is this: as I have already explained, I set out to write a tragedy in the form of a novel, but, as I wrote, I realized that the tragic motif, or indeed any really tragic event, slipped through my fingers as soon as I tried to formulate it. By this I mean that tragedy was impossible given the sort of background and the sort of characters I was dealing with, but if I had changed the background and characters then I would have turned my back on reality and created something artificial. In other words I began to see the impossibility of tragedy in a world in which non-materialist values seemingly lacked any right to exist, and where moral conscience had become so hardened that people acted from appetite only and were more and more like automata.

During the previous four years, his illness had forced him to spend his time in bed, and reading helped him pass the time in a tolerable way. "At that time," he recalls, "I was reading plays more than anything else—especially Molière, Goldoni and Shakespeare—and I gradually formed an ambition to write a novel combining the technique of drama and narrative. In 1926, I read James Joyce's *Ulysses*. Joyce seemed to me to have resolved the problem of the duration of time in the same way as the dramatists, that is to say, by bringing out its flexibility and conventionalism. So I conceived the idea of writing a novel describing minute by minute the life of a bourgeois family in Rome. *Ulysses* describes only one day. My ambition, if I remember correctly, was to apply to the novel Aristotle's principle of unity of time, place, and action." The extent to which Joyce influenced Moravia may well remain a question hard to resolve, particularly in view of the fact that he read *Ulysses* in the French translation of Valéry Larbaud, and could not have understood completely not merely the structural but also the linguistic achievement of Joyce.

By comparison, *The Time of Indifference* is a conventional novel, with an undistinguished, indeed banal plot and form. Yet, its conventionality of form and plot (which is nothing more than a variation of the overused and abused love triangle) is subtly turned into an asset. Never before had an Italian novelist dealt with a similar theme as effectively as Moravia, or created a tableau of decadence without moralizing.

The story of *Gli indifferenti* revolves around the doings of a middle-class Roman family. There is Mariagrazia Ardengo, an aging widow who for several years has been the unloved mistress of a cynical businessman, Leo Merumeci; Carla, her pretty daughter; her son, Michele, a law student with a definite flair for self-analysis. The dramatis personae are rounded out by Lisa, also an aging woman, who is presently hoping to become Michele's mistress.

The family's predicament is, first of all, of a practical sort. Its small fortune has dwindled away; its only remaining possession, the villa in which they live, is heavily mortgaged and is soon to be sold if the numerous debts incurred by the Ardengos are to be paid. On other counts the situation is hardly encouraging. The empty life led by the trio has brought them dangerously close to the point where each of them will lose completely man's most prized possession: his moral conscience. Fewer and fewer are the acts that succeed in shaking them: people and events slowly drown in the vast sea of their "indifference."

Their state of mind becomes total blindness in the face of their impending ruin. The first climax of the story, developed within a forty-eight-hour span, is reached when Carla allows herself to be seduced by her mother's lover. She consents to this in the faint hope that her life might take a different direction and become, if not happier, at least more meaningful. In her desperate search for some solid ground onto which she may anchor her vanishing hope, Carla brushes aside any question concerned with the moral or indeed even the practical propriety of her act. The yielding of her virginity proves to have been totally useless. Soon enough, Carla finds herself in an even worse predicament when her lover, having satisfied his purely libidinous passion, begins giving unmistakable signs of becoming bored with her naïve, yet all too human craving for affection, adventure, and security.

There is little that is really audaciously original about the plot. But then one could say much the same thing about a good many other famous novels, like Flaubert's *Madame Bovary*. *The Time of Indifference* goes well beyond what it presents: it unobtrusively raises questions other books, seemingly more sophisticated, fail to pose. It should be clear at once that, through a low-key presentation of trivial incidents and common, almost banale stories, Moravia places his characters in a state of crisis. Through their actions and behavior, he asks: "How are we to act in the face of reality" that no longer makes much sense to us? How are we supposed to conduct ourselves in a world where man finds it difficult, not to say impossible, to accept, and live by the large baggage of social, religious and moral beliefs inherited from the past?

It is this singular question that gives Moravia's work a homogeneity not easily found among many other writers. From the very beginning of his creative activity, Moravia found himself confronting the problem of "how man was to deal with reality," man "who found himself incapable of establishing a relationship with his own world, a world that had become dark and unplumbable—worse still, it had disappeared." In *Time of Indifference*, this inability, seized perhaps without full awareness of its scope and relevance in terms of Moravia's vision of life, is constantly presented as a kind of traumatic condition, a sort of paralysis of the will. The character of the novel who suffers most from this condition is Michele: his inability to act—which means to exercise his will in "choosing" his life, in acting responsibly and consciously in a manner that will permit him to control, to some degree, the course of his existence—cannot be overcome because there exists an unbridgeable gap between himself and the "world" out there, the world where life has become a farce. Michele sees all this, regrets it again and again, yet is impotent before it. Why? The world about him is disintegrating before his eyes: not the real world, of course, but the world of his feelings: love, trust, respect, affection, concern for his family and his friends, self-esteem, courage, purposefulness in facing the usual as well as the unusual problems and difficulties of existence.

More and more, as Michele pursues the path that leads him to a more thorough knowledge of himself and the world he inhabits, words begin to fail him. Words are no longer meaningful: they have become useless to communicate with other human beings, and equally useless in describing, and hence in seizing, reality. They have become hollow sounds, as false as reality itself: they no longer represent, comment on, and much less correct life; they have been turned into tools to deceive, to hide, to misrepresent what we truly are. Having prostituted man's highest, most important, and sacred gift, every possibility of tragedy is denied to the world. As Sanguineti observes, "the loss of the sense of the tragic, becomes, as Michele sees it, with great exactness and great clarity, the very loss of contact with reality, the symbol of a vital alienation endured: of indifference, of boredom."

Michele, aside from being the antihero of this singular story, provides the reader with a suitable vantage point from which the unfolding (and the implications) of the events may be observed. Conscious of the degrading life led by his family, he regrets the decay and senselessness of their doings; yet he cannot persuade himself that he is able, or capable, or indeed even willing, to change the situation to fit his vague concept of a dignified, purposeful, productive existence. What is certainly unusual about this, is that Michele's apparent incapacity to act responsibly, and ultimately restore a minimum amount of dignity to his, and their, lives, becomes an element of tension in the novel. Aware of his own indifference, he seems to relish it (because it makes activism impossible) as well as to suffer from it (because he knows it to be wrong). This condition materializes in a series of meaningless demonstrations of anger: typical of this situation are his frequent insults to Leo (for which he is time and again asked to apologize), or his hurling a heavy ashtray at him, missing his target and striking his mother instead.

As the novel moves toward the end, Michele is told by Lisa that Carla has become Leo's mistress and that the two may be caught, *in flagrante delicto*, in Merumeci's apartment. The young man realizes that this may be the last opportunity to test his sincerity and courage: Leo must be killed. Michele proceeds to purchase a revolver and, for a while, he even surrenders to his romantic imagination and imagines the consequences of his criminal act. He lives through the scene of the trial, the defense attorney's pleas, the judge's final pardon, the tears, the indignation, the shame of it all. When Leo opens the door of his apartment, Michele aims his gun and fires it. But the weapon does not fire. In his haste, Michele had curiously forgotten to load the revolver. A possibly tragic finale is turned into a farce, a cheap and shabby melodrama. And so Michele, who throughout the story had remained the voice of the author himself, articulating his disgust, his fears, his misgivings, his constant struggle to be sincere, in his attempt to retrieve the values he knows to be worthwhile, ends by joining the system and becomes Leo's partner, thus sealing the marriage of his mother's lover with his sister.

The whole novel has a special, almost Pirandellian quality about it. Things manage to look respectable, solid: the villa is located in the fashionable Roman district of Ludovisi. The streets are quiet, handsome, tree-lined, a far cry from city streets. But the villa is not really elegant, the air is far from being clean and fresh as one is led to expect, and the villa's owners are far from being happy. Heavy, gloomy drapes keep the light out, and everywhere we sense a feeling of decay. Inside the villa, five people find themselves enmeshed in an existence without much hope, trapped, as it were, in the quagmire of their schemes. They talk, but they do not communicate: indeed, their conversations (if such they can be called), read more like a catalogue of middle-class commonplaces, snobbish and crass remarks truly reflecting their insensitivity. Similarly, they think they love, but only fornicate. At one point, for example, Leo encourages Michele to visit Lisa, because, although no longer young, she is ready for a new lover, is still physically attractive, and won't cost him a lira! They are all puppets, with the exception of Leo who always plays the game conscious of what the stakes are, and manages to manipulate all with consummate skill. Given the theme of the novel, it was unavoidable that some readers would take it to be a relentless condemnation of the bourgeoisie, an intention Moravia disclaimed with these words:

"Only long after the publication of *Time of Indifference* . . . did I realize the real bearing of the book and begin to feel revulsion for the middle-class way of life as a whole. But I should point out that I began seeing that way of life as a moral, rather than a material, phenomenon. Comfort is always preferable to poverty, and I know many violently anti-middle-class people who would hardly be able to go on being what they are in any deep or sincere way if the material restrictions in which they are struggling were removed. They are anti-middle-class because they are poor, just as many middle-class people are anti-proletarian because they are rich. However useful they may be in the political struggle, their conclusions remove all interest from the attributes themselves. I think one can only be genuinely anti-middle-class on a wider plane, one that annihilates all social distinctions and aims at building a world for all men."

If *Gli indifferenti* examined the issue of man and reality, and dramatized the question of action, the problem of Moravia's second novel, *Le ambizioni sbagliate*, seems to be one of too much action. Where every action in the former moves deliberately toward the resolution of the drama, in the latter the complexity of the plot has become too complex and unwieldy. Maria Luisa

Tanzillo, the estranged wife of Marquis Matteo, growing impatient with her husband's unfaithfulness, tries to convince Sofia, her sister-in-law, and her fiancé, Pietro Monatti, to bring about a reconciliation. She asks Pietro to accompany her to visit her sickly brother Stefano, who lives at a *pensione* run by Professor Renato Malacrida. There she meets Carlino, a university student, whom she prods to become her lover. On their way home, Pietro and Maria Luisa stop at a pastry shop, where they meet Matteo and his mistress Andreina. When Andreina learns that Matteo is penniless, and is totally dependent on his wife's fortune, inherited after her first husband passed away, she joins with Pietro (whose mistress she becomes) and the two begin scheming to steal Maria Luisa's precious jewels with the help of her maid Rosa. But when the plan is changed, and murder is added to the plot, Pietro bows out, and Stefano (who started Andreina on her life as a courtesan) is brought into the picture. According to an old Roman law, it seems that in the event of Maria Luisa's death Stefano would be entitled to the inheritance. But Stefano refuses to go on with the plot, and runs away with Andreina's maid Cecilia. Andreina then decides to carry out the scheme by herself. As the novel comes to an end, we see Andreina running in the streets, presumably on her way to the police station to surrender herself, as the murder has been witnessed by Rosa and Stefano. The irony of the whole story is almost too obvious: no one gains anything from all the plottings and crimes committed: Maria Luisa is murdered; Andreina will end her days in jail; Stefano is left empty-handed, Matteo finds himself without a wife, or a mistress and, what is even worse, without money.

There can be little question that, when writing his second novel (which cost him more than five years' work) Moravia had an ambitious plan in mind, presumably to do for the Italian novel what Dostoyevsky had done for the Russian novel: a sustained, serious, complex work about the question of crime (such as murder and thievery), and the ensuing social and psychological repercussions. But, as even my bare outline of the plot of *Mistaken Ambitions* shows, the resulting book is a clumsy, awkward novel, often impressive, to be sure, but grossly overworked and full of technical flaws.

Moravia himself was disappointed by the rather unanimously negative reception accorded to his novel, and realized that, for him at least, "the best approach to fiction in our century was that of *The Time of Indifference*: very few characters and a fairly simple plot. I therefore decided," he concluded, "that henceforth I would adopt the viewpoint of only one character." The conclusion proved to be both correct and productive. For the next ten years, Moravia wrote several short stories (collected in five volumes) and two novellas, *La mascherata* (1941; *The Fancy Dress Party*, N.Y., 1952) and *Agostino* (1945; *Two Adolescents*, N.Y., 1950). The majority of his shorter works are excellent: without the necessity of being burdened by complicated plots, Moravia succeeds admirably in portraying a vast array of characters. To understand them it is necessary not merely to perceive what makes his fiction so absorbing, but to recognize in the way in which they act an objectified dramatization of some of the leading problems of contemporary existence.

What is the world Moravia writes about? Ever since his first novel, and with one or two brief interludes (the most notable being *Racconti romani*), Moravia has fictionalized the world of the middle class. His orientation is a matter of some interest since traditionally Italian novelists, the majority of whom come from the middle class, have dealt with the problems and mores of the working class. Svevo and Pirandello had little or no influence with respect to changing this pattern, although the ties Moravia has with both would indicate more than a mere coincidence of interests. From Svevo, who was in the process of being "discovered" at the time of *Gli indifferenti*, Moravia inherited the disinterested, clinical method of character analysis, while Pirandello transmitted something of his metaphysical curiosity about life, which is a pervasive feature of Moravia's fiction. Literary influences, especially in his early works, are numerous indeed (Manzoni and Verga, Boccaccio and Shakespeare, and, of course, Goldoni, among others); certainly enough such influences to justify amply the suggestion of R. W. B. Lewis that Moravia is "one of the most incorrigibly *literary* novelists of his generation." The passages and situations willfully lifted from the classics he has been reading since his adolescence are too obvious to be enumerated here. But Moravia expects his readers to understand that his overt borrowings have a definite place within the broader strategy of his fiction. What were in the classics occasions for lyricism and tragedy are cunningly turned into occasions for irony and ridicule—and hence unmistakable and necessary instruments to dramatize a world stripped of its meaning.

In the nightmare of our modern world, about which Moravia writes with forcefulness in his better creative moments, "the air is too foul to breathe." Michele, in *The Time of Indifference*, longs for the world of real tears and indignation— a world of sincerity and real feelings that has apparently vanished. We are all well acquainted with the new, efficient world of our century; and Moravia is right in reminding us that modern literature (Kafka, Camus, and Sartre are its typical, but not its only worthy representatives) gives us "the same sense of suffocation and claustrophobia. We seem to lack air; we want to free ourselves from whatever surrounds us; it is as if the sky itself were too low. All modern poetry, in different ways, expresses this feeling of suffocation. Poetry, the eternal Cassandra, warns man that his world has grown absurd." Michele himself "felt he was suffocating . . . everything around him was without weight and without value, fleeting as a play of light and shade."

It is fitting, too, that the special habitat of Moravia's characters should be Rome, seldom specifically mentioned by name, to be sure, but recognizable in the kind of activity and life that takes place. It is in the big cities, Boston or Bologna, Milan or San Francisco, Rome or New York, that modern man understands most intensely, amidst so many other men, how it feels and what it means to be alone. Today as yesterday Borgese's remark apropos of *Gli indifferenti* has retained its relevance and validity: "there is little of Rome here . . . the scene is made up of lights and draperies, as in certain *mise en scène*." But geography and history matter little in Moravia's fiction: and the locale of his tales, even when minutely described (as in *Two Women*, for example) is always raised to the symbolic value of a place somewhere, or anywhere in the Western world. There is enough in his fiction to make us "feel" Rome without our ever being certain we are there. In some instances (as in *Il conformista* [1951; *The Conformist*, N.Y., 1951] and *Two Women*) Moravia sets his story in a definite historical milieu, that of fascism and World War II. Unlike his contemporary novelists who have been effectively inspired by the war, Moravia rarely deals with history with an eye to exploring its phenomena and its chain of cause and effect. The historical dimension holds little or no interest for Moravia the novelist, who is too sophisticated to forget that history repeats itself with unending and disconcerting regularity. He prefers, rather, to deal with human vices, desires, frustrations, and the existential problems of individuals. He is therefore equally at home depicting characters living in Fascist Italy (as in *The Woman of Rome*, *The Conformist*, and *Two Women*) or in sixteenth-century Florence, as in the intriguing play *Beatrice Cenci*.

Generally speaking, Moravia's characters, much like Svevo's, are comfortably settled in society and seldom plagued by the harsh necessity of earning a living. In the majority of cases, their occupations are readily given: they are architects, students, lawyers, teachers, businessmen, government employees, writers who, even when unemployed, never worry about their future. Invariably, however, their professional life matters little because Moravia seldom focuses on the problems brought about by their jobs. There is also a large, colorful group of workers—those who, because of their occupation and standing in society, must be classified as the lower class—the *plebe*. The point of distinction between the middle and working classes is not an idle one since each group, well distinguished by its conventions and its socioeconomic structure, plays a particular role in Moravia's fiction.

To the best of my knowledge, the critic Fernandez has been the first to suggest that each social group incarnates certain problems. Thus, for instance, the relationship between mother and daughter is dramatized by characters belonging to the working class; the relationship between mother and son is always seen in a middle-class family; and, finally, the relationship between husband and wife is explored in situations involving only intellectuals. That the sympathy of the author goes unmistakably to the working class is something that may surprise us only momentarily. For the author, simple and unsophisticated as the workers generally are, they constitute the only group blessed with a special sort of ignorance and philosophical endurance, a wisdom and serenity invariably denied to the comparatively well-off, well-bred, literate bourgeoisie. Once again, no one better than Michele (in *Two Women*) articulates a view that has in time betrayed its polemical content vis-à-vis the intellectual. It is Rosetta who speaks first:

"Peasants don't know anything except the land, they are ignorant and live like beasts." He started laughing, and answered:

"Some time ago it wouldn't have been a compliment, but today it is. Today it's the people who read and write and live in towns and are gentlefolk who are really ignorant, the really uncultivated, the really uncivilized ones. With them there's nothing to be done, but with you peasants one can begin from the very beginning."

The absence of pressing financial problems does not prevent Moravia's heroes from being concerned with money. On the contrary, some of the early works (particularly *Le ambizioni sbagliate*) center on the struggle for money and for the kind of station in life only money can buy. Of course, the working people are also concerned with money; but for them the problem is of an entirely different nature, determining only whether or not they will be able to buy sufficient food the next day. Cesira, one of the *Two Women*, speaking of the peasants' attitude toward money, refers to it as "a kind of god . . . for them it is money that is the most important thing, partly because they haven't any, and partly because it is from money—from their point of view, anyhow—that all good things come." But beyond this first, realistic meaning, there lurks a greater one; for money is only seldom seen as a means to achieve power and security. Its meaning is frequently more Freudian: money symbolizes not so much what it *can* do (its purchasing power, so to speak) but what we are truly like. This is reflected in the varying attitudes we assume toward it. A greedy person or a miser, for example, is for Moravia both incapable of and unfit to love, since love is a feeling that flows from within and does not ordinarily expect anything tangible in return.

Money also becomes an instrument for establishing or maintaining a rapport with the world. The best illustration of this is provided by the youngster Luca, in the novella *La disubbidienza* (*Two Adolescents*), who accidentally sees his parents putting away some bonds and cash in a safe concealed behind a reproduction of Raphael's *Madonna*, the painting before which he customarily kneels down at night when he says his prayers. Luca is undergoing a critical period of his life, the time when an adolescent tries to find his place in his family's life amidst the confusion and difficulties presented by his other problems of adjustment. When he becomes aware that the money he himself had painfully saved from his allowances "bound him to the world and forced him to accept it, he felt a raging hatred for these objects and for his savings. . . . Those objects and that money were not merely objects and money, but living, tenacious strands in the woof of which his existence was woven." Since the youngster wishes to cut off his ties with a world he feels he can no longer love, his first impulsive act is to bury the small treasure of money he has saved, and thus "in burying the money he would also in a certain way be burying himself—or at any rate that part of himself that was attached to the money."

> He discovered that he felt a profound hatred for the money, the sort of hatred one might feel for a tyrant against whom one has rebelled. The idea, too, that money was held in such esteem by his parents and that he himself without knowing it had for so many years said his prayers in front of a safe full of money contributed to his resentment. . . . Luca . . . wanted to destroy [its value] not merely by his own desire to do so but in actual fact. Detested idol as he felt it to be, nothing less than this blasphemous tearing to pieces could serve utterly to desecrate it.

Although consistently projected against a background of material comfort, Moravia's heroes lack the feeling of security they so desperately need. If they are unable to connect with other human beings, it is because no relationship can exist if it is based on material considerations, thus making money is, as Donald Heiney perceptively points out, "an analogue to sexual power." In a world where an individual seeks to dominate, or "possess" another, money is what turns an already deplorable situation into a degrading and obscene one. The frequency and diversity with which Moravia deals with this issue is in itself indicative of its central position in his world view: we find it in *The Time of Indifference*, where Carla and Michele, and finally their mother as well, perceive Carla's marriage to Leo (irrespective of whether they are in love) as the factor that will save their family from total financial disaster; on in *La noia*, (1960; *The Empty Canvas*, N.Y., 1961) where its protagonist Dino, a well-to-do would-be painter, covers the body of his mistress Cecilia with banknotes, and offers her any amount of money if she will agree to live with him.

There is always a pervasive ironic twist whenever money enters into the picture (which is quite frequently), since money can only purchase the appearance of contentment, never truly genuine happiness. Moravia understands quite clearly the role that money plays in the world: after all, it is the money interests that finance and corrupt the politicians, who in turn govern the nations not according to what is best for all people, but what is best for those in power and those who helped those in power get where they are. The analogue is depicted at the family level: Mariagrazia Ardengo has no money, and must therefore resign herself to be at the mercy of Leo, who is rich; Maria Luisa of *The Wheel of Fortune*, is quite affluent and can well afford to take a young lover, while at the same time reproaching her husband for having done the same thing. Dino's mother (*The Empty Canvas*) is well-to-do and is presented as an astute businesswoman who expertly manages the properties of the family while her husband is away on business most of the time. Through money, she ultimately controls her son, who is vaguely trying to be independent, but cannot be, since his "hobby" produces no revenue. The two discuss their finances in the bathroom, where the safe is located, concealed behind a tile, just as the safe of Luca Mansi's parents (*Two Adolescents*) is hidden behind a religious painting. In both cases, and in general in much of Moravia's fiction, money is presented, with considerable justification, as one of the major causes of modern alienation.

Money, however, is not always the factor responsible for the crises in which Moravia's characters find themselves. The estrangement from which they seem to suffer in almost every case is rooted in a conspicuous lack of love: and the results are both painful and horrible to contemplate. Mothers are frequently estranged from their children, children are estranged first from their parents and then from each other, to the point where what used to be a normal or conventional rapport is expressed in terms of indifference, contempt, or even hatred. Adriana, the lowly prostitute of *The Woman of Rome*, is distressed by the hate her lover, Mino Diodati, shows for his family; Stefano, the sickly and penniless degenerate of *Mistaken Ambitions*, agrees that the death of his sister, Maria Luisa, "might be a good thing"; Luca Mansi, of *Two Adolescents*, realizes that once his love for his family and his friends, for his prized possessions and his studies, has disappeared, his strong *raison de vivre* is no more.

Love, robbed of its affective connotations, is then distilled into an activity that is hardly anything more than a purely sexual exercise. It is often on the purely physical aspect of man's relation with woman that Moravia dwells at length. In his fiction the cult of sexual love is seldom allowed to be transformed into a cult of true love.

A generation brought up under the influence of Freudian psychology and well read in the sexual behavior of men and women of all ages can hardly be shocked or annoyed by Moravia's supreme concern with sex. It is important to stress here, as Mr. Lewis has aptly done, that there is, in the last analysis, far less "sex" in Moravia than in most other contemporary writers. For him sex matters only as an important force in modern life, as a force that may afford freedom from the futility and boredom of our existence or one that may grant us a momentary consciousness of the "being" we otherwise lack in our spiritual world.

Now, what is extraordinary about Moravia's characters, and the world they inhabit, is not so much their sexuality, but the fact that, in Heiney's words, "the basic premise is the interaction of the individual will with its environment, including other human beings, and this conflict is characteristically presented in sexual terms." Love, rather than being a form of communication, an experience that binds people together, becomes a force that debases, and eventually alienates every person that practices it sexually; hence the discontent, the isolation, the wretchedness to which so many of Moravia's characters are condemned. They know how *to make* love, to be sure, but they do not know how *to love*. It is therefore refreshing that, granted the world being described, we should occasionally find a character like Adriana, the heroine of *The Woman of Rome*. Her love for the numerous men who come to her (perhaps to unburden the least lovable part of their personality) is transformed into a kind of pseudo-religion whose particular strength is in its Christian concept of Love as *Caritas*. The uniqueness of Adriana consists precisely in her being able to find in promiscuous love, generally deemed humiliating, the very strength to accept with cheerfulness an otherwise sordid existence.

In some cases, the initiation to sex opens the way to an emotional redemption, the beginning of a new, meaningful relation between the individual and the forces of life. The two youngsters portrayed in *Agostino* and *La disubbidienza* (*Two Adolescents*) find in the promised or realized sexual experience a reason to hope and accept what had previously filled them with nausea. But when the sexual encounter fails to open the door to a more harmonious relationship with the world, the future stability of the individual's own well-being is severely threatened. Moravia's fiction, as has frequently been remarked, reads much like a catalogue of failures, many of which begin at the sexual level. Beginning with Carla and her lover Leo, in the early work, *The Time of Indifference*, to Riccardo Molteni in *Il disprezzo* (1954; *A Ghost at Noon*, N.Y., 1955), or Dino (*The Empty Canvas*), and Francesco (*L'attenzione*, 1965; *The Lie*, N.Y., 1966), such failures are symptomatic of still larger failures as human beings. Moreover, as Dominique Fernandez has noted,

> The contrary of indifference will never be, for the Moravian hero, a straightforward and coherent moral conscience; only an acknowledgement—without reservations—of the sexual fact will permit them to rid themselves of their indifference and adhere once again in the strong manner to reality; and the novelist, making of the body the last truth, will at once have found the means to reduce the universe to a comprehensible universe and offer to the investigative capacity of his style an entirely explorable subject.

Through sexual integrity and through the spontaneous and unselfish giving of oneself it is possible to lessen the isolation to which man is condemned and to achieve a deeper, more satisfying understanding of our condition. The novel *Il disprezzo* (*A Ghost at Noon*) centers on a writer, Riccardo Molteni, who becomes a hack in order to earn more money. The drama itself pivots on the uncertain relationship between him and his wife, and climaxes in the disastrous end of what had been a relatively happy marriage. This pathetic situation is reached when Riccardo, anxious to buy the apartment his wife Emilia wants so much, first surrenders his artistic integrity by trying to reconcile the diverging interpretations of Battista, the producer, and Rheingold, the director, of a filmed version of Homer's *Odyssey*, and then allows Battista to make advances to Emilia, thus losing whatever respect she might have had for him:

During the first year of our married life my relations with my wife were, I can now assert, perfect. By which I mean to say that, in those years, a complete, profound harmony of the senses was accompanied by a kind of numbness—or should I say silence?—of the mind which, in such circumstances, causes an entire suspension of judgment and looks only to love for an estimate of the person. Emilia, in fact, seemed to me wholly without defects, and so also, I believe, I appeared to her. Or perhaps I saw her defects and she saw mine, but, through some mysterious transformation produced by the feeling of love, such defects appeared to us both not merely forgivable but even lovable, as though instead of defects they had been positive qualities, if of a rather special kind. Anyhow we did not judge: we loved each other. This story sets out to relate how, while I continued to love her and not judge her, Emilia, on the other hand, discovered, or thought she had discovered, certain defects in me, and judged me and in consequence ceased to love me.

Not much different from the case of Silvio Baldeschi, the would-be writer, self-defined dilettante, hero of *L'amore coniugale* (1949; *Conjugal Love*, N.Y., 1951), who at the outset of the story confesses readily that "there were only two things that could save me [from despair]: the love of a woman and artistic creation." The book eventually shows how Silvio, having temporarily suspended making love to his wife (when he decides that marital abstinence will prevent a disruption of his creative activity), is eventually betrayed by her and becomes conscious of his failure both as an artist and as a husband.

When the world cannot be comprehended through the love of the senses, Moravia's characters experience a range of emotions that range from violence to hate. Their world is desolate enough without love. The women and men are forced to enact their drama on a bare stage and although neither fear nor dread haunts their hearts they must accept what they are, without question.

The parable of a sick humanity is repeated time and again. Michele accepts indifference as a *modus vivendi*; Pietro (*Mistaken Ambitions*), having failed in his attempts to "redeem" Andreina, reverts to the role of the ambitious journalist that he really is;

Marcello Clerici (*The Conformist*) persists in his foolish conformity to the very end, and the lesson of history is of no avail.
To accept what we are and to make peace with our reality, so
that we may find through it the strength to go on living, appears
to be Moravia's implicit message. A moment of spiritual tranquility can only seldom be found by his characters. Religion rarely
offers any comfort to his struggling souls, and when it does it is
clearly expressed in terms of a form of superstition. Adriana
(*The Woman of Rome*) says: "I liked the Madonna because she
was so different from mother, so serene and tranquil, richly
clothed, with her eyes that looked on me so lovingly, it was as
if she were my real mother and not the mother who spent time
scolding me, and was always worn-out and badly dressed."

By and large, however, such reflections are unusual: as a rule,
it is anger and hate that reign in the narrative of Moravia with
an almost exasperating regularity: hate for the mother, for society,
for the whole wide world, whose history, as Mino Diodati sternly
proclaims in *The Woman of Rome*, is nothing but "a long yawn-
ing of boredom."

The characters' hate is basically reflective of their inability to
reconcile themselves with the reality of life. Incapable of shaking
off their moral indifference, unwilling to participate more fully
in life around them, they view life as a carrier of tedium and
wretchedness to be met with a philosophy of negatives: suicide,
murder, anger, spite, rage, sadism, rebellion. Luca Mansi (*Two
Adolescents*) having perceived that things and people show an
undue insubordination to his will, experiences a "violent rage."
He feels first that he should kill himself (as does indeed Silvio
Baldeschi in *Conjugal Love*). Having discarded the idea of suicide, the youngster decides to "disobey."

The word "disobey" pleased him because it was familiar.
Throughout his childhood and a great part of his boyhood he
had heard his mother say that he must be obedient, that he was
disobedient, that if he didn't obey she would punish him, and
other similar phrases. Perhaps by starting to be disobedient
again on a more logical, higher plane, he was merely redis-
covering an attitude of mind which was native to him but
which he had lost. So far he had been disobedient only in the

sphere of his school life, which was the fullest and most absurd part of his existence. But since the incident of the football game, he was discovering that this disobedience could be extended to other spheres as well: it could embrace other things which, because they were normal and obvious, had hitherto escaped him—the affections, for instance; and—an extreme case which immediately fascinated him—the actual fact of living.

Life is to be denied then, because it offers a preestablished order which Moravia's characters are often unfit, or unable, or unwilling to change—even in the smallest way. Hence the disorder, the streak of meanness and deep-running spite in their temperament.

Speaking from a philosophical perspective, two recent readers of Moravia (Joan Ross and Donald Freed) have noted how his "characters adventure into relationships and into the world looking not for another person, but for a showdown, an extreme situation that will open the channel for the vital current between mind-body-soul or kill themselves physically since they are already dead philosophically." If this observation is correct, it is only partly so. In point of fact, the situation is considerably more complex, and therefore elusive, than it may appear at first. Michele, of *The Time of Indifference*, longs for "the paradise of reality and truth," while *Agostino*, the hero of the postwar novella by the same tile, confronted by a reality largely shaped by violence and cruelty, "walked about for a little, naked on the soft, mirroring sand, and enjoyed stamping on it with his feet and seeing the water suddenly rise to its surface and flood his footprints. There arose in him a vague and desperate desire to ford the river and walk on and on down the coast, leaving far behind him the boys, Saro, his mother and all the old life. Who knows, if he were to go straight ahead and never turn back, walking, walking on that soft sand, might he not at last come to a country where none of these horrible things existed; a country where he would be welcomed as he longed to be, and where it would be possible for him to forget all he had learned, and then learn it again without all that shame and horror, gently and naturally as he felt that it might be possible."

The desire is always there: the desire to awaken from a terrible nightmare and live, for to live is what matters. "I am not alive . . . I am dreaming, this nightmare cannot possibly go on long enough to convince me that it is not a nightmare but reality; one day I shall wake up and recognize the world again, with the sun and the stars, the trees and the sky and all the other lovely things. Therefore I must have patience: the awakening is bound to come."

There are, to be sure, other terms for the "reawakening" to which Agostino refers: consciousness, awareness of what we are, what makes us unable to be ourselves, "authentic" human beings. The novels of Moravia, after *La ciociara* (*Two Women*) have become gradually more concerned with a problem stated and restated, implicitly or explicitly, in his work from 1929 to 1957: how can modern man, living in a progressively more alienating and absurd world find himself and thus lead a freer, more purposeful existence? In short, how can man renew a long lost contact with reality? Over and again, Moravia has addressed himself to these Hamletian questions by showing that where there is no love there cannot be real life, since love is "communion." As Moravia's contemporary novelist Ignazio Silone underscores, the spirit of a true community ought to be love, the feeling that we care deeply and unselfishly for each other.

The landscape of Moravia, however, is not marred by total unconcern for our fellow human beings. During his long literary career, Moravia has consistently striven to sum up the dilemma of modern man, used—and frequently abused—by other men. "To use man as a means and not as an end is the root of all evil," Moravia wrote in an essay entitled "L'uomo come fine" ("Man as an End in Himself"), from the volume *L'uomo come fine e altri saggi* (Milan, 1964; *Man as an End: A Defense of Humanism. Literary, Social and Political Essays*, N.Y., 1966). He continued: "The use of man as a means indicates a lack of respect for a man; and this presupposes that one does not sufficiently know what man actually is, or have a clear and adequate idea of what it signifies to be a man."

What it signifies to be a man. The order is a big one, to be sure, and in his own way Moravia has striven to achieve his own definition, however inadequate it may be. Behind the petty intrigues, the shabby conventions, the grotesque behavior, the sloth and indolence, and the futility and indifference that are the aspects of his fiction, there looms *that* purpose to which only a poet may aspire. It is a wicked, difficult life, the novelist implies, and it is impossible (and inconsequential, in the last analysis) to retrace our steps, so as to discover the reason at the root of our mistakes. Many of Moravia's characters are no longer concerned with finding out who or what is responsible for their faults: "The fault was everyone's; impossible to discover its source, the original cause of it," says Michele. The prostitute Adriana comes to much the same conclusion. "No one was guilty; and . . . everything was as it had to be; although everything was unbearable . . . everyone was innocent and guilty at the same time."

Through the years, the vision of Alberto Moravia has broadened. In *The Time of Indifference* we may see the indictment of a whole way of life of a given generation; in *The Conformist* (no matter how unsuccessful the work may be as a finished novel), one perceives the attempt to "explain" the evil of conformity and the worst plague it carries with it—the loss of identity. *Two Women* is, of Moravia's long novels, not only the most successful but the most human. It is also the finest tale about the war and the deepest statement about life made to this date by the novelist. The story consists of the trials and adventures of Cesira, the widow of a shopkeeper, and of her beautiful adolescent daughter Rosetta —two women of Rome's lower class. When the war begins to make itself felt in Rome, the two decide to leave for the country and finally take refuge in nearby Fondi. But aside from the few episodes at the beginning of the story much of the novel is essentially without plot. There are some extraordinarily effective descriptions of the months spent in a small hut atop a hill; of the women's friendship with Michele, an anti-Fascist intellectual, who is only distantly related to the host of intellectuals everpresent on the Moravian stage; there is the episode of Michele's final sacrifice, when he is slaughtered by the Germans; and finally, the shocking, deeply moving episode of Rosetta's loss of virginity when she is raped by the Moroccan troops, and her subsequent calm, dignified acceptance of her new condition. All that the two women go through—and it is quite a lot in terms of fear and trepidation by the end of the story—is not in vain. Cesira, the narrator of the story, confesses toward the end of the tale that she has discovered an important truth about life. She thinks about the episode of her innocent daughter:

> I said to myself that purity is not a thing that you can receive at birth as a gift of nature, so to speak; it is a thing that we acquire through the trials of life, and lose all the more disastrously for having been confident of possessing it; and, in short, it is almost better to be born imperfect and gradually become, if not perfect, at any rate better, than to be born perfect and to be then forced to abandon that first transient perfection for the imperfection that life and experience bring with them.

Of all the women adroitly depicted by Moravia, Cesira is the one who seems to have successfully synthesized the author's view of the human condition. Indeed, it seems almost paradoxical that the novelist, after having created a wasteland of corruption and confusion, of cruelty and violence, is a profound believer in life, in the miracle of life. With Henry James and the poet Giacomo Leopardi, Moravia has discovered that a poet cannot be concerned with dying. There is a passage (it happens to be the last page of *Two Women*) in which Cesira gives a poignant analysis of her experience:

> Sorrow. I thought of Michele, who was not with us in this eagerly longed-for moment of return and would never be with us again. I remembered the evening in the hut at Sant' Eufemia when he had read aloud to us the passage from the Gospel about Lazarus, and had been so angry with the peasants who had failed to understand anything, and had cried that we were all dead and waiting for resurrection, like Lazarus. At the time Michele's words had left me in doubt, but now I saw that Michele had been right, and that for some time now Rosetta and I had indeed been dead, dead to the pity that we owe to others and to ourselves. But sorrow had saved us at the last moment, and so in a way the passage about Lazarus held good for us too, since at last, thanks to sorrow, we had emerged from the war which had enclosed us in its tomb of indifference and wickedness, and had started to walk again along the path

of our own life, which was, maybe, a poor thing full of obscurities and errors but nevertheless the only life that we ought to live, as no doubt Michele would have told us if he had been with us.

The question of true love is connected, in the more recent phase of Moravia's development with the problem of "authenticity," a problem that is at the center of his last three works. The protagonist of *La noia* (*The Empty Canvas*) is once more another of a rich gallery of intellectuals and would-be artists: his name is Dino, he comes from a wealthy middle-class family, and he has turned to painting in the hope of "reestablishing contact with reality."

Dino belongs to a rather large nucleus of people who, for a variety of reasons are estranged from life. In all cases, in Moravia's novels, they are from the middle class: invariably educated, they have money, some aspirations, and are quite articulate. Almost always, they are pseudo-intellectuals: the two university students named Michele (*The Time of Indifference* and *Two Women*), Giacomo Diodati (*The Woman of Rome*), the two young students Luca and Agostino (*Two Adolescents*), writers of novels or screen plays (Silvio Baldeschi of *Conjugal Love* and Riccardo Molteni of *A Ghost at Noon*), journalists-novelists (Pietro Monatti of *Mistaken Ambitions* and Francesco Merighi of *The Lie*), or, as in *The Empty Canvas*, painters. Why they are at odds with society is often what their stories are about. But, if generalizations are permissible, they all seem to be repelled by the shabby social and moral values with which, often for financial reasons, they must live. Other times, they find themselves prisoners of a role for which they have been prepared, or are expected to play. At times, as in *La noia*, Moravia portrays a profound antagonism between mother and son rooted in the fact that the mother controls the purse strings and can therefore manipulate, or attempt to, her son's life. As in *Conjugal Love*, there is in Moravia's work an interesting exploration of the relationship of artistic creativity and human sexuality. In *The Empty Canvas*, as Donald Heiney cogently observes, "For the first time the nature of the parallel between art and sex is made explicit: in order to create a work of art it is first necessary to believe in the reality and meaningfulness of the external world just as in order to love it is necessary to believe in the reality and meaningfulness of the beloved object."

As usual with Moravia, *La noia* begins with a crisis: after working for over two months on an abstract painting, Dino realizes that the medium through which he could regain contact with "external things," and thus "escape boredom," is failing him. In a moment of anger, he slashes the painting on the easel, puts a new canvas in its place (a canvas that will remain "empty" throughout the story), and relapses into boredom. In the prologue of the book, Moravia, through Dino, defines "la noia" in these words: "Boredom . . . consists in a kind of insufficiency or inadequacy, or lack of reality. . . . The feeling of boredom originates for me in a sense of the absurdity of a reality which is insufficient, or anyhow unable, to convince me of its own existence."

How does one solve this problem? By connecting with another person, by becoming involved, engaged in some way in something important, practical, meaningful—like falling in love, for example, or having an affair. The opportunity presents itself when Dino meets Cecilia, a beautiful seventeen-year-old model and former mistress of an erotic painter, Balestrieri, whose studio is next to Dino's, and who has just passed away after having made love to Cecilia, a fact that may have hastened his death. Cecilia readily acceeds to Dino's advances, and the two become lovers, but not for long, however, as their relationship turns out, to no surprise of the reader, to be almost totally devoid of any real feelings, since it is based only on their sexual needs. Cecilia has become a sex object for Dino, and is courteous, but very cold toward him. Two months later Dino is once more becoming bored: the solution is to end the relationship. He goes to his mother, asks for a tidy sum of money on the pretext that he needs a vacation, and purchases an expensive handbag to give to Cecilia as a parting gift. But here things become suddenly more complicated than anyone had anticipated: Cecilia, usually punctual, does not come to their rendezvous. By breaking a pattern in their relationship, she injects an important note of surprise and shock into her lover's life, and acquires an unexpected dimension. So long as Cecilia could be taken for granted, *noia* overtook Dino. By breaking the pattern, on the other hand, she suddenly gains the power of making Dino suffer—and suffering, as Leopardi perceived, is the opposite of *noia*. As long as Cecilia refuses to be a mere object and chooses to be an individual, unique person with desires, needs, and mind, she cannot and will not be possessed by another human being.

The next day, quite by accident, Dino sees Cecilia with another man. When she comes to the studio, later that day, pressed by Dino, she reassures him by saying that Luciani, the name of her escort, is just an unemployed actor who wants her to be in a movie with him. Not completely satisfied with her explanation, Dino pursues the matter in the days that follow until Cecilia admits, in her own inimitably innocent way, that Luciani is her lover, whom she helps with the money Dino gives her. In fact, she asks him for some money so that she and Luciani can go to the island of Ponza for a brief vacation. It is at this point that Dino understands that the only way to possess her is to marry her even though such a step would bring boredom back into his life. Cecilia rejects his proposal, made at his mother's house, as she refuses the money with which he covers her body before their lovemaking. After Cecilia's departure with her lover, Dino goes for a drive in his car and crashes it into a tree in an attempt to take his life. He survives the accident, however, and reflecting upon his experience, as he lies in his hospital bed looking at a great cedar of Lebanon outside of his window, he reaches the conclusion that from now on he will be content with contemplating Cecilia, and life as well, so as not to become bored with her. Hopefully, he will go back to painting, and to a different existence.

Most of the points of *The Empty Canvas* are not new in Moravia's novels. But this time they are both lived and discussed, and the book is both a dramatization of some of the central themes of Moravia and a commentary upon them. Sex and money, two of the most potent bourgeois instruments to control "reality" (the reality of feelings and material things), are the chief causes of contemporary alienation. Dino's mother offers her son money (in the form of an allowance that will permit him to find himself while leading the life of a bohemian painter, or in the form of a new automobile and cash for his vacations), makes sex available to him by way of Rita, the house maid whose favors are for sale, and thus makes her request to come back "home" to manage the family's estate more enticing. Dino, for his part, realizes that "we were mother and son, and the tie that held us together was not love but money," proceeds to form a similar relationship with Cecilia who, although quite poor, is not at all greedy. The implications are quite clear: sex without money is as alienating as money with which people buy sex, and neither money nor sex are really instruments of knowledge.

What about art itself? Art, and more specifically literature, is most definitely a means to impose "order" on a chaotic world. The problem of the relationship between the literary artist and the creative act is one that fascinates Moravia. In several of his novels, from *Conjugal Love* to *A Ghost at Noon*, *The Lie*, and the more recent *Two: A Phallic Novel*, the hero is a writer, an artist manqué (despite his intelligence and creativity), a man experiencing great difficulties understanding what is happening around him and, more specifically, what is happening between himself and his wife. The schism between the artist and reality being portrayed in many of Moravia's stories is connected to a metaphysical and technical problem he himself began confronting in the late forties, during his writing of *The Woman of Rome*. It was then that, after considerable reflection, he decided to abandon the third-person technique he had uniformly used in his work for the first-person type of narrative. In his essay "Note sul romanzo" ("Notes on the Novel," from *Man as an End*), he articulated the problem in these words:

> The nineteenth-century novelist had believed in the existence of a language and a reality that were common and universal; now the novelist suddenly found himself confronted with the relativism of language and reality. It is from that time that we must date the impossibility of writing novels in the third person except by disguising the autobiographical "I" in a way false to science and objectivity; and from that time, too, the novel has become "fragmentary," if by that we understand the impossibility of an unchanging relationship between the author and reality.

Unhappy with the conventional form of the novel, Moravia turned to what he called the "essay-novel," of which *The Empty Canvas* is the first example, to rejuvenate a medium no longer capable to express, in its traditional mode, his ideas about the world. He continues in his essay on the novel:

By its very nature, the nineteenth-century novel was bound to reach the point of freeing itself from plot and character, as both are superfluous and incongruous in a scientific representation of objective reality. Plot and character become difficult if not impossible as the study of surroundings and social definitions gains ground, for surroundings and social definitions reduce man to the civil register level in which everything is known, foreseen, and conventional. . . . So we should view the increasing repudiation of, and contempt for, character and plot in good literature today as the last echo of the old naturalistic-impressionistic quarrel. The novel-as-essay is bound to take up the question of plot and character where it was abandoned and provide a new solution.

L'attenzione (1965; *The Lie*, N.Y., 1966), possibly Moravia's most absorbing and intriguing novel, has a number of affinities with *The Empty Canvas*: the hero of the story, told in the first person, is Francesco Merighi who, like Dino in the previous novel, is an intellectual and an artist at odds with reality. Dino slashed the painting on the easel in an act that dramatizes his inability to "seize" reality and communicate it through his creativity; Francesco, in *The Lie*, upon reading the draft of his novel on which he had worked six months, unable to accept the "air of falseness, unreality and unauthenticity emanating from every word of the manuscript," tears the three hundred pages he has written and throws them out of the window. Ten years later, his ambition to write his novel still very much alive, he decides to keep a diary of about two months of his life which he will write during one of his visits home from his trips abroad on assignment. His diary will be a record of personal, real incidents that will serve him to interpret, adapt, and reconstruct reality, without fundamentally altering it. From such a diary, he will extract the material for his novel.

The prologue of the novel presents other details vital to an understanding of Francesco's background and the theme of the book he is to write. Francesco is a successful journalist who, in 1947, during one of his regular assignments, met and eventually married Cora Mancini, a dressmaker and the daughter of humble peasants. The manuscript he has destroyed is a sort of fictionalized account of their brief love affair which lasted from the day they first met to their marriage. Almost immediately after their wedding, however, Francesco realized that he was no longer in love with his wife. Why? As Cora explains to him, several years later, what ended his love for her was his realization that she was "a lady like all other women, and you no longer liked me and stopped loving me." What we have in *The Lie* is the pattern followed by Marcello Clerici in *The Conformist*. After having shot a man who made homosexual advances to him, and fearing that he has killed him, Marcello's sole preoccupation in life is to "become" like the others, to be "normal" in every sense of the term. Thus, he joins the Fascist party, becomes a special agent, marries a woman of a lower social class, a "normal" woman, only to discover during their wedding night that she is not a virgin (virginity being a proof of purity and goodness) and that she has lesbian tendencies. In *The Lie* there is but one avenue left to Francesco: he leaves his job with a leftist newspaper and goes to work for a conservative paper not out of changed political persuasion, but only because his new post will permit him to travel extensively and spend only a few weeks home each year, thus evading—without giving the impression of doing so—his responsibilities as a husband and stepfather to Gabriella (or Baba, as she is nicknamed), Cora's daughter by a German soldier.

During the ten years before the beginning of the story, Francesco travels constantly, writing articles that enhance his reputation, and, by agreement with Cora, he continues living in the same apartment as though their relationship was quite normal in every respect.

The function of the prologue goes beyond that of merely giving the reader the background of the events that led Francesco to the idea of keeping a diary: it sets up, as it were, the psychological, aesthetic and artistic *raison d'être* of the theme and structure of the novel we see emerge from the diary. There is, for example, and despite his disclaimers, something suspicious about Francesco's shift from a leftist to a conservative newspaper, particularly since he mentions his not having changed his political ideology, but merely having "pushed it aside," like something which, no doubt, no longer had any importance in his life—a statement that says a good deal about his values. Yet, almost in the same breath, Francesco confesses that he is ashamed of what he is, claiming on one hand that he does not know why this should be so and, on the other hand, revealing the unpleasant personal mess in which he is trapped. The sudden loss of love is, to be sure, a typical situation in Moravia's novels: his heroes are often confronted with an inability to love, or feel loved. In some cases, they willingly put aside their love for the purpose of devoting their energies to creating something which gives permanence to their name.

In *The Lie*, as in other books, the attention of the novelist is centered on the reasons for the loss of love and the price the hero must pay for it. The nature of the story is such that it receives a treatment that is decisively intellectual. Once again, this is part of the burden Moravia and his characters must bear: they think too much and feel too little, and what they feel tends to be depicted too intellectually to be a moving experience for the reader. The choice of writing a diary, too, is a decision of an intellectual nature, since it is made on the grounds that a diary is, after all, more factual and, as such, less given to the flights of fancy common in fiction. But even a diary, however objective a writer may try to be, ultimately requires a choice, consciously and at times unconsciously made, of what will or will be not included. Moreover, as the story unfolds, we are informed that the writer of the diary has taken considerable liberty with his material, some of which is invented (much as in a work of fiction) and is therefore a lie—thereby hopelessly compromising the integrity of the truthfulness of the diary. We know then that the border line between truth and fiction—the diary and the novel—has been crossed, and that we, the readers, must accept the whole thing as part of the structural apparatus of the book the narrator is writing, without his knowing where the project will take him.

The diary begins on a startling note: Francesco, just back from one of his trips abroad (to Iran, this time), returns home, feeling more like a visitor than a man who belongs there, and finds an anonymous letter informing him that his wife's dressmaking business is nothing but a façade of her house of assignation, a lucrative business which has made her financially independent. It was also Cora (as we learn when the story unfolds) who, for several months after Francesco stopped making love to her, kept him supplied with women and went as far as offering her adolescent daughter Baba to him to satisfy his sexual needs. The situation, as the reader of modern Italian literature has surely realized, is

Pirandellian. The central experience of *Six Characters in Search of An Author* revolves around a man who goes to a house of assignation and almost makes love to his stepdaughter (without realizing who she is), an experience that paves the way to a series of tragic events. But here the similarities end.

In Pirandello's work there is invariably a plea not to increase people's sufferings by accepting their desire to hide behind a mask. In Moravia's novels, the world is full of inauthentic people, performing, or acting out life not living it, passively accepting the roles society has imposed upon them. Their inauthenticity ultimately is rooted in their value system: corruption, of one sort or another, breeds corruption. Francesco's intellectualism and immaturity led him to marry Cora, in the hope that by marrying a woman of the people he could reject the values of his middle-class background and achieve genuineness. He becomes deaf to love and is driven by the excitement of a possible liaison with his stepdaughter, with whom he thinks he has fallen in love. Cora's money, derived mostly from her illicit trading in human flesh, corrupts her family: once simple peasants, they are now crass business people who have accepted the materialistic system of the middle class. Deception and duplicity abound in the novel: the wife of Consolo (Francesco's new editor at the newspaper) makes advances to Francesco, as does Popi, the mistress of his brother Massimiliano, a well-to-do stockbroker who plans on getting rid of her, as one does an automobile two or three years old.

The events of the story of the book are relatively few and not terribly interesting. Indeed, one might say that the real center of attention of *The Lie* is not its hero or heroine, but the novel itself. In this respect, the diary soon turns into something larger and more vibrant than a mere record of two months of Francesco's life. It begins to incorporate its writer's drafts of his "work in progress," the eventual chapters of the novel he will write, and some discussions at the theoretical and structural level of the validity of the "invented" parts of the story in the guise of dialogues or ruminations between Francesco the man and Francesco the novelist. The line separating reality from fiction, or truth from falsehood, becomes increasingly more blurred to the point that we no longer can tell one from the other.

This, of course, is part of the strategy of the narrator-novelist-protagonist, whose diary ultimately becomes the story of the novel (the "novel's novel," as it were), in a manner somewhat reminiscent of Gide's *Les Faux-Monnayeurs* (1926; *The Counterfeiters*, N.Y., 1951). Life is artificial, or inauthentic: art (and, more specifically, the novel) supposedly mirroring life, cannot therefore be anything else but artificial. In a manner calculated to remind us of *The Empty Canvas* and of Dino's special predicament, Francesco strives to write "a novel without a story, without a series of events, without drama, a novel in which nothing happens." The goal is akin to Dino's possession through contemplation. With a difference, however: a novel, whether disguised as a diary or anything else, has to be written, it cannot be merely contemplated. At the risk of losing much of its purity and perfection, and its "authenticity," it cannot be held within a writer's head: it must be committed to the printed page. The choice of the device of the diary becomes clear: not having to depend on a plot, or "action," of a novel, it comes closest to that idea of "noninvolvement," or lack of action, through which the artist's thought can best be transmitted.

The end of the novel not only ties up, in a manner of sorts, several loose threads, but it provides us with the key to the structure of the work. The entry dated "Tuesday, December 15," reports a conversation between Francesco and Baba, in the course of which we learn that six years before Baba had been taken by her mother to her villa for the specific purpose of offering her to Francesco. When he arrived, Baba had in fact recognized him by catching a glimpse of his face in the mirror in front of the divan on which she was seated waiting for him, her shoulders turned to the wall. Francesco had left the house of assignation in a hurry, but had always regretted the fact that he had failed to confront Cora and take her to task for manipulating her daughter as an object, a means to keep him as her husband, in name if not in fact.

It is this incident in particular that caused Francesco to have shame of his past, a shame he feels at the beginning of the book (in the prologue) but the reasons for which he professes to ignore —momentarily, at least. The last entry in the diary (dated two days later) is written five hours before his departure for the United States. Cora's house of assignation has been raided by the police, and she herself is gravely ill with what was thought to be tuberculosis, but is really cancer of the lungs, from which she will die.

Francesco declares that the meeting with Baba described in the previous entry and his confession never took place, nor did all the things which he said he had done. But this proves to be one of the two alternatives that are open to him: the other one insists that the conversation with Baba really did take place exactly as it appears in the penultimate entry in the diary. But the most important part of it all is that writing the diary has served the narrator to deepen his experience of life, while at the same time, as a novelist, he has faced the problem of representing both his guilt and of his sense of guilt.

The brief epilogue tells of Francesco's return to Rome from the United States after he learns that his wife is dying. He arrives in time for the funeral, meets and says good-bye to Baba, whose marriage to a student is imminent, rereads his diary and realizes that its substance (the record of the events of the two months at home and his observations on the problem of the novel) is hardly suited as material for the novel he wanted to write. He concludes that there is nothing that could be said to constitute the structure of a narrative work. Yet, he also perceives that he has completed not so much a novel in the conventional sense of the term, with characters and action and a plot, but the story of a novel, or, more exactly, the "story of the novel I intended to write." For this reason, Francesco decides to publish his diary which, appropriately enough, will be entitled *L'attenzione*.

In the concluding remarks of his essay on Moravia, Luciano Rebay wrote: "Certainly with *La noia* and *L'attenzione* Moravia has reached an extreme limit in his development as a novelist, and he is well aware of it." The history of criticism of Moravia shows that with practically every work he has published he has compelled his readers (the present one included) to wonder about the direction of his art and his ability to pursue a productive course. Not everyone has been particularly impressed by or satisfied with the results. Olga Ragusa, for example, in a perceptive overview of Moravia's fiction, has chosen to make his "voyeurism" the "point" that may provide the key to his fiction. (I should add here that R. W. B. Lewis in his "Eros and Existence" was the first to suggest what has become lately both a motif and a strategy, if not, as I personally believe, a fundamental flaw in Moravia's art.) Ragusa's conclusion is hardly positive: "Moravia has by and large been unable to renew himself"; "his work which is traditional in structure and unimaginative in language will never benefit from the prestige-given attention of 'close' reading."

Io e lui (1971, literally "He and I," translated as *Two: A Phallic Novel*, N.Y., 1972) has confirmed the critics' misapprehensions if not necessarily their harsh judgment of Moravia's art. Four years in the writing, *Two*, with its many flaws, may well be considered the inevitable conclusion of Moravia's previous essay-novels, *The Empty Canvas* and *The Lie*. Structurally and thematically, its links with the two novels are both numerous and apparent.

The story is told in the first person by the protagonist Federico (or Rico, as he is called throughout the book), a thirty-five-year-old screenwriter, whose lifelong ambition is to direct a film. He hopes to accomplish his goal just as soon as the script on which he has been working with a young revolutionary by the name of Fabrizio is completed. The title of the film is to be *L'espropriazione* [Expropriation]. Rico's personal life is a mess: feeling "desublimated" or "underneath," two terms that recur *ad nauseam* in the novel, he has been separated for the last six months from his wife Fausta, formerly a prostitute, and their son, Cesarino. His professional relationship with his collaborator Maurizio is equally strained, not to say disastrous, and Rico is experiencing serious problems with the ideological and practical sides of his project. Protti, who is supposed to be the film producer, is not entirely pleased with the creative treatment of the script, while Maurizio insists that the film's theme be dealt in a manner that addresses itself more clearly to the "political" resolution of the story.

In addition, Maurizio insists that only by contributing five million lire to the radical left revolutionary group whose activities are the substance of the screenplay will Rico be able to be assured the job of director. The generous contribution, he claims, will persuade the group that Rico has given up his bourgeois values, and has espoused the stance of the revolutionaries. Although Rico disagrees strongly on this point, so great is his ambition to direct the film that he agrees to make the necessary contribution and change the ending of the film to suit the ideological premises of Maurizio, and his Maoist girlfriend Flavia, the daughter of the producer Protti.

He also agrees to take part in a dialogue with the revolutionary group during which he will publicly renounce his ideological values and a session of self-criticism while the audience's response is controlled by the colors green, orange, or red flashed by something that looks like a traffic light. The session, effectively described in what are probably the best pages of the novel, turns out to be a demeaning, humiliating, and unproductive experience for Rico. Frustrated by the adverse reaction of the group, he decides to give up the project altogether and let the revolutionary group keep the contribution he made to assure himself of their approval and Maurizio's cooperation in the future. The end of the book ends on a more positive note. Rico and Maurizio agree, after all, to make the film that cost so much anguish, but not before Rico tries to seduce Protti's aging wife, Malfana, a star of the silent movies who has been in retirement for a long time (the seduction fails to come off because "he" refuses to cooperate) and attempts to set fire to the villa, during a party given while Protti is away on business.

These are the main incidents of the story, which includes a rather bizarre affair between Rico and Irene, an attractive divorcée who works as a secretary in one of the Arab diplomatic missions, and whom Rico has met at the bank and has followed, and then driven home. Disappointed by her experiences with her former husband, Irene tells Rico that she has turned to masturbation, ritually performed in front of a mirror in her bedroom, to satisfy her sex needs without fearing failure since the act requires no other participant. Rico thinks he has fallen in love with Irene, despite the fact that he has received no encouragement from her, and almost decides to live with her and her daughter Virginia on her terms. After spending one night in her bed, however, and having experienced an unhealthy attraction to her child, afraid of being unable to curb his strange feelings and, at the same time, not happy with the kind of relationship that looms ahead, he has a change of heart and goes back to his wife Fausta, literally dragged by "him" who has now become Rico's true master.

Two is an overlong (the Italian edition is over four hundred pages), repetitive, belabored book. Written in the erotic-satyrical tradition that spans from Petronius's *Satyricon* to Philip Roth's *Portnoy's Complaint* and Gore Vidal's *Myra Breckinridge*, it only rarely succeeds in being comical and in evoking real laughter. The insistence on the unusual size of Rico's genitals (to which he gives the name of Federicus Rex, with its rather obvious implications) after a while loses the spontaneity necessary in comic situations: the confrontations between "he" (Rico) and "the Other" (his penis) soon become tedious and monotonous. And several passages of the book are downright tasteless to say the least, as are the frequent discussions of Federico's "desublimation." This is not meant to slight those parts of the novel that are felicitous and at once stimulating and enjoyable: the vivacity of certain episodes, particularly those that seem to have been inspired by Moravia's own confrontations with the young Turks of the self-styled Gruppo 63, and the programmed response of the young radicals called to witness Rico's recantation, are quite successful and are fine examples of the novelist's humor and irony.

What is wrong with the book—the central flaw as it were—is intimately connected with the basic void in Moravia's vision: and that void, as anyone who has followed his career knows, is the absence of love. Not sexual, or lustful, or unconventional love, which is found in varying quantities in Moravia's *oeuvre*, beginning with his sadistic, insipid short stories "Tired Courtesan" and "Crime at the Tennis Club" (both dating back to the mid-twenties), and his first novel, *Gli indifferenti*, to his most recent *Two*, but love that is goodness, generosity, compassion, understanding. Without such love, no real, meaningful communication between two human beings can take place. In the last analysis, as Olga Ragusa noted, Moravia's characters, by and large, remain content with seeing without feeling, a stance that yields only voyeurism, the act of looking at a sexual experience without participating in it: looking, therefore, for the mere sake of looking, with no joy or pleasure.

What of Moravia's accomplishments? There is no doubt that, probably more than any other living Italian writer, Moravia must be given credit for putting the Italian novel back on the international cultural map. His books, whatever their flaws, have proved to be not merely reflections of the character of Italian society, but effective dramatizations of the existential preoccupations of most nations of the Western world. Throughout fifty years of literary activity—a record not easy to match—the author has shown a steady, disciplined effort to be at once thematically consistent and willing to experiment, if only to a limited degree, with new concepts. He has moved from his first novel, *The Time of Indiffer-*

ence, conceived much like a play, to the concept of the novel-within-a-novel of *The Lie*. While some readers have expressed reservations about the attention sex has received in his books, few have denied Moravia's gift for keeping his reader's interest high, thanks to his directness of approach and simplicity of style in a country where literature has traditionally been written for a cultural elite.

Several years ago, after the publication of *Two Women*, I expressed the hope that Moravia would continue to pursue the path traced by the moving story of Cesira and Rosetta, move on to higher perspectives so as to broaden his vision and give us new, deeper understanding of life by throwing new light on other sides of the human experience. The books Moravia has written since that time have not fulfilled such expectations. And thus, a judgment of his *oeuvre* remains, for the time being, mixed. On the basis of his work to date, it would be unreasonable and unrealistic to expect many surprises from our subject, who reached his peak in the early sixties. Nonetheless, even if his "work in progress" should not add substantially to his *vision du monde*, we should be grateful for the many novels (and short stories) he has written, for they have enriched the quality of imaginative writing in Italy and our perceptions of contemporary existence.

Selected Bibliography

General Works on Italian Literature

Apollonio, Mario. *I contemporanei*. New rev. ed. Milan: La Scuola, 1970.
Astaldi, Maria Luisa. *Nascita e vicende del romanzo italiano*. Milan: Garzanti, 1939.
Baldacci, Luigi. *Letteratura e verità*. Milan: Ricciardi, 1968.
Barberi-Squarotti, Cesare. *La narrativa italiana del dopoguerra*. Milan: Cappelli, 1965.
Barilli, Renato. *La barriera del Naturalismo*. Milan: Mursia, 1964.
Bertacchini, Renato. *Figure e problemi di narrativa contemporanea*. Bologna: Cappelli, 1961.
Bo, Carlo. *Riflessioni critiche*. Florence: Sansoni, 1953.
Cecchi, Emilio. *Letteratura italiana del Novecento*. 2 vols. Ed. by Pietro Citati. Milan: Mondadori, 1971.
———, and Sapegno, Natalino, eds. *Storia della letteratura italiana*. Vol. 9. *Il Novecento*. Milan: Garzanti, 1969.
Contini, Gianfranco. *La letteratura dell'Italia unita: 1861–1968*. Florence: Sansoni, 1968.
David, Michel. *La psicanalisi nella cultura italiana*. Turin: Borlinghieri, 1966.
De Michelis, Euralio. *Narratori al quadrato*. Pisa: Nistri-Lischi, 1962.
———. *Narratori antinarratori*. Florence: La Nuova Italia, 1972.
De Robertis, Giuseppe. *Altro Novecento*. Florence: Le Monnier, 1962.

————. *Scrittori del Novecento*. Florence: Le Monnier, 1940.

De Tommaso, Pietro. *Narratori italiani contemporanei*. Rome: Ateneo, 1965.

Falqui, Enrico. *La letteratura del ventennio nero*. Rome: La Bussola, 1948.

————. *Novecento letterario*. Ser. 1–8. Florence: Vallecchi, 1954–66.

————. *Prosatori e narratori del Novecento italiano*. Turin: Einaudi, 1950.

————. *Tra racconti e romanzi del Novecento*. Messina: D'Anna, 1950.

Fernandez, Dominique. *Il romanzo italiano e la crisi della coscienza moderna*. Milan: Lerici, 1960.

Ferretti, Gian Carlo. *La letteratura del rifiuto*. Milan: Mursia, 1960.

————. *Letteratura e ideologia*. Milan: Feltrinelli, 1954.

Forni, Mizzau M. *Tecniche narrative e romanzo contemporaneo*. Milan: Mursia, 1965.

Gadda, Carlo Emilio. *I viaggi la morte*. Milan: Garzanti, 1958.

Gargiulo, Alfredo. *Letteratura italiana del novecento*. Florence: Le Monnier, 1958.

Guarnieri, Silvio. *Cinquant'anni di letteratura italiana*. Florence: Parenti, 1955.

————. *Condizione della letteratura*. Rome: Edit. Riuniti, 1975.

Guidotti, Mario. *Lo scrittore disintegrato*. Florence: Vallecchi, 1961.

Heiney, Donald. *America in Modern Italian Literature*. New Brunswick, N.J.: Rutgers University Press, 1964.

Lombardi, Olga. *La giovane narrativa*. Pisa: Nistri-Lischi, 1963.

————. *Narrativa italiana nelle crisi del novecento*. Rome: Sciascia, 1971.

Manacorda, Giuliano. *Storia della letteratura italiana contemporanea: 1940–1965*. Rome: Edit. Riuniti, 1974.

————. *Vent'anni di pazienza. Saggi sulla letteratura italiana contemporanea*. Rome: Edit. Riuniti, 1975.

Mauro, Walter. *Cultura e società nella letteratura italiana*. Rome: Ateneo, 1964.

————. *Realtà mito e favola nella narrativa italiana del novecento*. Milan: Sugar, 1974.

Muscetta, Carlo. *Realismo e controrealismo*. Milan: Del Duca, 1958.

Pacifici, Sergio. *A Guide to Contemporary Italian Literature: From Futurism to Neorealism*. Carbondale: Southern Illinois University Press, 1972.

————. *The Modern Italian Novel: From Capuana to Tozzi*. Carbondale: Southern Illinois University Press, 1972.

————. *The Modern Italian Novel: From Manzoni to Svevo*. Carbondale: Southern Illinois University Press, 1967.

————, ed. *From Verismo to Experimentalism: Essays on the Modern Italian Novel*. Bloomington: Indiana University Press, 1969.

Pancrazi, Pietro. *Ragguagli di Parnaso*. Vols. 2–3. Milan: Ricciardi, 1967.

Personé, Luigi. *Scrittori italiani contemporanei*. Florence: Olschki, 1968.

Petronio, Giuseppe, and Martinelli, Luciana. *Il Novecento Letterario in Italia*. Vols. 2, 3. Palermo: Palumbo, 1974, 1975.

Pomilio, Mario. *Contestazioni*. Milan: Rizzoli, 1967.

Pullini, Giorgio. *Il romanzo italiano del dopoguerra: 1940–1960*. Milan: Schwarz, 1961.

————. *Volti e risvolti del romanzo italiano contemporaneo*. Milan: Mursia, 1967.

Rosa, Alberto Asor. *Scrittori e popolo*. Rome: Samona & Savelli, 1964.

Russo, Luigi. *I Narratori (1850–1957)*. Milan: Principato, 1958.

Salinari, Carlo. *La questione del realismo*. Florence: Parenti, 1960.

————. *Preludio e fine del realismo*. Naples: Morano, 1967.

Scaramucci, Ines. *Romanzi del nostro tempo*. Milan: La Scuola, 1956.

Solmi, Sergio. *Scrittori negli anni*. Milan: Il Saggiatore, 1963.

Varese, Claudio. *Cultura letteraria contemporanea*. Pisa: Nistri-Lischi, 1951.

Venè, Gian Franco. *Letteratura e capitalismo in Italia dal '700 ad oggi*. Milan: Sugar, 1963.

Reference Works

Dizionario critico della letteratura italiana. 3 vols. Turin:
    UTET, 1973. Milan: Mondadori, 1959.
Dizionario enciclopedico della letteratura italiana. Bari: Laterza
    & UNEDI, 1966.

Selected References

The following is a highly selective list of essays and books which
I found to be particularly helpful and stimulating in the course
of writing this book. In view of the fact that this study has been
prepared for the English-speaking student of Italian letters, special
care has been taken to include whenever possible the best critical
material in English. In some cases, certain titles have been listed,
for the sake of convenience, in a shortened version. Complete
information pertaining to such works will be found in the Selected
Bibliography. The following abbreviations have been used:

FI   *Forum Italicum*
IQ   *Italian Quarterly*
Ital.   *Italica*
LIC   *Letteratura italiana: I contemporanei*. Vols. 1, 2, 3.
              Milan: Marzorati, 1963–69.
LICr   *Letteratura italiana: Le correnti*. Vol. 2. Milan: Mar-
              zorati, 1956.
MLN   *Modern Language Notes*
SdLI   *Storia della letteratura italiana*. Vol. 9. *Il Novecento*.
              Ed. by Emilio Cecchi and Natalino Sapegno.

BACKGROUND OF THE MODERN ITALIAN NOVEL

There is an abundance of material in both English and Italian
on the purely historical situation in Italy from the end of the last
century to the Second World War. In English, one might begin
with a brief, but lucid account by Massimo Salvadori, *Italy*
(Englewood Cliffs, N.J.: Prentice-Hall, Inc., 1965) and Salvatore
Saladino's *Italy from Unification to 1919* (N.Y.: Thomas Y.

Crowell, 1970). Denis Mack Smith's *Italy: A Modern History* is still the best and deepest treatment of the subject. Edward T. Tannenbaum's *The Fascist Experience: Italian Society and Culture, 1922–1945* (N.Y.: Basic Books, 1972) is an ambitious and, on the whole, comprehensive analysis, whose major flaw is the absence of a satisfactory bibliographical apparatus. In Italian, Luigi Salvatorelli and G. Mira, *Storia d'Italia nel periodo fascista* (Turin: Einaudi, 1964) is quite satisfactory; Ruggero Zangrandi's *Il lungo viaggio attraverso il fascismo* (Milan: Feltrinelli, 1962), is indeed, as the subtitle promises, "a contribution to the history of a generation" brought up under Fascist rule. Among the works focusing on the relationships between history and culture, Eugenio Garin's *La cultura italiana tra '800 e '900* (Bari: Laterza, 1963) is a wise, philosophical study of the period; Giuseppe Petronio's and Luciana Martinelli's *Novecento letterario in Italia*, vols. 1–3 (Palermo: Palumbo, 1975) are enlightening, as are the perceptive notes and articles by Elio Vittorini collected in *Diario in pubblico* (Milan: Bompiani, 1970).

For a more thorough understanding of the role played by Italian reviews in contemporary Italian writing, the following should be of particular interest: Augusto Hermet, *La ventura delle riviste* (Florence: Vallecchi, 1941); Riccardo Scrivano, "Da *La Ronda* a *Solaria*," in *Riviste, scrittori e critici del Novecento* (Florence: Sansoni, 1965); Sergio Pacifici, "The Reviews," in his *A Guide to Contemporary Italian Literature: From Futurism to Neorealism* (Carbondale: Southern Illinois University Press, 1972), pp. 270–92, still the only recent comprehensive survey in English of the Italian literary scene between 1910 and 1962.

Other helpful treatments (in English) of the contemporary Italian novel are: Paul West's "Italy," in his volume *The Modern Novel* (N.Y.: Hillary House, 1967) vol. 2, pp. 354–82; Louis Tenenbaum's "The Italian Novel: Traditions and New Paths," in *Contemporary European Novelists*, ed. by Siegfried Mandel (Carbondale: Southern Illinois University Press, 1968), pp. 126–57; Dante Della Terza, "The Neorealists and the Form of the Novel," *IQ* 10 (1966): 3–20 and "Italian Fiction from Pavese to Pasolini," *IQ* 3, no. 11 (1959): 29–41; Italo Calvino, "Main Currents in Italian Fiction Today," *IQ* 4, nos. 13–14 (1950): 3–14; Frank Rosengarten, "The Italian Resistance Novel: 1945–1962," in Pacifici, ed., *From Verismo to Experimentalism*, pp.

212–38; Sergio Pacifici, "From Engagement to Alienation: A View of the Contemporary Italian Novel," *Ital*. 40, no. 3 (1964): 236–58.

For a more thorough understanding of literary developments of recent years the following studies are particularly valuable: Carlo Bo, *Inchiesta sul neorealismo* (Turin: RAI, 1951); Silvio Guarnieri, *Cinquant'anni di narrativa in Italia* (Florence: Parenti, 1950); Carlo Salinari, *La questione del realismo* (Florence: Parenti, 1960); Cesare Barberi Squarrotti, *La narrativa italiana del dopoguerra* (Bologna: Cappelli, 1965); Giorgio Pullini, *Il romanzo italiano del dopoguerra* (Milan: Schwarz, 1961); Giuliano Manacorda *Storia della letteratura italiana: 1940–1965* (Rome: Edit. Riuniti, 1975); Norberto Bobbio's long essay, "Profilo ideologico del Novecento," in *Storia della letteratura italiana*, vol. 9, ed. by Emilio Cecchi and Natalino Sapegno (Milan: Garzanti, 1969), pp. 121–230, is fundamental to a study of the period; and Dominique Fernandez's *Il romanzo italiano e la crisi della coscienza moderna* (Milan: Lerici, 1960). The overview by Sergio Antonelli, "Dal Decadentismo al Neorealismo," *LICr*, pp. 897–936, is clear and useful. For the "Problema del Mezzogiorno," see the bibliographical notes on Alvaro, Brancati, and Lampedusa. For the literature of the Underground, the reader should turn to Angelo Paoluzi, *La letteratura della Resistenza* (Rome: 5 Lune, 1956), and the essay by Raffaele Crovi, "Meridione e letteratura," in *Menabò*, vol. 3 (Turin: Einaudi, 1960), pp. 267–302). Finally, no reader should neglect two excellent studies from a nonliterary point of view: Gian Franco Vene's *Letteratura e capitalismo in Italia dal '700 ad oggi* (Milan: Sugar, 1963), and Michel David's *La psicanalisi nella cultura italiana* (Turin: Borlinghieri, 1966).

ENRICO PEA

Pea's popularity seems to have reached its peak in the forties, as attested by the critical attention received by his work, particularly two book-length assessments, Umberto Olobardi's *Saggi su Tozzi e Pea* (Pisa: Vallerini, 1940) and Aldo Borlenghi's *E. P.* (Padova: CEDAM, 1943). More recently, Ernesto Travi has written a long study, *Umanità di E. P.* (Milan: Vita e Pensiero, 1965) concentrating on the spiritual and religious aspect of Pea's work.

In addition to the many reviews and notices listed in Travi's monographic study, there are a number of long, highly intelligent, and serious essays on Pea: Eurialo De Michelis's *Narratori antinarratori* (Florence: La Nuova Italia, 1952), pp. 1–30; Giuseppe A. Peritore's "In margine al 'romanzo breve' di E. P.," in *Belfagor* 6 (1972): 660–77; Felice Del Beccaro's "E. P.," *Belfagor* 9, no. 1 (1954): 46–61; Silvio Guarnieri's "E. P.," in *Cinquant'anni di narrativa in Italia* (Florence: Parenti, 1955), pp. 485–541; and Mario Alicata's "Motivi di E. P.," in *Scritti letterari* (Milan: Il Saggiatore, 1968), pp. 168–85. Aldo Borlenghi's "E. P.," in *LIC*, vol. 1, pp. 377–96, is a clear survey of the development of Pea as a writer, while Carlo Bo's "Torniamo a P.," *L'approdo letterario* 15, no. 47 (1969): 29–46, is a sensitive discussion of, among other things, the influence of the Bible on the poetry, theatre, and narrative of Pea.

The magazine *Rassegna Lucchese*, no. 7, 1951, devoted an entire issue to Pea, with articles, notes, and tributes by Ungaretti, Piccioni, Binni, Borlenghi, and others. See also works by Cecchi, De Robertis, Russo, Pancrazi, as cited in "General Works on Italian Literature."

BRUNO CICOGNANI

Short, useful reviews of Cicognani's work may be found in Russo, De Robertis, Cecchi, Gargiulo, and Falqui, as cited in "General Works on Italian Literature." Among the more sustained critical overviews, the following are particularly useful: Luigi Baldacci, "B. C." in *Letteratura e verità* (Milan: Ricciardi, 1968), pp. 129–41; Luigi M. Personè, *Scrittori italiani moderni e contemporanei* (Florence: Olschki, 1968), pp. 183–203; and Personè's commemorative piece "B. C. grande narratore," *L'osservatore politico e letterario* 18, no. 1 (1972): 35–46; Silvio Guarnieri, *Cinquant'anni di narrativa in Italia* (Florence: Parenti, 1955), pp. 218–27. On the more personal side, there are two articles the reader may find interesting for the light they cast on Cicognani the man: Armando Meoni, "Ricordo di B. C.,"

Nuova Antologia (1972), pp. 45–51; and Cesare A. Padovani, "La difficile amicizia di B. C.," *L'osservatore politico e letterario* 18, no. 1 (1972): 35–46. The essay by Piero Rebora, "B. C." in *LIC*, vol. 1, pp. 279–90, is disappointingly short, Domenico Mondrone, S.I., devotes several pages to Cicognani in his *Scrittori al traguardo*, 3d ed. (Rome: La Civiltà Cattolica, 1947), vol. 1, pp. 35–86. Among the less recent estimates, see Giuseppe Ravegnani's *I Contemporanei* (Turin: Bocca, 1930), pp. 225–32, "Le figurine di c."; and Thomas G. Bergin's "B. C.," *Ital.* 19, no. 1 (1942): 22–25.

ALDO PALAZZESCHI

There are two important monographs on Palazzeschi, one by Giorgio Pullini, generous, traditional in its positive evaluation of his subject (*A. P.* [Milan: Mursia, 1972]), the other, by Mario Miccinesi (*A. P.* [Florence: La Nuova Italia, 1972]), far more critical of the quality and achievement of Palazzeschi. Among the general surveys, Aldo Borlenghi's "A. P." in *LIC*, vol. 1, pp. 625–48, and Luigi M. Personè's "A. P.," in *Scrittori italiani moderni e contemporanei* (Florence: Okschki, 1968), pp. 205–29, and Giorgio Pullini's "Gli ottant'anni di A. P.," in *Volti e risvolti del romanzo italiano contemporaneo* (Milan: Mursia, 1971), pp. 50–57, are instructive. Other useful essays include: Silvio Guarnieri, "A. P.," in *Cinquant'anni di narrativa in Italia* (Florence: Parenti, 1955), pp. 325–45; Carlo Bo, "P.," in *L'eredità del Leopardi* (Florence: Parenti, 1964), pp. 183–203; Lanfranco Orsini, "La parabola di P.," in *La cantina di Auerbach* (Naples: ESI, 1971), pp. 59–95; Luigi Baldacci's harsh but intelligent "A. P.," in *Letteratura e verità* (Milan: Ricciardi, 1963), pp. 142–69; Claudio Marabini's "A. P.," in *Gli anni sessanta: narrativa e storia* (Milan: Rizzoli, 1969), pp. 135–66, concentrates on post–World War II Palazzeschi; Sergio Solmi's "P. poeta e romanziere," in *Scrittori negli anni* (Milan: Il Saggiatore, 1963), pp. 153–62. The magazine *Galleria* 24 (1974) with contributions by numerous critics (Baldacci, De Michelis, Pullini, and others) and writers (Quasimodo, Betocchi, P. P. Pasolini, and others) is dedicated to Palazzeschi on the occasion of his ninetieth birthday.

In English, there are G. Singh's "A. P.," in Pacifici, ed., *From Verismo to Experimentalism*, pp. 81–101, and Thomas G. Bergin's "The Enjoyable Horrendous World of A. P." *Books Abroad* 46, no. 1 (1972): 55–60. See also: Russo, Cecchi, De Robertis, Gargiulo, Pancrazi, Falqui, as cited in "General Works on Italian Literature."

CORRADO ALVARO

Judging from the amount of critical material on Alvaro, it is undeniable that he remains, two decades after his passing, one of the most respected and esteemed of contemporary novelists. Among the many monographs on his work, Luigi Reina's *Cultura e storia di C. A.* (Naples: Guida, 1973), A. Balduino's *C. A.* (Milan: Mursia, 1965), and Domenico Cara's sensitive monograph *C. A.* (Florence: La Nuova Italia, 1974), are intelligent and thorough. Vincenzo Paladino's *L'opera di C. A.* (Florence: Le Monnier, 1968), although not profound, commends itself for its simplicity, as does Walter Mauro's *Invito alla lettura di C. A.* (Milan: Mursia, 1973). Mauro's interest in Italian literature and culture of the South produced a volume, *Cultura e società nella narrativa meridionale* (Rome: Ediz. dell'Ateneo, 1965), that contains several perceptive pages on Alvaro. Raffaele Crovi's essay, "Meridione e Letteratura," in *Il menabò* (Turin: Einaudi, 1960), vol. 3, pp. 267–303, is pretty much required reading on the South and the novel in our day. Giuliano Manacorda's piece on A., previously published in the Marxist magazine *Società* (1954), may be read in Luigi Russo's *I Narratori: 1850–1957* (Milan: Principato, 1958), pp. 286–304. Other useful and perceptive insights on A. may be found in Carlo Salinari's *Preludio e fine del realismo in Italia* (Naples: Morano, 1967), pp. 100–105; Riccardo Scrivano, "C. A." *LIC*, vol. 2, pp. 1093–1111; A. Mele, "Crisi della società in A.," in *Sei narratori del novecento* (Naples: I.E.M., 1971), pp. 45–81; Michele Prisco, "A. e il personaggio," *La ragioni narrative* 1, no. 2 (1960): 74–90. See also Cecchi, Barberi-Squarotti, and Falqui, as cited in "General Works on Italian Literature."

VITALIANO BRANCATI

There are two monographs on the work of Brancati: Enzo Lauretta's informative *Invito alla lettura di Brancati* (Milan: Mursia, 1973); and the subtle and academically correct study by Vanna Gazzola Stacchini, *La narrativa di V. B.* (Florence: Olschki, 1970), with an ample bibliography. The following essays contain many insights into the narrative work of Brancati: Piero de Tommaso, "V. B.," in *Narratori italiani contemporanei* (Rome: Ateneo, 1965), pp. 37–58; Livia Jannuzzi, "V. B.," in *LIC*, vol. 3, pp. 1413–28; Mario Pomilio, "Situazione di B." (originally published with the title "La doppia crisi di B.," *Ragioni narrative* 1, no. 1 (1960): 68–99), in *Contestazioni* (Milan: Rizzoli, 1967), pp. 9–33; Mario Alicata, "V. B. I–II," in *Scritti letterari* (Milan: Il Saggiatore, 1968), pp. 154–64; and Giuseppe Peritore, "Punti di vista sulla narrativa di V. B.," *Belfagor* 26, no. 2 (1972): 273–89. The December 1955 issue of *Galleria* is completely dedicated to Brancati, and contains essays by Emilio Cecchi ("Comicità e mestizia di B."), Arnoldo Bocelli ("La narrativa di B."), and Alberto Moravia ("Il destino di B."). In addition, the volumes by Cecchi, De Robertis, Falqui, Pullini, as cited in "General Works on Italian Literature," should be consulted. In English, there are Robert S. Dombrowski, "Brancati and Fascism: A Profile," *IQ* 13, no. 49 (1969): 41–63; Louis Tenenbaum's articles "V. B. and Sicilian Eroticism," *Books Abroad* 31, no. 3 (1957): 223–36, and "V. B. 1907–1954," *Cesare Barbieri Courier* 7, no. 1 (1964): 3–10 (with a translation into English of the first chapter of *Don Giovanni in Sicilia*); and Claire L. Huffman's perceptive "V. B.: A Reassessment," *FI* 6, no. 3 (1972): 697–714.

GIUSEPPE TOMASI DI LAMPEDUSA

In the light of its extraordinary success, it is not surprising that the bibliography on *The Leopard* and its author should be unusually large and stimulating. From the biographical point of view, Francesco Orlando's precious slim book, *Ricordo di Lampedusa* (Milan: Scheiwiller, 1965) is indispensable. There are two monographs on L. well worth reading: Giancarlo Buzzi's *Invito alla lettura di G. T. di L.* (Milan: Mursia, 1972–73), and Simonetta Silvestroni's *G. T. di L.* (Florence: La Nuova Italia, 1973). Giorgio Bassani's introductory essay to the original edition of *The Leopard* is required reading. Of the numerous interpretations of the quality and meaning of *The Leopard* published shortly after the appearance of the novel, Giuseppe De Rosa's *"Il Gattopardo," Civiltà Cattolica*, April 8, 1959, pp. 169–82, Mario Alicata's "Il principe di L. e il Risorgimento siciliano," in *Scritti letterari* (Milan: Il Saggiatore, 1968), pp. 337–53, and Elio Vittorini's "Impariamo a conoscere gli scrittori italiani," *Il Giorno*, February 24 and March 12, 1959, may be said to represent the spectrum of political-literary views on the novel by Lampedusa. The question of Sicily in the novel is the subject of a penetrating analysis by Leonardo Sciascia (himself an excellent novelist) in *"Il Gattopardo,"* in *Pirandello e la Sicilia* (Caltanisetta: Sciascia, 1961), pp. 147–60. Other critical essays worthy of attention are: Luigi Russo's "Analisi del *Gattopardo," Belfagor* 14, no. 5 (1960): 513–30; Gualtiero Todini's "T. di L.," *Belfagor* 25, no. 2 (1960): 163–84; Furio Felcini's piece, "G. T. di L.," in *LIC*, vol. 3, pp. 249–66, is a good overview of Lampedusa. In English, there are several superb critical pieces: David Nolan, "Lampedusa," in *Irish Studies* (1966), pp. 403–14; Jeffrey Meyers, "Symbol and Structure in *The Leopard," IQ* 9, nos. 34–35 (1965): 50–70; Archibald Colquhoun, "A Note by the Translator," *Two Stories and a Memory*, by G. T. di L. (New York: Pantheon Books, 1962), pp. 19–39. A persuasive interpretation in psychological-philosophical key is offered by Richard F. Kuhns, "Modernity and Death," in *Contemporary Psychoanalysis* 5, no. 2 (1969): 95–119; John Gilbert's "The Metamorphosis of the Gods," in *MLN* 81, no. 1 (1966): 22–31, is absorbing, as is Stanley G. Eskin's piece "Animal Imagery in *Il Gattopardo," Ital.* 39, no. 3 (1962): 189–96. Of special importance in the debate on Lampedusa, particularly with respect to his connection with Stendhal, is Louis Aragon's celebrated piece *"Le Guépard* et la *Chartreuse," Les Lettres francaises*, 18–24 February 1960, pp. 1, 8. Olga Ragusa's piece on "Stendhal, Tomasi di Lampedusa, and the Novel" (now collected in *Narrative and Drama: Essays in Modern Italian Literature from Verga to Pasolini.* [The Hague and Paris: Mouton, 1976], pp. 1–34) goes well beyond the fascinating aspects of the two writers into structural observations of unquestionable validity. Her excellent survey of Lampedusa is followed by a highly selected bibliography of criticism in Italian, French, and English.

DINO BUZZATI

While Buzzati enjoyed wide popular interest and success, the critics have not always been too generous in their evaluation of his work. Two monographic studies, Fausto Gianfreschini's *D. B.* (Turin: Borla, 1966) and Antonia Veronese Arslan's *Invito alla lettura di D. B.* (Milan: Mursia, 1974) go a long way toward justifying a favorable critical evaluation. Luigi Persone's essay "D. B." (*Scrittori italiani moderni e contemporanei* [Florence: Olschki, 1968], pp. 271–88) is a perceptive interpretation of Buzzati's work published shortly before his death and concentrating on his earlier books. Claudio Marabini's "D. B." (*Gli anni sessanta: Narrativa e storia* [Turin: Rizzoli, 1966], pp. 113–24), also focuses on Buzzati's later fiction. For earlier estimates, see Pietro Pancrazi, *Scrittori d'oggi*, ser. 4 (Bari: Laterza, 1946), pp. 166–70; Emilio Cecchi *Di giorno in giorno* (Milan: Garzanti, 1954), pp. 95–98; Enrico Falqui, *Prosatori e narratori* (Turin: Einaudi, 1950), pp. 377–83; Giorgio Pullini, *Narratori italiani del Novecento* (Padua: Liviana, 1959), pp. 74–76, 339–52; Renato Bertacchini, "D. B.," *LIC*, vol. 2, pp. 1395–1411, is a rapid overview of our novelist. In English, Gian-Paolo Biasin's essay "The Secret Fears of Men: D. B.," *IQ* 4, no. 22 (1962): pp. 78–93, is effective and perceptive.

CARLO LEVI

Although Carlo Levi enjoys wide esteem in his country and abroad, and has always been considered a colorful and interesting artist, writer, and politician, only in recent years has his literary work been carefully scrutinized by the critics. Mario Miccinesi's *Invito alla lettura di C. L.* (Milan: Mursia, 1973) is a favorable, sympathetic evaluation of Levi's writing. The same cannot be said of Giovanni Falaschi's *C. L.* (Florence: La Nuova Italia, 1971), a monograph whose validity is partly vitiated by a hostile ideological posture. Both books carry a fairly extensive bibliography. Marcello Aurigemma's essay "C. L.," in *LIC*, vol. 3, pp. 393–423, is a brief overview of Levi's work. Much emphasis has been devoted to the "Southern" quality of most of Levi's books: perceptive discussions on this, and other facets of our author may be found in Mario Alicata's "*L'orologio* di C. L." and "Il meridionalismo non si può fermare a Eboli," in *Scritti letterari* (Milan: Il Saggiatore, 1968), pp. 260–65 and 309–30; Walter Mauro's *Cultura e società nella narrativa meridionale* (Rome: Ediz. dell'Ateneo, 1965), pp. 109–12, 328–31; Carlo Muscetta's biting essay "Leggenda e verità di C. L.," in *Letteratura militante* (Florence: Parenti, 1953), pp. 94–108; Alberto Asor Rosa dedicates several pages to Levi in his *Scrittori e popolo* (Rome: Savona & Savelli, 1965) and questions Levi's interpretation of the peasant world that is the focus of much of his work. For two engaging discussions of *L'orologio*, the reader might turn to Pancrazi's and Russo's books, as cited in "General Works on Italian Literature," as well as the studies of Cecchi, Pullini, and others, also cited.

The May–December 1967 issue of *Galleria* is completely dedicated to Levi (and contains some good pieces by Mario Petrucciani and Dominique Fernandez, among others). In English, the reader will find the following titles perceptive and valuable: Donald Heiney, "Emigration Continued: Levi, Alvaro, and Others," in *America in Modern Italian Literature* (New Brunswick, N.J.: Rutgers University Press, 1964), pp. 126–31; Lawrence Grant White, "Time and the Man," *Sat. Rev. of Lit.*, June 30, 1951; and Harold Rosenberg, "Politics as Dancing," *Tradition of the New* (New York: Horizon Press, 1959), pp. 119 ff.

CARLO EMILIO GADDA

By critical consensus, the best (but also most difficult) student of Gadda is Gianfranco Contini, whose essays, introductions, and notes are a veritable mine of interpretations and explanations: "Note private sul *Castello di Udine*", in *Esercizi di lettura* (Florence: Parenti, 1939), pp. 149–66; "Introduction," in C. E. Gadda's *L'Adalgisa*. (Turin: Einaudi, 1963), pp. vii–ix; "Introduction," in C. E. Gadda's *La cognizione del dolore* (Turin: Einaudi, 1963), pp. 7–28, now collected in *Varianti e linguis-*

tica (Turin: Einaudi, 1971). For a more elementary, but adequate introduction to Gadda, Ernesto Ferrero's slim monographic study, *Invito alla lettura di C. E. G.* (Milan: Mursia, 1974) is quite useful. Adriano Seroni's study, *C. E. G.* (Florence: La Nuova Italia, 1969) is commendable. For shorter overviews of Gadda, see Angelo Guglielmi's "C. E. G.," *LIC*, vol. 2, pp. 1051–69; and Olga Ragusa's fine essay "Gadda, Pasolini, and Experimentalism: Form or Ideology?" in Pacifici, ed., *From Verismo to Experimentalism*, pp. 239–69).

Guido Baldi's volume, *C. E. G.* (Milan: Mursia, 1973) is a more temperate and enthusiastic appreciation of our subject. Gian Carlo Roscioni's *La disarmonia prestabilita* (Turin: Einaudi, 1975) contains excellent insights into the art of Gadda and is a genuine stylistic as well as a philosophical commentary no serious student should miss; nor should one miss Pietro Citati's excellent "Il male invisibile," *Il Menabò* 6 (1963): 12–41. Other valuable essays are: Leone Piccioni's "L'arte di G.," *Sui contemporanei* (Florence: Fabbri, 1953), pp. 39–52; Renato Barilli, "Gadda e la fine del Naturalismo," in *La barriera del naturalismo* (Milan: Mursia, 1964), pp. 105–30.

On Gadda's language and style, the reader may turn to Giacomo Devoto, *Studi di linguistica* (Florence: LeMonnier, 1950), pp. 57–90; Cesare Segre, *Lingua stile e società* (Milan: Feltrinelli, 1963); Pier Paolo Pasolini's fine pages in *Passione e ideologia* (Milan: Garzanti, 1960), pp. 170–83; Piero Gelli, "Sul lessico de G.," *Paragone* 20, no. 230 (1969): 52–77; and the more difficult comments of Guido Guglielmi, "Lingua e metalinguaggio di G.," in *Letteratura come sistema e come funzione* (Turin: Einaudi, 1967), pp. 128–37. Alberto Arbasino's interviews and notes on G. in *Sessanta posizioni* (Milan: Feltrinelli, 1970), pp. 185–210, are amusing and informative in the best sense of the word. In English, aside from the essay by Ragusa already cited, the following are highly readable and insightful: Robert Bongiorno, "Prose Texture as Content in *Quer Pasticciaccio Brutto de Via Merulana*," *Romance Notes* 14 (1972): 49–56; Robert S. Dombrowski, "The Meaning of Gadda's Diary," *Ital.* 47 (1970): 373–86; and "Some Observations on the Revision of *Quer Pasticciaccio*," *MLN* 86, no. 1 (1971): 61–72; Pietro Citati, "Gadda's Critical Essays," *The London Magazine* 3, no. 7 (1953): 57–62; and Pietro Pucci, "The Obscure Illness," *IQ* 11, no. 42 (1967):

43–62. Among the more recent particularly useful and stimulating studies of Gadda are: Robert S. Dombrowski's monograph *Introduzione allo studio di C. E. G.* (Florence: Vallecchi, 1974); and Gian-Paolo Biasin's "The Pen, the Mother," in *Literary Diseases: Theme and Metaphor in the Italian Novel* (Austin: University of Texas Press, 1975), pp. 127–55.

CESARE PAVESE

Since his suicide in 1950, so much has been written on Pavese in Italy and abroad, that it is almost embarrassing to make a choice. The only "authorized" biography of our novelist is David Lajolo's *Il vizio assurdo: Storia di Cesare Pavese* (Milan: Il Saggiatore, 1960). Armanda Guiducci's *Invito alla lettura di C. P.* (Milan: Mursia, 1974) is the easiest introduction to P., but her longer *Il mito P.* (Florence: Vallecchi, 1967) is far more stimulating and insightful. Gianni Venturi's *C. P.* (Florence: La Nuova Italia, 1974) is intelligent and methodical; Ruggero Puletti's *C. P. la maturità impossibile* (Padua: Rebellato, 1961) puts his subject in a European context. Franco Mollia's *C. P.* (Florence: La Nuova Italia, 1963, 2d rev. ed., 1974) is excellent. Dominique Fernandez's long chapter on P. in her *Il romanzo italiano e la crisi della coscienza moderna* (Milan: Lerici, 1960), pp. 117–67, originally published in French in 1958, is one of the finest assessments by a non-Italian critic; by the same author, I also recommend *L'échec de P.* (Paris: Grasset, 1967). In English, Gian Paolo Biasin's *The Smile of the Gods: A Thematic Study of C. P.'s Work* (Ithaca, N.Y.: Cornell University Press, 1968) is fundamental; Donald Heiney's *Three Italian Novelists: Moravia, Pavese, Vittorini* (Ann Arbor: University of Michigan Press, 1968), pp. 147–213, is revealing, thanks to the critic's sensitive comparative approach. Leslie Fiedler's essay, "Introducing C. P.," *Kenyon Review* 14 (1954): 536–54, deserves the credit for having been responsible for calling the attention of American readers to Pavese. The connection between P. and American literature is the subject of Richard H. Chase's "C. P. and the American Novel," *Studi americani* 3 (1957): 347–69; Peter Norton's "Cesare Pavese and the American Nightmare," *MLN* 77 (1962): 24–36; Nemi d'Agostino's "P. e l'America," *Studi americani* 2 (1956): 399–

413; Vito Amorusi's "Cecchi, Vittorini, Pavese e la letteratura americana," *Studi americani* 6 (1960): pp. 9–71; Donald Heiney's "The Moon and the Bonfires," in *America in Modern Italian Literature* (New Brunswick, N.J.: Rutgers University Press, 1964), pp. 171–86; and L. K. Barnett's "Notes on P.'s Critical Views of American Literature," *FI* 8 (1974): 381–89. Giose Rimanelli has written copiously on P. Of his essays, the most challenging are: "Myth and De-Mythification in C. P.'s Art," *IQ* 13, no. 49 (1969): 3–39; "P's *Diario*: Why Suicide? Why Not?" in *Italian Literature: Roots and Branches: Essays in Honor of Thomas Goddard Bergin* (New Haven: Yale University Press, 1976), pp. 383–405.

Among the finest studies of particular books or problems in Pavese's art are: R. Rupert Roopnaraine's "Structure of Self and Art in P.'s *Il Carcere*," *IQ* 66 (1973): 25–46; Louis Tenenbaum's "Character Treatment in P.'s Fiction," *Symposium* 15 (1961): 131–38; Bruce Merry's "Artifice and Structure in *La Luna e i falò*," *FI* 5, no. 3 (1971): 351–58; John Freccero's "Mythos and Logos: *The Moon and the Bonfires*," *IQ* 4, no. 16 (1961): 3–16, and Linda Hutcheon's "Pavese's Intellectual Rhythm," *IQ* 15, nos. 60–61 (1972): 5–26.

ELIO VITTORINI

Vittorini's narrative work has recently appeared in a superlative two-volume edition, published by Mondadori (Milan, 1974), with a long, perceptive preface by Maria Conti, and an unusually thorough, international bibliography prepared by Raffaela Rotondi (vol. 2, pp. 973–1011).

Several monographic studies on V. have appeared in recent years: Sergio Pautasso, V. (Turin: Borla, 1967); Sandro Briosi has published two small, but useful and intelligent volumes, *E. V.* (Florence: La Nuova Italia, 1970) and *Invito alla lettura di E. V.* (Milan: Mursia, 1973). Among essays, the following are instructive: Renato Bertacchini, "E. V.," *LIC*, vol. 2, pp. 1507–26; Piero de Tommaso, "E. V.," *Narratori italiani contemporanei* (Rome: Ateneo, 1965), pp. 59–92; two essays on *Conversazione in Sicilia*, by Franca Bianconi Bernardi, are particularly original —"Parola e mito in C. in S.," *Lingua e stile* 1 (1966): 161–90, and "Simboli e immagini nella C. di V.," *Lingua e stile* 2 (1967): 27–46.

In English, the reader may begin with the general introductory essay by C. A. McCormick, "E. V.," *IQ* (1967), pp. 39–61; R. W. B. Lewis, "E. V.," *IQ* 4, no. 15 (1960): 55–61. Joy Hamnuchen Potter has written with much insight on "V.'s Literary Apprenticeship: 1926–1929," *FI* 3, no. 3 (1969): 375–85; "The Poetic and Symbolic Function of Fable in *Erica*," *Ital.* 48, no. 1 (1971): 51–70; "An Ideological Substructure in *C. in S.*" *Ital.* 52, no. 1 (1975): 59–69; and "Patterns of Meaning in *C. in S.*," *FI* 9, no. 1 (1975): 60–73. Other essays include: Bruce Merry, "V.'s Multiple Resources of Style," *Mosaic* 5 (1972): 93–108; G. Cambon, "E. V.: Between Poverty and Wealth," *Wisc. Stud. in Cont. Lit.* 3 (Winter 1962): 20–24; Nicolas V. Polletta, "*C. in S.*: Literature as Nostalgia," *Ital.* 41 (1964): 415–29; Edwina Vittorini, "V.'s *Uomini e no*: An Epic of the Resistance?" *Durham Univ. Journal* 62 (1970): 65–80; Marilyn Schneider, "Circularity as Mode and Meaning in *C. in S.*," *MLN* 90 (1975): 93–108. The best, most comprehensive, and detailed study of V. in English is still Donald Heiney's *Three Italian Novelists: Moravia, Pavese, Vittorini* (Ann Arbor: University of Michigan Press, 1968), pp. 147–213. On V.'s work as a student of American letters, see Vito Amoruso's long and detailed essay "Cecchi, Vittorini, Pavese e la letteratura americana," in *Studi americani* 6 (1960): 9–71. The May–August 1968 and July–August 1973 issues of the review *Il Ponte* are dedicated to Elio Vittorini, and contain numerous critical and biographical essays, articles, and notes by distinguished writers, scholars, and friends of their subject. The magazine of the Italian Radio and Television, *Terzo Programma* (no. 3, 1966) published a homage section dedicated to V., which includes an essay by Geno Pampaloni, "V.: la narrativa e la letteratura," and other contributions.

For other estimates, see Cecchi, Venè, David, Guarnieri, Solmi, Manacorda, Pullini, and others, as cited in "General Works on Italian Literature." Donald Heiney's English translation of Vittorini's preface to the Italian edition of *The Red Carnation* appeared in *The Western Humanities Review* 9 (1955): 197–208, with the title: "Truth and Censorship: The Story of *The Red Carnation*."

ALBERTO MORAVIA

There is no shortage of criticism on Moravia on either side of the Atlantic. For a swift, but comprehensive survey of Italian and American studies, one should turn to Ferdinando Alfoni, "A. M. nel pensiero critico italiano e americano," *Città di vita* (1971), pp. 61–72. Oreste Del Buono's *M.* (Milan: Feltrinelli, 1972) is a collection of selections of biographical and critical material, complemented by an anthological selection of typical Moravian narrative; Edoardo Sanguineti's *A. M.* (Milan: Mursia, 1962) is an incisive and penetrating study, perhaps one of the best produced in Italy on our subject. Fulvio Longobardi's monograph, *M.* (Florence: Il Castoro, 1969) is illuminating, as is Alberto Limentani's *A. M. tra esistenza e libertà* (Venice: Neri Pozza, 1962). The recent monograph, *A. M.*, by Giancarlo Pandini (Milan: Mursia, 1973) is comprehensive and pedagogically useful in its detailed treatment of M.'s works and the themes of his fiction as well as the critical views of his work. For early assessments, the following should be consulted: Giuseppe A. Borgese's review of *Gli indifferenti*, in *Il corriere della sera* (July 21, 1929); Eurialo De Michelis, *Introduzione a M.* (Florence: La Nuova Italia, 1934, rev. 1954); Luigi Russo, "A. M.: Scrittore senza storia," *I Narratori: 1850–1957* (Milan: Principato, 1958), pp. 367–76; Francesco Flora, "A. M.," *Scrittori italiani contemporanei* (Pisa: Listri-Nischi, 1952), pp. 197–231); Gaetano Trombatore, "Il punto su Moravia," in *Società* 7 (1951): pp. 610–24. Among the more recent original essays and notes, Renato Barilli's "M. Dall' Indifferenza' alla 'noia,'" in *La barriera del Naturalismo* (Milan: Mursia, 1964), pp. 64–104; Ines Scaramucci's "A. M.," in *LIC*, vol. 2, pp. 1455–88. Giorgio Pullini's "A. M." in his *Il romanzo italiano del dopoguerra* (Milan: Schwarz, 1961), pp. 69–116, has been reprinted several times without having been updated. The various introductory essays by Geno Pampaloni to the special edition of Moravia's work being published by Bompiani, commend themselves for their acumen and clarity. In English, the long essay by Luciano Rebay, *A. M.* (New York: Columbia University Press, 1970) is useful as an introduction to our subject; the essay by R. W. B. Lewis, "Eros and Existence," *The Picaresque Saint: Representative Figures in Contemporary Fiction* (New York: Lippincott, 1959), pp. 35–56, is full of insights that have retained all their validity despite the passing of time. Joan Ross and Donald Freed have written an absorbing study of the philosophical strain in M.'s work, *The Existentialism of A. M.* (Carbondale: Southern Illinois University Press, 1972); Olga Ragusa's "A. M.: Voyeurism and Story-Telling," *Southern Review* 4 (Winter 1968): 127–41, is a devastating appraisal of Moravia. Jane Cottrell's *A. M.* (N.Y.: Ungar, 1976) is a modest but useful survey of Moravia's literary work. Donald Heiney's "A. M.," in *Three Italian Novelists: Moravia, Pavese, Vittorini* (Ann Arbor: University of Michigan Press, 1968), pp. 1–82, is an excellent, carefully thought out, incisive analysis of his subject's fiction. Other commendable essays in English are: Frank Baldanza's "The Classicism of A. M.," *Modern Fiction Studies* 3 (1958): 309–20, and his more recent "Mature M.," *Contemp. Lit.* 9, no. 4 (1968): 506–21; Eenelm Foster, "A. M.," *Blackfriars* 43 (1962): 221–30; and Giose Rimanelli, "M. and the Philosophy of Personal Existence," *IQ* 41 (1967): 39–68. In French, Dominique Fernandez's *Le roman italien et la crise de la coscienze moderne* (Paris, Grasset, 1958), available in the Italian translation published by Lerici, of Milan, in 1960 (*Il romanzo italiano e la crisi della coscienza moderna*, trans. by Franca Lerici), is a ground-breaking study that deserves to be read by students of the modern novel in Italy. Finally, the volume *Mas As An End: A Defense of Humanism. Literary, Social and Political Essays* (New York: Farrar, Straus & Giroux, 1966) should be consulted for the autobiographical and theoretical pieces Moravia has written over the years. An unusually penetrating interview-essay on Moravia has been included in Ferdinando Camon's volume *Il mestiere di scrittore: Conversazioni critiche* (Milan: Garzanti, 1973), pp. 11–32. An earlier interview by Ben Johnson and Maria De Dominicis appeared in the *Paris Review*, no. 6 (1955), pp. 17–37.

Index

(*Continued from front flap*)

Pacifici's monumental work is unique in English presentations of twentieth-century Italian writing, above all for its admirable range; moreover, it combines important information with expert evaluation. One of the work's most important achievements is the bibliography, which not only contains a full list of recent works on Italian literature but also presents useful critical commentary on these books and essays.

Students of modern Italian and comparative literature will find this third volume of a classic trilogy—and the series as a whole—indispensable.

Sergio Pacifici is Professor of Italian and Comparative Literature at Queens College of the City University of New York. He received his Ph.D. degree from Harvard University. Among his numerous books and translations are *The Poet and the Politician and Other Essays* by Salvatore Quasimodo (co-translated with Thomas G. Bergin), and *A Guide to Contemporary Italian Literature: From Futurism to Neorealism*.

Harry T. Moore is Research Professor Emeritus, Southern Illinois University at Carbondale. Among his recent books are *Twentieth-Century French Literature*, *Twentieth-Century German Literature*, and *Age of the Modern and Other Literary Essays*. He is the author of the highly acclaimed *The Priest of Love: A Life of D. H. Lawrence* (previously titled *The Intelligent Heart*), a revision of the classic biography containing considerable material about Lawrence made available since first publication.